Case-Based Oral and Maxillofacial Surgery

Case-Based Oral and Maxillofacial Surgery

Editor: Jeffrey Young

AMERICAN
MEDICAL PUBLISHERS
www.americanmedicalpublishers.com

AMERICAN
MEDICAL PUBLISHERS
www.americanmedicalpublishers.com

Cataloging-in-Publication Data

Case-based oral and maxillofacial surgery / edited by Jeffrey Young.
p. cm.
Includes bibliographical references and index.
ISBN 979-8-88740-623-7
1. Mouth--Surgery. 2. Maxilla--Surgery. 3. Dentistry, Operative. 4. Face--Surgery.
5. Jaws--Surgery. I. Young, Jeffrey.
RK529 .E87 2023
617.522 059--dc23

American Medical Publishers,
41 Flatbush Avenue,
1st Floor, New York,
NY 11217, USA

ISBN 979-8-88740-623-7 (Hardback)

Contents

Preface

This book has been a concerted effort by a group of academicians, researchers and scientists, who have contributed their research works for the realization of the book. This book has materialized in the wake of emerging advancements and innovations in this field. Therefore, the need of the hour was to compile all the required researches and disseminate the knowledge to a broad spectrum of people comprising of students, researchers and specialists of the field.

Oral and maxillofacial surgery is a specialized branch of dentistry that focuses on the diagnosis and surgical management of conditions affecting the face, jaws, mouth and neck. Some of the key procedures which are undertaken within this area of medicine are orthognathic surgery, management of facial trauma, and the extraction of impacted teeth. Orthognathic surgery aims to correct severe abnormalities of the jaw and facial structures, including problems with biting, chewing, speech, and facial balance. The management of facial trauma involves treating facial injuries resulting from accidents, sports-related incidents or assaults. Treatment of oral and facial infections also lies within this field of medicine. In this book, using case studies and examples, constant effort has been made to make the understanding of the difficult concepts of oral and maxillofacial surgery as easy and informative as possible, for the readers. It will help new researchers by foregrounding their knowledge in this area of medicine.

At the end of the preface, I would like to thank the authors for their brilliant chapters and the publisher for guiding us all-through the making of the book till its final stage. Also, I would like to thank my family for providing the support and encouragement throughout my academic career and research projects.

Editor

1

PEEK Implants: An Innovative Solution for Facial Aesthetic Surgery

Rocco Narciso,[1] **Emanuela Basile,**[2] **Davide Johan Bottini,**[3] **and Valerio Cervelli**[4]

[1]*Plastic Surgery Resident, Graduate School of Plastic Reconstructive and Aesthetic Surgery, "Tor Vergata" University, Rome, Italy*
[2]*Department of Plastic and Reconstructive Surgery, Policlinico Casilino Hospital, Rome, Italy*
[3]*Reconstructive and Aesthetic Surgery University "Tor Vergata" of Rome, Department of Plastic and Reconstructive Surgery, Policlinico Casilino Hospital, Rome, Italy*
[4]*Department of Surgical Sciences, University "Tor Vergata", Rome, Italy*

Correspondence should be addressed to Rocco Narciso; ro.narciso@hotmail.it

Academic Editor: Claudio Feo

The authors present a case report showing their experience with the use of PolyEtherEtherKetone (PEEK) implants as an innovative solution for the skeleton and soft tissues' reshaping in facial aesthetic plastic surgery. This technique offers the surgeon a reliable and effective way to answer patients' request of increasing volume and reshaping the malar area. A fifty-year-old patient complaining about hypoplasia of the malar area, after undergoing three operations of silicon implants' placement and replacement, was still unsatisfied about the symmetry and feeling through the skin of the lower lid, the rim of the prostheses. The authors suggested the use of bone-anchored PEEK implants, to increase the volume and reshape the malar area by a skeleton and soft tissue camouflage. The treatment was planned and previewed on the preop 3-dimensional CT scans for the customization of the implants. Although no cases are reported in international literature on the use of this material in facial aesthetic surgery, this technique seems to offer a safe and effective solution for the treatment of patients asking to increase and modify the shape of their malar area. Custom made PEEK implants are already used in craniofacial reconstructive bony surgery with good results, and 3D CT scan planning is widely used in these cases. No complications were reported in the case reported and the outcomes seem to the authors and to the patient being, finally, satisfactory.

1. Introduction

The PolyEtherEtherKetone (PEEK) implants are a recent answer to the research of reliable material for facial and skeleton reshaping and camouflage [1]. Different kinds of material can be chosen, and the following are the most popular used today for facial skeleton implantation:

MedPor (high-density porous polyethylene), silicone, titanium, aluminia ceramics, methyl methacrylate, lipofilling, and hydroxyapatite [2].

These implants are utilized to reconstruct several bony and soft-tissue defects, including the frontal and temporal areas; orbital walls; infraorbital margin; zygomatic, paranasal, and nasal regions; and mandible [2].

Craniofacial surgeons often use these materials, performing cranial vault and craniofacial posttraumatic and oncologic bone-defect reconstructions [3].

During surgical planning, the research was oriented to a material that could have a solid structure, a malleable shape, good biocompatibility, and low rate of infection.

The experience with other solution as the methacrylate demonstrates an increase probability of infections and a challenging preoperative implant measures assessment [2]. The PEEK, instead, had less chance of infection and allow an access as the intraoral that is a nonsterile route. The implants are printed with a 3D printer and it is very simple to obtain an implant that perfectly fit the searched volume and shape.

The authors present the case of a patient who underwent three operations of silicon implants' placement and replacement and was still unsatisfied about the symmetry and the feeling of the rim of the prostheses. The patient was treated by the replacement of the old prostheses with PEEK custom made bone anchored implants in the zygomatic area. Customization of the prostheses was planned to preview the shape and the volume to obtain, on the preoperative 3-dimensional CT scans. PEEK has been chosen but rarely described in literature for the reconstruction of the malar regions [4] and is an innovative solution in the field of facial aesthetic surgery.

2. Case Presentation

The patient is a fifty-year-old man who received three different surgery procedures for an improvement in projection and reshaping of the malar areas.

In 2014, were positioned bilaterally silicone implant CSM (Combined Malar Shell®) for malar area in the subcutaneous tissues, from an intraoral access, with concomitant malar e submalar lipostructure.

In the 2016, was positioned a new TSM (Terino Malar Shell®) implant near to preexisting one for each side, from an intraoral access.

In 2018, all the protheses were removed and were implanted Hanson SM 12-3® prosthesis for each side.

The authors visited the patient in 2019; he complained about the mobility of the implants and about a subcontinuous nuisance in the infraorbital regions.

The operation performed to achieve the result was the bilateral positioning in the malar area of two custom made PEEK bone-anchored implants. An intraoral and subperiosteal plane approach for both the malar areas places the new prostheses, after removing the old silicone implants.

Based on the preop CT scan, the PEEK PSIs (patient-specific implant) were planned and manufactured previewing the size, shape, and the precise location of the prostheses; even the size and inclination and the type of screw could be planned, in order to achieve a fast and correct placement of the implants.

Under general anesthesia, the surgical placement was obtained with an incision performed in the upper oral vestibule on preexisting scars and through an intraoral subperiosteal approach. The two preexistent silicone implants were removed, and then, subperiosteal soft tissue detachment is allowed to place the implants on the bone surface and to anchor with screws in the programmed position (Figure 1). The patient was discharged after one night of recovery with an oral antibiotic and analgesic oral therapy.

The follow-up schedule (Table 1) included stitch removal fourteen days after surgery. The postoperative edema showed a great reduction after 2 weeks and a complete resolution after 2 months. A CT scan was performed after 3 months, and photos were taken after 6 and 12 months.

3. Discussion and Conclusion

The authors found a satisfactory result, not only aesthetic but also functional with an improvement of the symptoms complained by the patient.

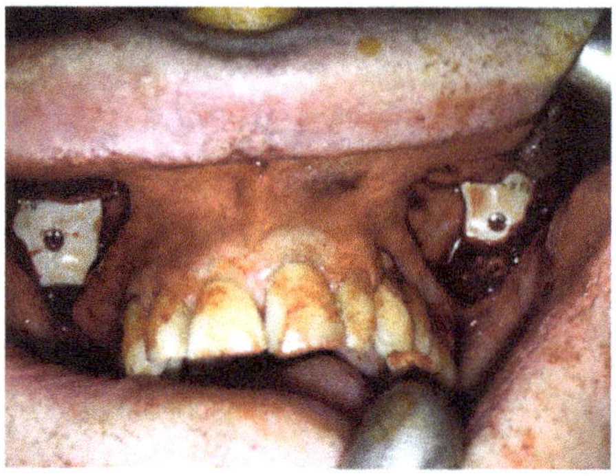

Figure 1: The new PEEK implants fixed into the subperiosteal pocket bilaterally.

Table 1: Follow-up schedule.

14 days	Stitch removal
2 months	Edema resolution
3 months	CT scan control
6 months	Photo control
12 months	Photo control

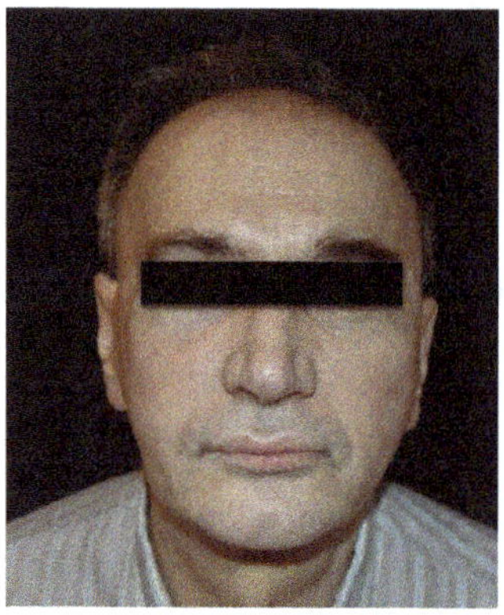

(a)

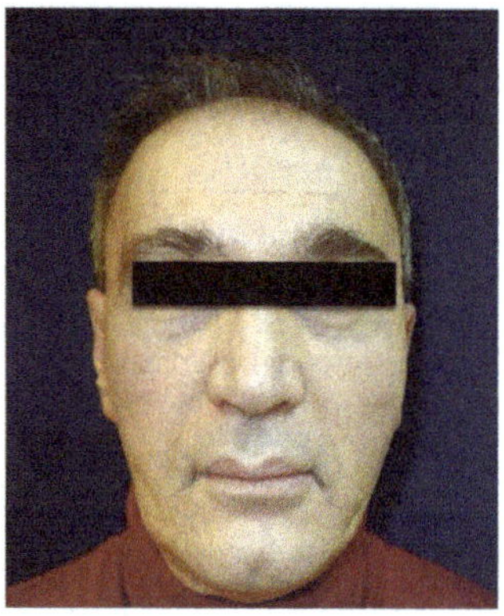

(b)

Figure 2: The presurgery picture (a) and the postsurgery picture (b). Published with the patient's consent.

The preoperation pictures and the follow-up pictures after 1 year are shown in the paper (Figure 2).

In the literature, there are several papers that describe the use of the PEEK implants, in orthopedic surgery [5], in maxillo-facial surgery [6, 7], in oral implantology and prosthodontics [8], and in neurosurgery [9]. This material is gaining positive replay for its high biocompatibility and low weight.

Furthermore, the PEEK PSIs can be trimmed with a cutting burr in the operating room if it is needed to be reshaped or if the aesthetic result is not satisfying, despite of the customization process that could not be enough.

PEEK has many advantages compared with other alloplastic implant materials. PEEK has radiographic translucency [10] and does not produce artefacts on radiographic imaging. PEEK is also nonallergenic and nonmagnetic and does not develop exothermic reactions as methyl methacrylate does [3]. Furthermore, PEEK is comparable to cortical bone regarding its elasticity.

The fixation is possible with the traditional screws. The availability of a custom made prothesis allows a significant reduction of the surgery time [4].

The PEEK is widely used in maxillo-facial surgery, but it was never described in aesthetic surgery.

In our case, we found a satisfactory result, not only aesthetic but also functional with an improvement of the symptoms complained by the patient.

Consent

Informed consent from the patient was obtained for the case report, and written informed consent obtained for the accompanying photographs.

References

[1] J. M. Foletti, N. Lari, P. Dumas, P. Compes, and L. Guyot, "PEEK customized implant for skull esthetic reconstruction," *Revue de Stomatologie et de Chirurgie Maxillo-Faciale*, vol. 113, no. 6, pp. 468–471, 2012.

[2] Y. A. Rojas, C. Sinnott, C. Colasante, J. Samas, and R. G. Reish, "Facial implants: controversies and criticism. A comprehensive review of the current literature," *Plastic and Reconstructive Surgery*, vol. 142, no. 4, pp. 991–999, 2018.

[3] A. M. Shah, H. Jung, and S. Skirboll, "Materials used in cranioplasty: a history and analysis," *Neurosurgical Focus*, vol. 36, no. 4, article E19, 2014.

[4] R. N. Hussain, M. Clark, and A. Berry-Brincat, "The use of a polyetheretherketone (PEEK) implant to reconstruct the midface region," *Ophthalmic Plastic & Reconstructive Surgery*, vol. 32, no. 6, pp. e151–e153, 2016.

[5] D. Liu, J. Fu, H. Fan et al., "Application of 3D-printed PEEK scapula prosthesis in the treatment of scapular benign fibrous histiocytoma: a case report," *Journal of Bone Oncology*, vol. 12, pp. 78–82, 2018.

[6] S. Järvinen, J. Suojanen, E. Kormi et al., "The use of patient specific polyetheretherketone implants for reconstruction of maxillofacial deformities," *Journal of Cranio-Maxillo-Facial Surgery*, vol. 47, no. 7, pp. 1072–1076, 2019.

[7] G. Saponaro, P. Doneddu, G. Gasparini et al., "Custom made onlay implants in peek in maxillofacial surgery: a volumetric study," *Child's Nervous System*, vol. 36, no. 2, pp. 385–391, 2020.

[8] S. Najeeb, M. S. Zafar, Z. Khurshid, and F. Siddiqui, "Applications of polyetheretherketone (PEEK) in oral implantology and prosthodontics," *Journal of Prosthodontic Research*, vol. 60, no. 1, pp. 12–19, 2016.

[9] M. Punchak, L. K. Chung, C. Lagman et al., "Outcomes following polyetheretherketone (PEEK) cranioplasty: systematic review and meta-analysis," *Journal of Clinical Neuroscience*, vol. 41, pp. 30–35, 2017.

[10] T. Nieminen, I. Kallela, E. Wuolijoki, H. Kainulainen, I. Hiidenheimo, and I. Rantala, "Amorphous and crystalline polyetheretherketone: mechanical properties and tissue reactions during a 3-year follow-up," *Journal of Biomedical Materials Research Part A*, vol. 84, no. 2, pp. 377–383, 2008.

2

Feminizing the Face: Combination of Frontal Bone Reduction and Reduction Rhinoplasty

C. J. Salgado, H. AlQattan, A. Nugent, D. Gerth, W. Kassira, C. S. McGee, and L. Wo

Division of Plastic, Reconstructive, Transgender, and Aesthetic Surgery, University of Miami Leonard M. Miller School of Medicine, Miami, FL, USA

Correspondence should be addressed to C. J. Salgado; csalgado2@med.miami.edu

Academic Editor: Gaetano La Greca

Gender affirmation surgeries in male-to-female patient transitioning include breast augmentation, genital construction, and facial feminization surgery (FFS). FFS improves mental health and quality of life in transgender patients. The nose and forehead are critical in facial attractiveness and gender identity; thus, frontal brow reduction and rhinoplasty are a mainstay of FFS. The open approach to reduction of the frontal brow is very successful in the feminization of the face; however, risks include alopecia and scarring. Endoscopic brow reduction, in properly selected patients, is minimally invasive with excellent outcomes avoiding these risks. Since both reduction rhinoplasty and frontal brow reduction are routinely performed in FFS, a combined approach provides superior control over the nasal radix and profile when performing surgery on the frontal bone region first followed by nose reduction. We present a case series of four transwomen undergoing frontal bone reduction in combination with a reduction rhinoplasty. All had excellent results with one DVT that resolved with treatment. Transgender patients frequently require multiple operations during their transition increasing their hospital stay and costs. This combined approach offers superior control over the nasofrontal angle and is not only safe but reduces hospitalizations and costs and is a novel indication to reduce gender dysphoria.

1. Introduction

With increasing coverage of medically necessary procedures for transgender patients by health insurances and major industries, more patients have benefited from a decrease in their dysphoria and ultimately their quality of life. Gender affirmation surgeries in male-to-female transition patients include breast augmentation, genital construction, and facial feminization [1]. Facial features serve an integral role in identifying an individual's gender, with certain characteristics perceived as feminine or masculine [2]. The approach to analysis and planning of facial feminization surgery involves division of the face into the upper, middle, and bottom thirds. Feminization of the bottom third of the face can be addressed by procedures to decrease the angle of the mandible, lip augmentation through the use of fillers, and narrowing of the chin via genioplasty. The nose, as the centerpiece of the middle third of the face, is an important component of facial attractiveness and gender identity. Thus, reduction rhinoplasty is a mainstay of facial feminization surgery, while cheek augmentation and widening of the zygomatic complex can be employed to achieve a more feminine heart-shaped contour of the face [3]. The upper third of the face is considered to be the most significant portion in recognizing female gender. The male brow and forehead are typically more pronounced, especially in the glabella and superior orbital rim regions [2–4]. The open approach via a bicoronal incision or a pretrichial incision for exposure of the frontonasal-orbital complex has been the most common approach for modification of this bone. Patient satisfaction rates are high with open forehead contouring procedures, but open approaches impart risks such as alopecia, scarring, paresthesias, and, rarely, damage to the frontal branches of the facial nerve [5–7].

Endoscopy has been used in craniofacial surgery for the last 20 years primarily in the trauma setting for fracture reduction [8]. Endoscopic-assisted facelifts and forehead lifts

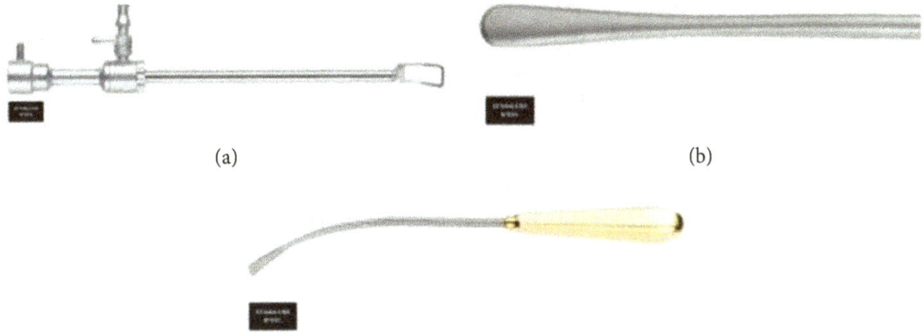

(a) (b) (c)

Figure 1: (a) Endoforehead fenestrated cannula. (b) Endoscopic straight periosteal elevator. (c) Endoscopic curved periosteal elevator.

have also recently been described as well [9]. Guyuron et al. published a series on endoscopic reduction of frontal bossing in 10 patients, with excellent aesthetic outcomes and no postoperative complications at follow-up [10].

Having performed both modification of the frontal bone and reduction rhinoplasty individually in this patient population, we noticed that when using a combined approach, performing the brow reduction prior to the reduction rhinoplasty, one is allowed superior control over the nasal radix and profile of the nose in one stage. We present a case series and our technique in transgender patients undergoing either open or endoscopic frontal bone reduction in combination with a reduction rhinoplasty for facial feminization.

2. Materials and Methods

2.1. Surgical Technique: Endoscopic Brow Reduction. Following a preoperative lateral cephalogram, an assessment is made of the anterior table of the frontal sinus. Preoperative facial bone CT provides significantly more detail on the anatomy of the glabellar region and the possible varying thickness of the anterior table in this region. Patients with an anterior table thickness of greater than 5 mm are amenable to burring with a notable difference in their facial aesthetics. These are candidates for an endoscopic brow procedure, particularly, if a hairline lowering procedure is not needed. A 30-degree 4 mm endoscope attached to an endoforehead fenestrated cannula (Figure 1(a)) and straight and curved periosteal elevators (Figures 1(b) and 1(c)), as well as an angled Midas Rex high-speed surgical drill (Medtronic), attached to a round cutting burr are the typical instruments used in the endoscopic brow reduction technique. We perform these cases under general anesthesia using an oral RAE tube with the patient's occiput positioned in a Mayfield horseshoe headrest. This allows for optimal exposure and access to the surgical site. For the endoscopic access ports, we place two incisions approximately 1-2 cm posterior to the frontal hairline in an anteroposterior direction, each in the paramedian position equidistant from each other. Once the endoscope and fenestrated cannula is introduced under the flap, we dissect anteriorly in a subgaleal and then subperiosteal plane to approach the supraorbital rim. Care must be taken not to violate the supraorbital nor supratrochlear pedicles during this

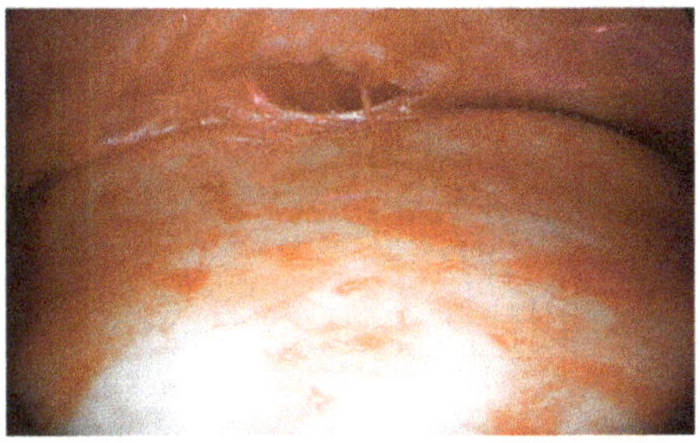

Figure 2: Intraoperative endoscopic view.

dissection. The most prominent area of protuberance is typically just superior to the glabellar region in the paramedian plane. We then proceed to burr the anterior table of the frontal sinus with numbers 4 and 3 cutting burrs, followed by a number 3 diamond burr for more refined contouring at 20,000 rpm. An irrigating tube is used to prevent thermal injury to the bone. Once the underlying bone becomes translucent, the endpoint is reached and no further reduction can be performed without entering the frontal sinus cavity. Constant motion of the drill and avoidance of aggressive drilling 10–20 mm lateral to the midline help to minimize the risk of exposure of frontal sinus mucosa as these areas of bone tend to be thinner (Figure 2) [11].

Once sufficient contouring has been achieved, assessment of the eyebrow position is performed, and if a brow lift is indicated, forehead skin can be removed accordingly. We perform a concurrent septorhinoplasty, usually with a second surgical team. Dorsal nasal hump reduction, nasal bone osteotomies, submucosal septal cartilage resection, nasal tip refinement via cephalic trimming, and columellar strut grafts are standard in our technique. Turbinate outfracture, spreader grafts, and lateral crural strut grafts are performed as needed, depending on the patient's nasal airway. A soft-pressure dressing is applied and maintained in position for 24 hours, along with head elevation while at rest for 3 days to minimize associated edema.

2.2. Surgical Technique: Open Brow Reduction. Following a preoperative lateral cephalogram, an assessment is made of the anterior table of the frontal sinus. Patients with an anterior table thickness of greater than 5 mm are amenable to burring with a notable difference in their facial aesthetics. If a hairline lowering procedure is also needed, then these are candidates for an open approach. A pretrichial incision extending across both temporal areas and the midline is marked and infiltrated with a local anesthetic and epinephrine. Our incision is slightly beveled anteriorly, and subgaleal dissection is carried out to the midportion of the forehead where we then transition to a subperiosteal dissection. Periosteal elevators are used to elevate the periosteum and create a pericranial flap that extends to the supraorbital rim to be used if needed. We extend the dissection to include the lateral orbital wall to obtain a clear view of the frontal bone with unhindered access. The supraorbital and supratrochlear neurovascular bundle must be identified and preserved during this dissection. The areas of most protuberance are identified and burred down as previously described in the endoscopic brow reduction technique.

If the patient's anterior table is too thin for burring (less than 5 mm), then a frontal bone setback is performed. We drill circumferentially around the frontal sinus, and the anterior table of the frontal bone is removed as two main segments due to their fusion in the midline. The intersinus septum and midline air cells are divided. The anterior table segments are transferred to a back table where they are further contoured using a burr and then plated to a titanium mesh. Simultaneously, the remaining supraorbital rim and periorbital contour is further refined using burring techniques. Finally, the anterior plate segments are secured to the margin of the frontal sinus using 4-5 mm screws. A scalp reduction is then performed by undermining the posterior incision in the subgaleal plane and advancing the scalp flap anteriorly to lower the hairline. The excess skin is excised off the forehead flap. The soft tissue of the brow and galea is secured with suture to the titanium mesh to create a temporal brow lift bilaterally. The scalp incision is closed in layers with absorbable sutures.

To evaluate postoperative success, patients were asked to qualitatively rate their satisfaction as ranging from "not satisfied," "satisfied," and "very satisfied" at follow-up. We saw every patient in the follow-up clinic, with a mean follow-up of 21 months.

3. Results

3.1. Case 1. A 27-year-old male-to-female transgender patient presented to our clinic desiring a more feminine face. She had previously undergone a rhinoplasty and was specifically concerned with her brow and residual nasal asymmetry. On physical exam, she had a prominent superior orbital rim, right nasal septum deviation, a dorsal hump, and airway obstruction on the right side with a droopy tip (Figures 3(a) and 3(b)). Preoperative lateral cephalograms confirmed a thick anterior table of the frontal sinus making her an ideal candidate for endoscopic reduction (Figure 3(c)). Three weeks postoperatively, she was seen in the clinic with a significant improvement in the supraorbital bossing and a softer more feminine nose. Postoperative lateral cephalograms demonstrated thinning of the supraorbital prominence with a less acute angle at the superciliary arches (Figure 4(a)). At 3-month, 2-year, and 4-year follow-ups, she developed no complications, had an excellent aesthetic result, and was satisfied with the procedure (Figures 4(b) and 4(c)).

3.2. Case 2. A 41-year-old male-to-female transgender patient presented to our clinic inquiring about facial feminization and gender confirmation bottom surgery. On examination of her face, she had a prominent supraorbital ridge, brow descent with wrinkling of the forehead, and a large masculine nose (Figures 5(a) and 5(b)). Preoperative lateral cephalograms confirmed a thick anterior table amenable to burring. Open frontal bone burring, frontal brow lift, and rhinoplasty were performed. At 2-week follow-up, she had excellent healing with pleasing results (Figures 6(a) and 6(b)) and postoperative lateral cephalograms demonstrated adequate thinning of the supraorbital prominence. She also underwent gender confirmation bottom surgery during the same hospitalization, 9 days prior to her facial feminization surgery. Her hospitalization was complicated by bilateral upper extremity DVTs which further work-up revealed Factor V Leiden. She was treated with a three-month course of anticoagulation with no long-term complications. At 8- and 16-month follow-ups, she continues to have no complications and is very satisfied with her results.

3.3. Case 3. A 62-year-old male-to-female transgender patient presented to our clinic desiring a more feminine face. She had previously undergone gender confirmation bottom surgery with penile skin inversion in addition to hormonal therapy. Her areas of main concern were frontal bossing and the asymmetry of her nose. On physical exam, she had right nasal septum deviation with left-sided internal nasal valve collapse and a bulbous tip. Additionally, she reported a history of left nasal obstruction and recurrent sinus infections. CT of the preoperative facial bones confirmed a thin anterior table of the frontal sinus making her not suitable for an endoscopic approach. Open frontal bone set back with septorhinoplasty was planned. One week postoperatively, she was seen in the clinic for the removal of her intranasal and extranasal splints. CT of the postoperative facial bones with 3D reconstruction demonstrated a less acute angle at the superciliary arches with an anterior table set back (Figures 7(a) and 7(b)). Follow-ups at 3 and 10 months demonstrated excellent results with no complications and patient satisfaction.

3.4. Case 4. A 28-year-old male-to-female transgender patient presented to our clinic desiring a more feminine face. She had previously undergone gender confirmation bottom surgery with penile skin inversion in addition to breast augmentation and hormonal therapy. Her greatest areas of concern were the brow, nose, and chin. On examination of her brow, she had eyebrows at the level of the superior orbital rim with supraorbital bossing. Her nasal tip was slightly bulbous with a wide dorsum in addition to a bony prominence in the symphyseal and parasymphyseal regions. Preoperative lateral cephalogram confirmed a thick anterior table of the frontal sinus making her a suitable candidate for endoscopic

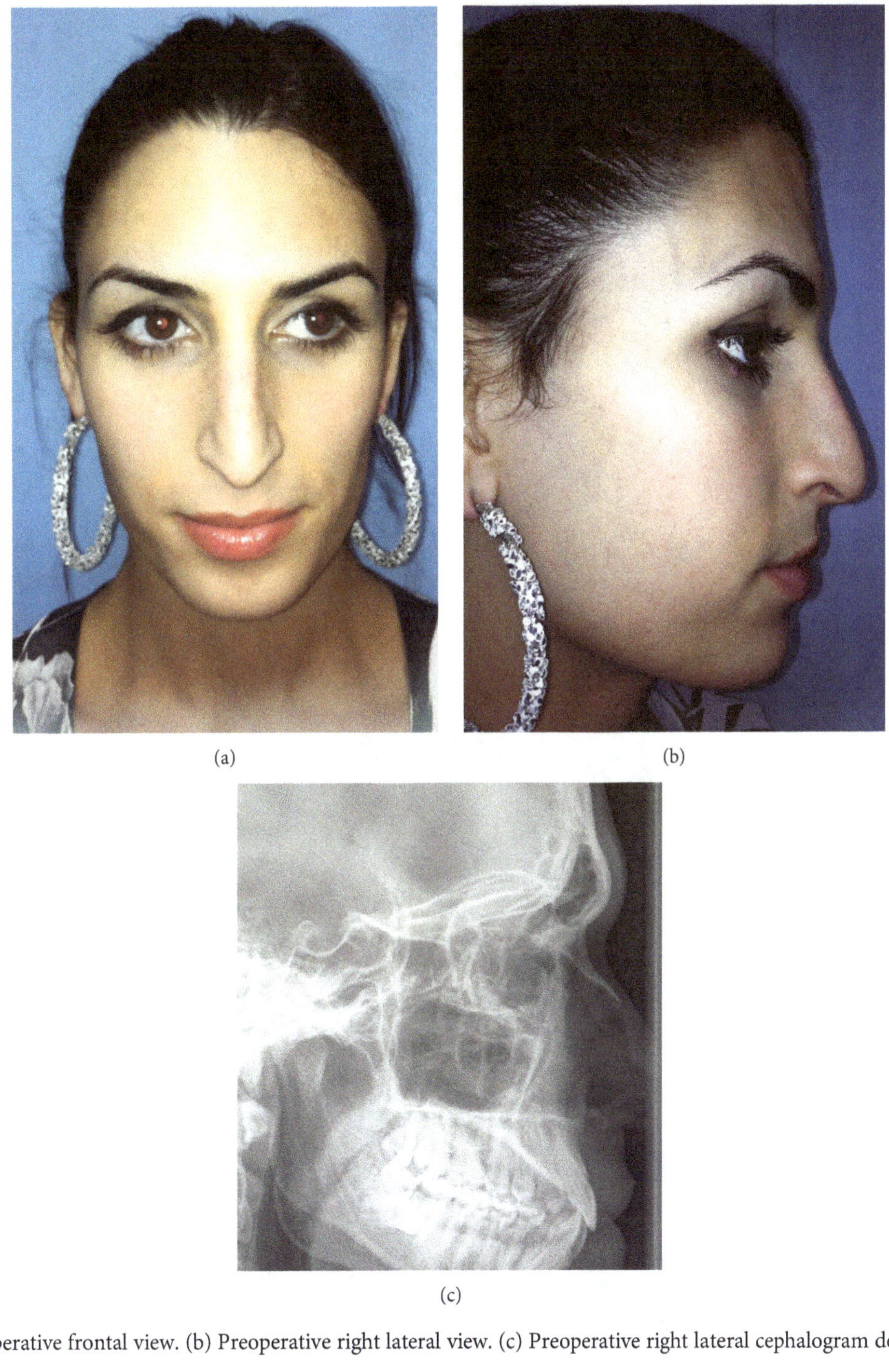

Figure 3: (a) Preoperative frontal view. (b) Preoperative right lateral view. (c) Preoperative right lateral cephalogram demonstrating a thick anterior table.

reduction. Rhinoplasty in combination with endoscopic frontal bone reduction and transoral mandibular osteoplasty was performed. Follow-up at two weeks confirmed excellent wound healing, and her intranasal and extranasal splints were removed. She was very satisfied with her results at one year.

4. Discussion

Masculine features of the upper third of the face include frontal bossing, a posteriorly displaced hairline, and heavier, straighter eyebrows. Facial feminization of this portion of the face typically involves bony contouring to reduce frontal bossing, brow lift, and lowering of the hairline. The implementation of forehead sculpturing in plastic surgery dates back to 1987 and has traditionally employed an open surgical technique via a coronal forehead flap or pretrichial approach [4]. While the open approach has been safe and efficacious, it may leave the patient with a cosmetically unappealing scar and may increase the risk for alopecia and forehead paresthesias [12].

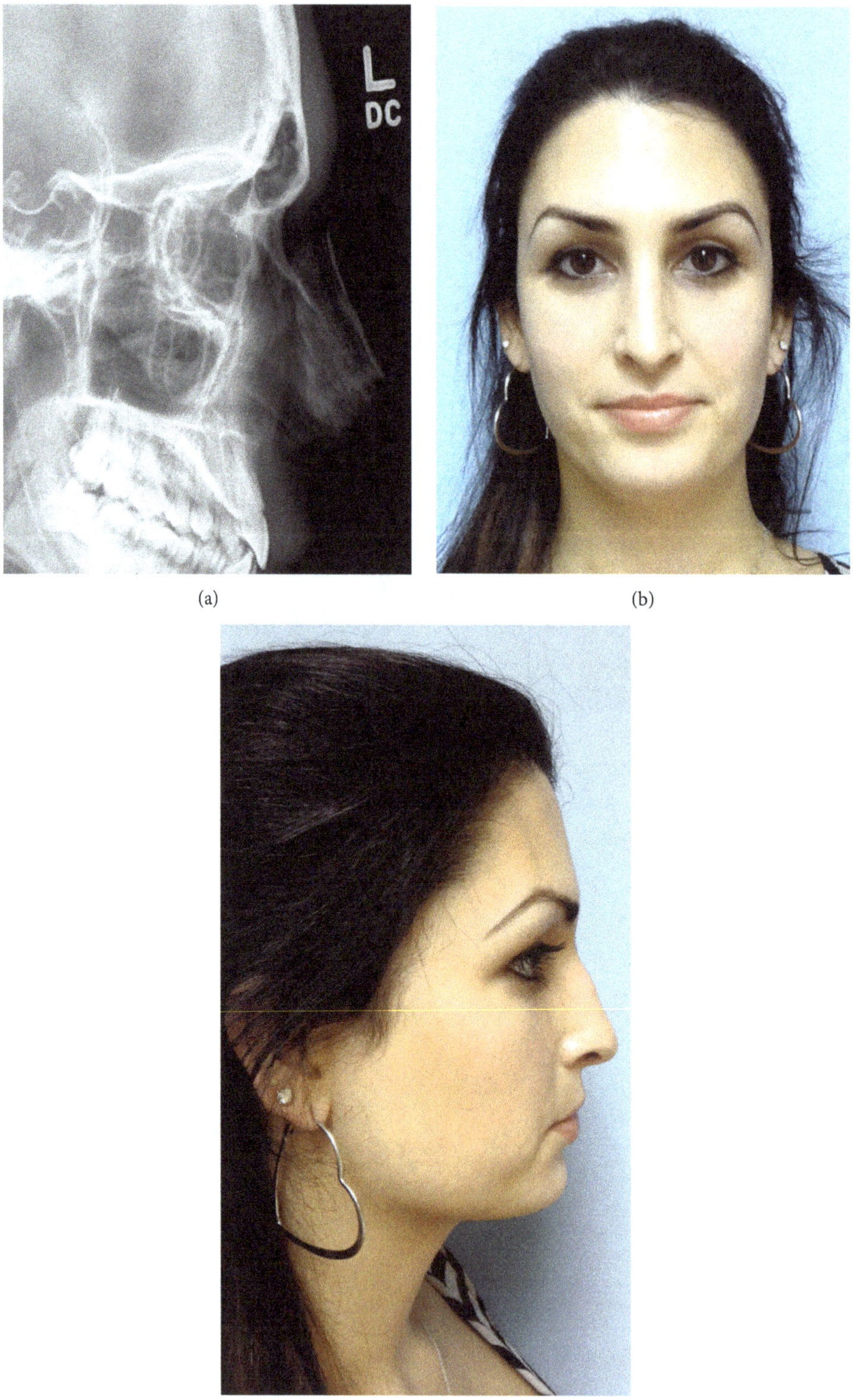

(a) (b) (c)

Figure 4: (a) Postoperative right lateral cephalogram. (b) Postoperative frontal view at 2 years. (c) Postoperative right lateral view at 2 years.

A minimally invasive approach to the anterior table of the frontal sinus has become a useful option for the reduction of frontal sinus fractures in the trauma setting [8]. Endoscopic assistance allows magnified visualization with the benefit of smaller scars, reduced risk of nerve injury, decreased length of hospital stay, and less soft tissue dissection as compared to open techniques [10, 13]. Song et al. reported a sentinel case of endoscopic frontal bone contouring in a 42-year-old Korean woman in 1995 [14]. A recent retrospective report on the success of the endoscopic

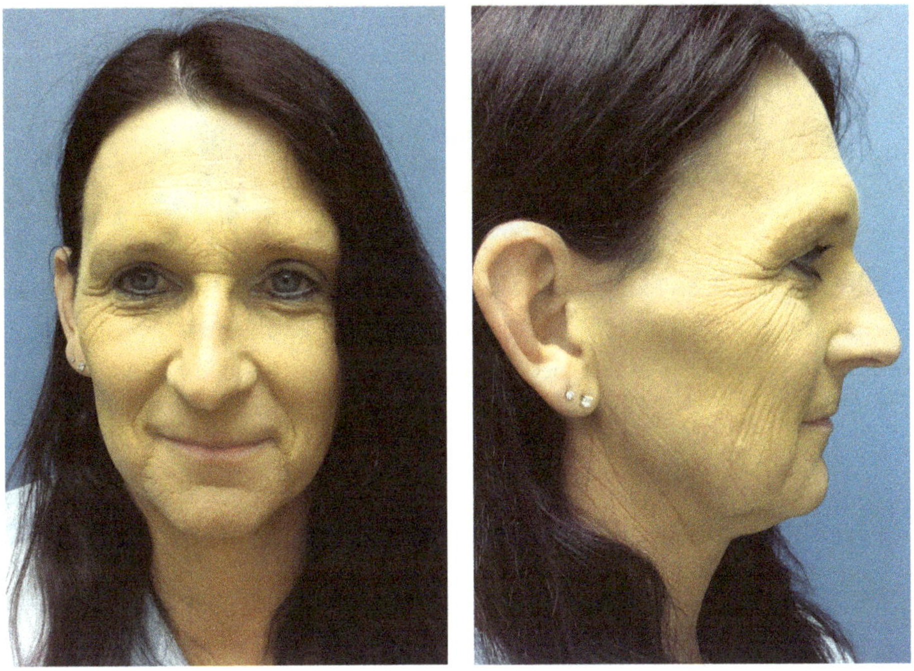

(a) (b)

Figure 5: (a) Preoperative frontal view. (b) Preoperative right lateral view.

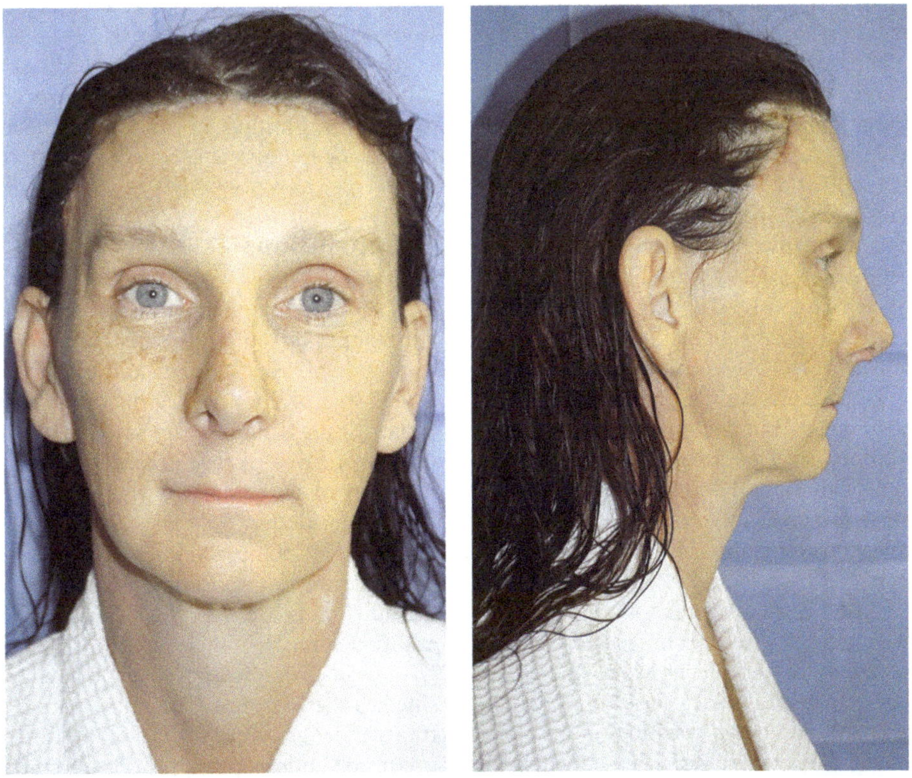

(a) (b)

Figure 6: (a) Postoperative frontal view at 2 weeks. (b) Postoperative right lateral view at 2 weeks.

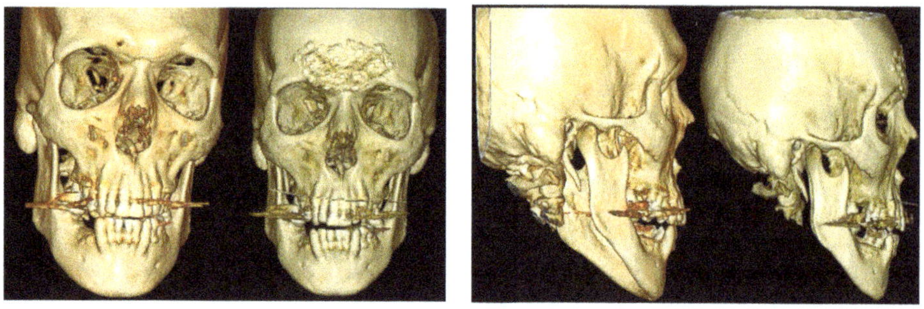

(a) (b)

FIGURE 7: (a) Preoperative and postoperative anterior view of facial bones using CT with 3D reconstruction. (b) Preoperative and postoperative right lateral view of facial bones using CT with 3D reconstruction.

approach to correct female frontal bossing has lent support to the efficacy, decreased morbidity, and positive aesthetic outcomes. Additionally, endoscopic contouring can be performed under a local anesthetic leading to same day discharge and reduced costs [10].

Of significant importance in the successful outcome of endoscopic reduction of the anterior table is preoperative planning. Lateral cephalograms help assess the thickness of the anterior table and supraorbital ridge in relation to the frontal sinus in order to prevent penetration into the sinus. Males tend to have a more pronounced frontal sinus and are particularly at risk for sinus penetration [11]. Patients ideally suited for endoscopic correction are those with mild-moderate frontal bossing and adequate (>5 mm) anterior table thickness. Those with a thin anterior table are better suited for a traditional open frontal bone setback secured with miniplates or titanium mesh. Additionally, if the patient required a lowering of the hairline or a frontal brow lift, then an open approach is used.

Technical challenges of the operation do include a learning curve with regard to the use of the drill under limited access of the endoscopic ports. Entry into the frontal sinus must be avoided by continuously checking the degree of reduction and bone translucency by inspection and palpation [10]. The endoscopic approach is even more challenging when a nasofrontal angle correction is also desired. For example, orbital opening or burring of the frontomalar region cannot be accomplished endoscopically using incisions above the hairline. In these scenarios, an open approach can be used. Care must also be taken to protect the supraorbital and supratrochlear nerves during the dissection when using either technique [15].

Reduction rhinoplasty is also of chief importance in facial feminization surgery, especially in regard to the profile view. The stereotypical female nose has increased concavity at the dorsum and a wider nasofrontal angle with a slightly upturned nasal tip resulting in a more obtuse nasolabial angle. Thus, these areas are targeted to increase the nasolabial and nasofrontal angle. Additionally, the overall size of the nose should be in harmony with the rest of the face. This usually means contouring the nasal dorsum and tip to create a more delicate petite nose [16]. While the middle and lower thirds of the nose can be addressed without any concurrent operations, the radix and nasofrontal angle are more difficult to control without also altering the glabella and brow region. While a deep radix can be augmented and the nasofrontal angle softened via rhinoplasty alone, creation of a significantly widened nasofrontal angle can only be achieved with frontal bone reduction in combination with rhinoplasty [17]. We believe that, based on our operative experience, concurrent nasal and frontal bone feminization is not only safe but also a more powerful and convenient technique. We routinely see patients in consultation that are out of state, and, therefore, by reducing the number of operations for these patients, we are able to address their facial feminization needs more expeditiously. Furthermore, health care costs may also be better controlled. As these patients are now frequently covered for their procedures under insurance plans, limiting the number of hospital stays via concurrent operations is a benefit in that regard as well.

5. Conclusions

Gender affirmation surgery is a rapidly developing field that necessitates ongoing refinement. Patients typically require a multitude of reconstructive and medically necessary surgeries tailored to the patient's own needs. The feminization of facial features significantly impacts the mental health and quality of life of male-to-female transgender individuals. It has been shown that those who have undergone a transition without facial feminization surgery have significantly lower quality of life compared to those who have [16]. The success of such surgeries depends on a thorough understanding of the differences between the male and female skeletal contour and structure.

The open surgical approach to a reduction of frontal bossing has been described for many years in the male-to-female transgender literature with favorable outcomes. However, the use of the endoscopic approach for supraorbital rim reduction in facial feminization offers patients a less invasive option and is a novel indication in this patient population. Furthermore, combining reduction rhinoplasty with frontal brow reduction in a single operation is safe and efficacious with potentially reduced healthcare costs.

References

[1] K. Wylie, "Gender related disorders," *BMJ*, vol. 329, no. 7466, pp. 615–617, 2004.

[2] J. H. Spiegel, "Facial determinants of female gender and feminizing forehead cranioplasty," *The Laryngoscope*, vol. 121, no. 2, pp. 250–261, 2011.

[3] S. D. Morrison, K. S. Vyas, S. Motakef et al., "Facial feminization: systematic review of the literature," *Plastic and Reconstructive Surgery*, vol. 137, no. 6, pp. 1759–1770, 2016.

[4] L. Capitan and D. Simon, "Facial feminization: a global approach," in *Gender Affirmation: Medical and Surgical Perspectives*, C. J. Salgado, S. Monstrey, and M. L. Djordjevic, Eds., pp. 3–31, Thieme Publishers Inc., New York, NY, USA, 2017.

[5] S. Manolidis and L. H. Hollier, "Management of frontal sinus fractures," *Plastic and Reconstructive Surgery*, vol. 120, no. 7, pp. 32S–48S, 2007.

[6] K. K. Kim, R. Mueller, F. Huang, and B. E. Strong, "Endoscopic repair of anterior table: frontal sinus fractures with a Medpor implant," *Otolaryngology-Head and Neck Surgery*, vol. 136, no. 4, pp. 568–572, 2007.

[7] E. B. Strong, G. M. Buchalter, and T. H. M. Moulthrop, "Endoscopic repair of isolated anterior table frontal sinus fractures," *Archives of Facial Plastic Surgery*, vol. 5, no. 6, pp. 514–521, 2003.

[8] H. D. Graham 3rd and P. Spring, "Endoscopic repair of frontal sinus fracture: case report," *The Journal of Cranio-Maxillofacial Trauma*, vol. 2, no. 4, pp. 52–55, 1996.

[9] B. C. Drolet, B. Z. Phillips, E. A. Hoy, J. Chang, and P. K. Sullivan, "Finesse in forehead and brow rejuvenation: modern concepts, including endoscopic methods," *Plastic and Reconstructive Surgery*, vol. 134, no. 6, pp. 1141–1150, 2014.

[10] B. Guyuron, M. Lee, K. Larson, and B. Amirlak, "Endoscopic correction of frontal bossing," *Plastic and Reconstructive Surgery*, vol. 131, no. 3, pp. 388e–393e, 2013.

[11] M. K. Lee, O. Sakai, and J. H. Spiegel, "CT measurement of the frontal sinus—gender differences and implications for frontal cranioplasty," *Journal of Cranio-Maxillo-Facial Surgery*, vol. 38, no. 7, pp. 494–500, 2010.

[12] S. W. Cho and H. R. Jin, "Feminization of the forehead in a transgender: frontal sinus reshaping combined with brow lift and hairline lowering," *Aesthetic Plastic Surgery*, vol. 36, no. 5, pp. 1207–1210, 2012.

[13] G. Mensink, A. Zweers, and J. P. R. van Merkesteyn, "Endoscopically assisted reduction of anterior table frontal sinus fractures," *Journal of Cranio-Maxillo-Facial Surgery*, vol. 37, no. 4, pp. 225–228, 2009.

[14] I. C. Song, J. N. Pozner, A. E. Sadeh, and M. S. Shin, "Endoscopic-assisted recontouring of the facial skeleton: the forehead," *Annals of Plastic Surgery*, vol. 34, no. 3, pp. 323–325, 1995.

[15] O. M. Ramirez, "Endoscopic techniques in facial rejuvenation: an overview. Part I," *Aesthetic Plastic Surgery*, vol. 18, no. 2, pp. 141–147, 1994.

[16] K. L. Eckstrand and J. M. Ehrenfeld, *Lesbian, Gay, Bisexual, and Transgender Healthcare: A Clinical Guide to Preventive, Primary, and Specialist Care*, Springer, Cham, Switzerland, 2016.

[17] R. J. Bellinga, L. Capitan, D. Simon, and T. Tenorio, "Technical and clinical considerations for facial feminization surgery with rhinoplasty and related procedures," *JAMA Facial Plastic Surgery*, vol. 19, no. 3, pp. 175–181, 2017.

3

Human Amniotic Membrane Positioning in the Surgical Treatment of Temporomandibular Joint Degenerative Disorder

Luca Guarda-Nardini,[1] Diletta Trojan,[2] Giulia Montagner,[2] Elisa Cogliati,[2] Matteo Bendini,[3] and Daniele Manfredini[4]

[1]*Section of Dentistry and Maxillofacial Surgery, Treviso Hospital, Treviso, Italy*
[2]*Treviso Tissue Bank Foundation, Treviso, Italy*
[3]*Section of Neuroradiology, Treviso Hospital, Treviso, Italy*
[4]*School of Dentistry, Department of Neuroscience, University of Padova, Padova, Italy*

Correspondence should be addressed to Diletta Trojan; dtrojan@fbtv-treviso.org

Academic Editor: Mario Ganau

Background. Temporomandibular joint (TMJ) arthritis is a degenerative pathology that may cause pain and dysfunction. Nonsurgical therapy is the traditional treatment of TMJ diseases but if ineffective, TMJ surgery can be performed and may include arthroplasty with interposition of autograft. The encouraging results reported with the use of human amniotic membrane (HAM) in different surgical fields have highlighted its potential, but approaches providing the positioning of HAM within the intra-articular space of arthritic TMJs have never been investigated. *Case Presentation.* A 48-year-old woman was presented with limited mouth opening and pain with palpation at the left joint. A severe TMJ degeneration was diagnosed, and a surgical treatment was necessary. In the present case report, the authors describe the application of a cryopreserved HAM patch within the joint space as a disc-replacing film during major surgeries for discectomy and arthroplasty. Three months after the intervention, the patient reported an overall improvement in chewing efficiency as well as the absence of pain. *Conclusions.* According to the regenerative effects of HAM, the design of trials on the topic should be encouraged for its possible inclusion within the field of TMJ disease practice.

1. Introduction

Temporomandibular disorders (TMDs) are the most frequent orofacial pain condition having multifactorial aetiology and affecting the intra-articular structures of the TMJs or the masticatory muscles [1]. They comprised a number of signs and symptoms: masticatory muscle and/or TMJ pain, articular sound during mandibular movement, and abnormalities of the mouth opening path, such as reduction or deviation of the range of joint motion. TMJ degenerative disorders have a complicated aetiology; a decreased adaptive capacity in the articulating structures or sustained physical stress may cause the degenerative remodeling of TMJs [2]. The traditional treatment of TMJ diseases is primarily based on nonsurgical options such as physical therapy, nonsteroidal anti-inflammatory drugs, or arthrocentesis with lubrification [3–5], while surgical treatment of TMJ diseases is only rarely indicated.

The choice of the treatment intervention depends primarily on the diagnosis. Structural disorders (e.g., overt or occult trauma, primary or secondary tumors, degenerative disorders, and infective diseases) [6–11] must be differentiated from nonstructural pain syndromes (e.g., neuropathic pain, myofascial pain, and psychological amplification) [12–14]. Amongst the former, surgery-demanding conditions must be clearly identified.

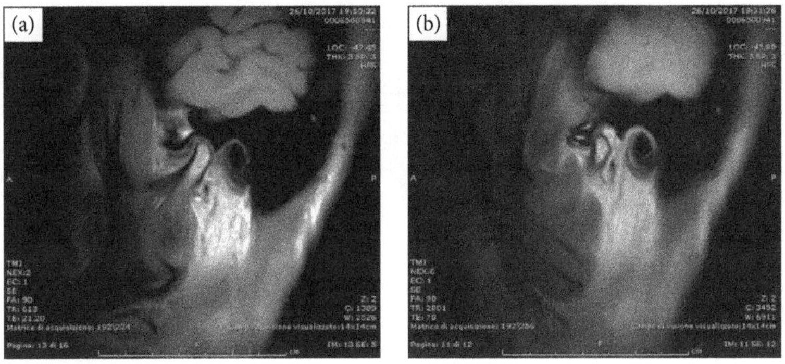

(a) (b)

Figure 1: MRI performed in closed (a) and open mouth (b) position during the first visit (T0).

Within these premises, TMJ arthroplasty with interposition of autograft (i.e., dermis, muscle-temporal fascia, and ear cartilage) is one of the primary surgical treatments [15–17]; however, the use of an autologous tissue might be associated with the morbidity of the second surgical site.

Human amniotic membrane (HAM) is the innermost layer of the fetal membranes with anti-inflammatory, antimicrobial, antifibrotic immunomodulatory properties, epithelialization and cell differentiation-modulating capacities, and low immunogenicity [18–20]. The extensive use and the encouraging results reported with the use of HAM in different surgical fields including maxillofacial surgery have highlighted its potential [21, 22].

The placenta is usually sourced from donors undergoing caesarean sections and processed shortly after retrieval. The HAM is carefully detached from the chorion and rinsed with sterile saline solution to remove residual blood. The membrane is flattened on a nitrocellulose membrane filter (Merck Millipore), with its stromal/mesenchymal side facing down, in contact with the filter. Afterwards, the HAM is immersed in a cocktail of antibiotics including vancomycin 100 μg/ml (Hospira), meropenem 200 μg/ml (Fresenius Kabi Italia), and gentamicin 200 mg/ml (Fisiopharma) at +4°C for 24 h in sterile conditions, validated for human tissues [23]. HAM was cut in $3 \times 3\ cm^2$ patches and cryopreserved. Microbiological analyses are performed at several stages throughout the process and only HAMs without microbial contamination were considered suitable for implants. The so-obtained tissue is positioned within the joint space.

The positioning of human amniotic membrane (HAM) within the intra-articular space of arthritic TMJs has never been investigated, but increasing amount of evidence highlights the potential positive effects of HAM on a number of surgical conditions, even included the interpositional arthroplasty for TMJ ankylosis [24, 25].

Based on these premises, HAM positioning within the intra-articular space of temporomandibular joints with severe inflammatory-degenerative disorders was suggested [26]. The purpose of this article is to report a case of patient with a diagnosis of TMD who underwent major surgery with the application of a cryopreserved HAM patch.

2. Case Presentation

A 48-year-old female came to our observation due to a limitation in mouth opening range. She also reported crepitus sounds at the left TMJ as well as pain, exacerbated by function (e.g., chewing) and increasing in intensity over the past three months. Clinical assessment showed a limited mouth opening (i.e., 22 mm) and pain with palpation at the left joint and all the main masticatory muscles, more severe on the left side. At the first appointment (T0), mandible manipulation was performed to achieve a forced opening of about 40 mm. A magnetic resonance (MRI) was prescribed to assess the disc-condyle relationship as the possible source of limitation in mouth opening and to gather some pictorial evaluation of the presence of joint effusion (Figure 1). Despite the clinical suspicion of TMJ arthritis, computerized tomography was not prescribed at this stage due to the expected low impact on treatment planning decisions.

MRI showed a regularly shaped condyle, with an anteriorized disc at closed mouth. At the maximum mouth opening, the condylar translation is reduced and the disc is not recaptured. Joint effusion of severe entity is also present. A conservative approach to provide pain relief and to manage muscle tension was provided, based on counseling, a home program of self-exercise and a stabilization appliance to wear at night. After three months, symptoms improved only partially, with a reduction of pain with muscle palpation but a steady pain at the left joint.

Based on that, a cycle of five arthrocentesis plus viscosupplementation with hyaluronic acid (Sinovial, IBSA) has been performed weekly. Clinical data has been recorded at each time point before each injection and 15 days after the last one (Table 1).

After one month from the last arthrocentesis plus viscosupplementation, the patient still showed some pain and, more important, still felt a limitation in the unassisted mouth opening and right laterotrusion. A diagnosis of TMJ intermittent locking on the left side was thus performed, and given the difficulties to stabilize clinical symptoms and mouth opening with the usual conservative approaches, the patient was planned for a surgical removal of the TMJ disc with concurrent HAM positioning (Figure 2).

Table 1: Clinical data collected before each injection (T0-T4) and 15 days after the last injection.

Parameters	T0	T1	T2	T3	T4	15 days after the last injection
Masticatory capacity (scores from 0 to 10)*	3	3	5	7	7	7
Chewing-related pain (scores from 0 to 10)**						
min	0	0	0	0	0	0
max	6	9	6	6	6	6
Phonation-related pain (scores from 0 to 10)**						
min	0	0	0	0	0	0
max	8	8	8	1	5	5
Rest-related pain (scores from 0 a 10)**						
min	0	0	0	0	0	0
max	0	7	0	0	3	3
Level of functional limitation$	4	4	1	1	3	3
Efficacy evaluation***	-	1	2	3	1	1
Tolerability evaluation***	-	2	3	3	3	3
Mouth-opening ability						
Spontaneous	23 mm	23 mm	30 mm	33 mm	25 mm	25 mm
Forced	23 mm	42 mm	35 mm	33 mm	25 mm	27 mm
Right laterality	0	0	0	10 mm	10 mm	10 mm
Protusion	5 mm	5 mm	5 mm	5 mm	3 mm	3 mm
Left laterality	10 mm	10 mm	10 mm	10 mm	10 mm	10 mm

*Scores from 0 = inability to chew and only the consumption of semiliquid foods is possible to 10 = optimal chewing capacity of any type of food. **NRS scores from 0 = no pain to 10 = intolerable pain. $0 = none; 1 = tolerable; 2 = moderate; 3 = intense; 4 = serious. ***0 = light; 1 = tolerable; 2 = moderate; 3 = good; 4 = excellent.

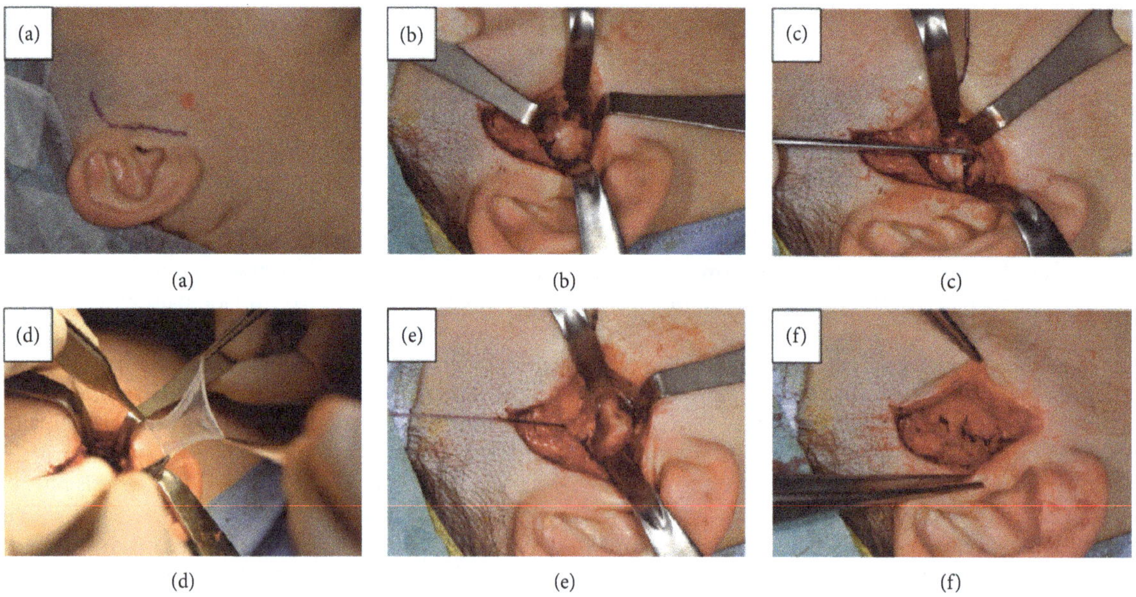

Figure 2: (a–f) condyle remodelling and meniscectomy of TMJ with HAM graft.

TMJ surgery provided condyle remodelling and discectomy (Figures 2(a)–2(c)), after which a HAM patch is positioned within the intra-articular space (Figure 2(d)), and stratified stitching is performed to avoid postoperatory scars (Figures 2(e) and 2(f)).

Three months after the intervention, the patient showed no negative exitus or postsurgical side effects. Jaw range of motion was increasing, both as for unassisted mouth opening (38 mm) and right laterotrusion (8 mm). The patient reported an overall improvement in chewing efficiency as well as the absence of pain (Table 2).

Five months after surgery, a new MRI was performed (Figure 3). The images showed the physiological excursion of the TMJ condyle during mouth opening (Figure 3(b)).

TABLE 2: Three-month follow-up assessment. Clinical data.

Parameters	3 months after surgery
Masticatory capacity (scores from 0 to 10)*	8
Chewing-related pain (scores from 0 to 10)**	
min	0
max	0
Phonation-related pain (scores from 0 to 10)**	
min	0
max	0
Rest-related pain (scores from 0 to 10)**	
min	0
max	2
Level of functional limitation$	2
Efficacy evaluation***	3
Tolerability evaluation***	3
Mouth-opening ability	
Spontaneous	38 mm
Forced	38 mm

*Scores from 0 = inability to chew and only the consumption of semiliquid foods is possible to 10 = optimal chewing capacity of any type of food. **NRS scores from 0 = no pain to 10 = intolerable pain. $0 = none; 1 = tolerable; 2 = moderate; 3 = intense; 4 = serious. ***0 = light; 1 = tolerable; 2 = moderate; 3 = good; 4 = excellent.

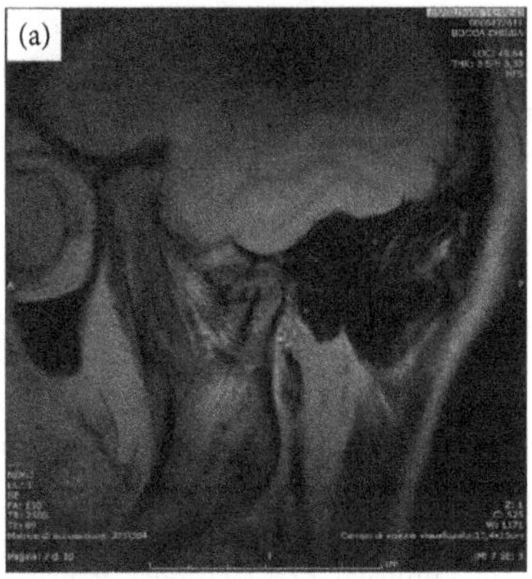

(a)

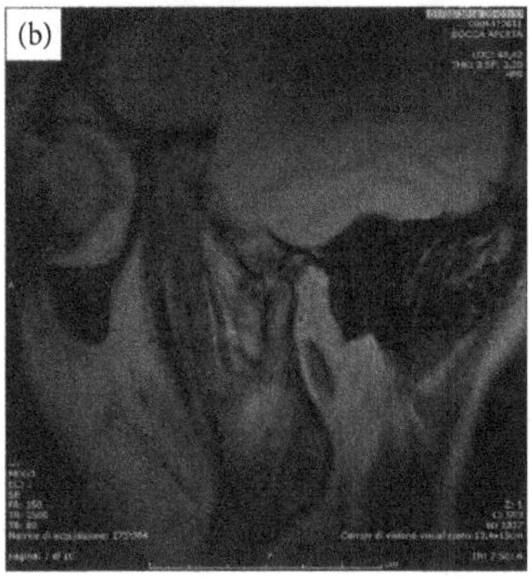

(b)

FIGURE 3: MRI at the five-month follow-up. Closed (a) and open mouth position (b) showing the HAM patch. The HAM patch covers the condyle head; the translation is improved.

3. Discussion

This case report demonstrates that in the surgical treatment of TMJ arthrosis, the interposition of HAM in the intra-articular space resulting from an arthroplasty intervention represents a promising solution. In fact, three months after the intervention, the patient reported the absence of pain, an increased masticatory capacity, and an improvement of the range of mouth opening.

Since the etiopathogenesis and symptoms of TMJ diseases are variable, several different treatments are adopted. In rare selected cases, surgical treatments are necessary, including meniscectomy, condylectomy, and arthroplasty with interposition of autologous tissues [15–17].

The benefits of HAM positioning in TMJs with severe inflammatory-degenerative disorders could be related with its anti-inflammatory and antimicrobial properties and low immunogenicity [18–20]. In addition, thanks to its properties, it has been demonstrated that the application of HAM to wounds markedly reduces patients' experienced pain intensity [27]. Moreover, amniotic membrane is able to reduce postoperative adhesion [28].

Within the limits of the present case report, a promising suggestion concerning the use of HAM for TMJ surgery has been provided. Case series providing a longer follow-up should be encouraged, as well as the assessment of less invasive strategies for HAM positioning. In particular, future clinical trials might aim at comparing the effectiveness of HAM with respect to standard interpositional surgical intervention. Imaging techniques trying to assess the intra-articular changes associated with the use of human membrane are also recommended for a better comprehension of the course of degenerative disorders in patients undergoing this treatment.

References

[1] M. Romero-Reyes and J. M. Uyanik, "Orofacial pain management: current perspectives," *Journal of Pain Research*, vol. 7, pp. 99–115, 2014.

[2] E. Tanaka, M. S. Detamore, and L. G. Mercuri, "Degenerative disorders of the temporomandibular joint: etiology, diagnosis, and treatment," *Journal of Dental Research*, vol. 87, no. 4, pp. 296-307, 2008.

[3] M. L. McNeely, S. Armijo Olivo, and D. J. Magee, "A systematic review of the effectiveness of physical therapy interventions for temporomandibular disorders," *Physical Therapy*, vol. 86, no. 5, pp. 710-725, 2006.

[4] D. Manfredini, F. Piccotti, and L. Guarda-Nardini, "Hyaluronic acid in the treatment of TMJ disorders. A systematic review of the literature," *CRANIO®*, vol. 28, pp. 166–176, 2010.

[5] M. A. Moldez, V. R. Camones, G. E. Ramos, M. Padilla, and R. Enciso, "Effectiveness of intra-articular injections of sodium hyaluronate or corticosteroids for intracapsular temporomandibular disorders: a systematic review and meta-analysis,"

Journal of Oral & Facial Pain and Headache, vol. 32, no. 1, pp. 53–66, 2018.

[6] K. Miyauchi, K. Sano, M. Nagai et al., "Occult fractures of articular eminence and glenoid fossa presenting as temporomandibular disorder: a case report," *Oral Surgery, Oral Medicine, Oral Pathology, Oral Radiology, and Endodontology*, vol. 101, no. 6, pp. e101–e105, 2006.

[7] F. Paparo, M. Massarelli, R. Cordeschi, V. Sciannameo, and F. Spallaccia, "Chondromatosis of the temporomandibular joint as a consequence of persistent long-lasting joint dysfunction: late diagnosis of a rare occurrence," *Journal of Craniofacial Surgery*, vol. 27, no. 7, pp. e636–e637, 2016.

[8] S. Lohiya and J. Dillon, "Septic arthritis of the temporomandibular joint—unusual presentations," *Journal of Oral and Maxillofacial Surgery*, vol. 74, no. 1, pp. 87–94, 2016.

[9] H. J. Park, B. C. Kim, E. J. Choi, S. R. Samayoa, and H. J. Kim, "Tuberculosis of the temporomandibular joint: a case of misdiagnosis," *Journal of Oral & Facial Pain and Headache*, vol. 28, no. 2, pp. 165–170, 2014.

[10] L. Guarda-Nardini, E. Stellini, A. Di Fiore, and D. Manfredini, "A rare case of misdiagnosed silent lung cancer with solitary metastasis to the temporomandibular joint condyle," *Journal of Oral & Facial Pain and Headache*, vol. 31, no. 2, pp. 180–185, 2017.

[11] J. Emanuelsson, C. M. Allen, K. Rydin, and M. Sjöström, "Osteoblastoma of the temporal articular tubercle misdiagnosed as a temporomandibular joint disorder," *International Journal of Oral and Maxillofacial Surgery*, vol. 46, no. 5, pp. 610–613, 2017.

[12] L. Prisco, M. Ganau, F. Bigotto, and F. Zornada, "Trigeminal neuralgia: successful antiepileptic drug combination therapy in three refractory cases," *Drug, Healthcare and Patient Safety*, vol. 3, pp. 43–45, 2011.

[13] L. Guarda-Nardini, F. Piccotti, G. Ferronato, and D. Manfredini, "Myositis ossificans traumatica of the temporalis muscle: a case report and diagnostic considerations," *Oral and Maxillofacial Surgery*, vol. 16, no. 2, pp. 221–225, 2012.

[14] B. B. Horswell and J. Sheikh, "Evaluation of pain syndromes, headache, and temporomandibular joint disorders in children," *Oral and Maxillofacial Surgery Clinics of North America*, vol. 30, no. 1, pp. 11–24, 2018.

[15] M. Bayat, A. Badri, and N. Moharamnejad, "Treatment of temporomandibular joint ankylosis: gap and interpositional arthroplasty with temporalis muscle flap," *Oral and Maxillofacial Surgery*, vol. 13, no. 4, pp. 207–212, 2009.

[16] A. Holmlund, B. Lund, and C. K. Weiner, "Mandibular condylectomy with osteoarthrectomy with and without transfer of the temporalis muscle," *British Journal of Oral and Maxillofacial Surgery*, vol. 51, no. 3, pp. 206–210, 2013.

[17] J. Yazdani, M. Ali Ghavimi, S. Pourshahidi, and H. Ebrahimi, "Comparison of clinical efficacy of temporalis myofascial flap and dermal graft as interpositional material in treatment of temporomandibular joint ankylosis," *Journal of Craniofacial Surgery*, vol. 21, no. 4, pp. 1218–1220, 2010.

[18] E. Inge, Y. P. Talmi, L. Sigler, Y. Finkelstein, and Y. Zohar, "Antibacterial properties of human amniotic membranes," *Placenta*, vol. 12, no. 3, pp. 285–288, 1991.

[19] Y. Hao, D. Ma, D. Hwang, W. Kim, and F. Zhang, "Identification of antiangiogenic and antiinflammatory proteins in human amniotic membrane," *Cornea*, vol. 19, no. 3, pp. 348–352, 2000.

[20] N. J. Koizumi, T. J. Inatomi, C. J. Sotozono, N. J. Fullwood, A. J. Quantock, and S. Kinoshita, "Growth factor mRNA and protein in preserved human amniotic membrane," *Current Eye Research*, vol. 20, no. 3, pp. 173–177, 2000.

[21] C. R. Kothari, G. Goudar, N. Hallur, B. Sikkerimath, S. Gudi, and M. C. Kothari, "Use of amnion as a graft material in vestibuloplasty: a clinical study," *British Journal of Oral and Maxillofacial Surgery*, vol. 50, no. 6, pp. 545–549, 2012.

[22] M. Ragazzo, D. Trojan, L. Spagnol, A. Paolin, and L. Guarda Nardini, "Use of amniotic membrane in the treatment of patients with BRONJ: two case reports," *Journal of Surgical Case Reports*, vol. 2018, no. 4, 2018.

[23] A. Serafini, E. Riello, D. Trojan et al., "Evaluation of new antibiotic cocktails against contaminating bacteria found in allograft tissues," *Cell and Tissue Banking*, vol. 17, no. 4, pp. 619–628, 2016.

[24] M. Akhter, N. Ahmed, M. R. Arefin, M.-U. Sobhan, M. R. Molla, and M. Kamal, "Outcome of amniotic membrane as an interpositional arthroplasty of TMJ ankylosis," *Oral and Maxillofacial Surgery*, vol. 20, no. 1, pp. 63–71, 2016.

[25] F. Bauer, L. M. Hingsammer, K. D. Wolff, and M. R. Kesting, "Temporomandibular joint arthroplasty with human amniotic membrane: a case report," *Eplasty*, vol. 13, article e17, 2013.

[26] L. Guarda-Nardini, D. Trojan, A. Paolin, and D. Manfredini, "Management of temporomandibular joint degenerative disorders with human amniotic membrane: hypothesis of action," *Medical Hypotheses*, vol. 104, pp. 68–71, 2017.

[27] I. Mermet, N. Pottier, J. M. Sainthillier et al., "Use of amniotic membrane transplantation in the treatment of venous leg ulcers," *Wound Repair and Regeneration*, vol. 15, no. 4, pp. 459–464, 2007.

[28] C. T. Walker, J. Godzik, U. K. Kakarla, J. D. Turner, A. C. Whiting, and P. Nakaji, "Human amniotic membrane for the prevention of intradural spinal cord adhesions: retrospective review of its novel use in a case series of 14 patients," *Neurosurgery*, vol. 83, no. 5, pp. 989–996, 2018.

4

Surgical Management of the Peripheral Osteoma of the Zygomatic Arch: A Case Report and Literature Review

Umberto Autorino, Claudia Borbon, Maria Chiara Malandrino, Giovanni Gerbino, and Fabio Roccia

Division of Maxillofacial Surgery, Surgical Science Department, Città della Salute e delle Scienza Hospital, University of Turin, Corso A.M. Dogliotti 14, 10126 Torino, Italy

Correspondence should be addressed to Claudia Borbon; cla.borbon@gmail.com

Academic Editor: Giulio Maccauro

An osteoma is a benign, slow-growing, osteogenic neoplasm with a low recurrence rate that is typically characterized by the proliferation of a compact or cancellous bone. It can be peripheral, central, or extraskeletal. Usually asymptomatic, peripheral osteomas in the maxillofacial region commonly arise in the paranasal sinuses and mandible and rarely occur in the zygomatic arch, with only six previously documented cases in the literature. Here, we present the management of a solitary peripheral osteoma of the right zygomatic arch in a 72-year-old woman and a review of the literature.

1. Introduction

Osteoma is a benign, slow-growing, osteogenic neoplasm characterized by the proliferation of a compact or cancellous bone [1]. It was first recognized as a tumor by Jaffe [2]. The etiology of these lesions remains unknown, but several explanations have been suggested for its origin including embryologic, traumatic, inflammatory, metaplastic, and genetic causes [1, 3–5]. It is more common in females, with a mean age at diagnosis of about 50 years [4, 5]. They can occur as solitary or multiple lesions, the latter of which can be seen in cases of Gardner syndrome [6].

Osteomas almost exclusively affect the maxillofacial skeleton, particularly the paranasal sinuses and mandible, and can be classified based on the location from which they arise. Central osteomas arise centripetally from the endosteum, peripheral osteomas are caused by centrifugal growth of the periosteum, and extraskeletal soft tissue osteomas develop within the muscles [1, 4, 5, 7]. The majority of these lesions are peripheral varying from 41.9% [4] to 49% [1], while central osteomas in the craniofacial skeleton are uncommon. Peripheral osteomas of the craniofacial region occur in the frontal, ethmoid, and maxillary sinuses with no sex or age predilection [3, 8–12].

Clinically, peripheral lesions appear as unilateral, pedunculated, and asymptomatic mushroom-like masses and can produce pain, trismus (when there is nerve involvement), limited mandibular movement, malocclusion, swelling, and facial asymmetry [3, 8, 10–13].

Computer tomography (CT) is the current gold standard for the diagnosis and surgical management of an osteoma. A peripheral osteoma is seen as an oval, radiopaque, well-circumscribed mass attached to the cortex by a broad base or pedicle [3, 10, 13, 14]. Differential diagnosis should include fibrous dysplasia, exostosis, chondroma, ossifying fibroma, condensing osteitis, osteoblastoma, Paget's disease of the bone, osteosarcoma, or odontoma if the lesion occurs near the teeth [15]. Histologic classification can differentiate between two types of peripheral osteomas: compact osteomas, which are composed of mature lamellar bone that do not contain any fibrous component, and trabecular osteomas composed of cancellous trabecular bone and bone marrow surrounded by a cortical margin [3, 10, 13]. Osteomas have a low recurrence rate when treated using adequate surgical techniques. Although excision is recommended for growing or symptomatic lesions, there have been no reports of malignant transformation in the literature [1, 3–5, 10, 13].

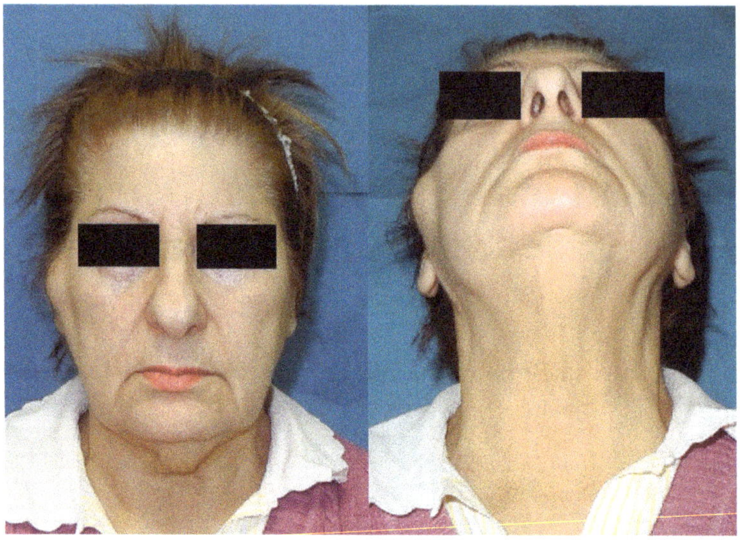

Figure 1: Clinical preoperative view showing preauricolar swelling on the right side of the face.

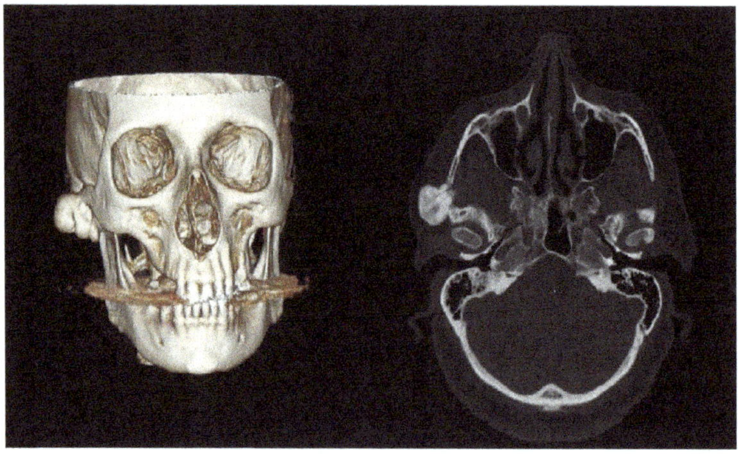

Figure 2: Axial CT scan and three-dimensional reconstruction image showing a well-defined, pedunculated, and radiopaque mass of the right zygomatic arch.

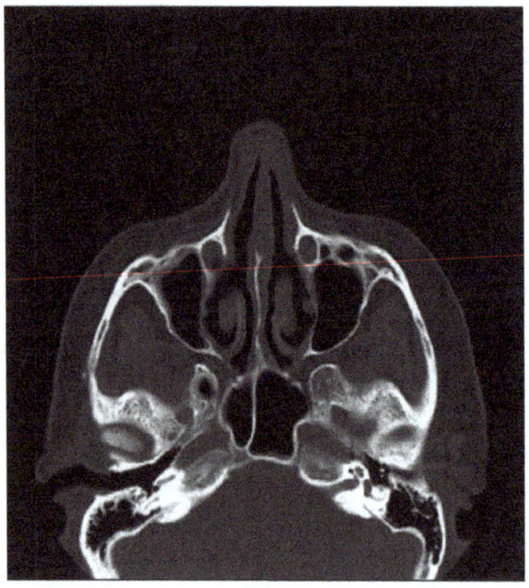

Figure 3: Postoperative axial CT scan.

We describe a rare case of peripheral osteoma in the zygomatic arch and present a review of the literature.

2. Case Report

A 72-year-old woman was referred to the division of Maxillofacial Surgery, Città della Salute e della Scienza Hospital, University of Turin (Torino, Italy), for an enlarged preauricular mass on the right side of her face. The lesion had slowly been growing for 3 years (Figure 1). There was no previous history of facial trauma. Her medical history was only remarkable for arterial hypertension and diabetes mellitus type II. Examination revealed a solitary, smooth, nontender, firm, bony asymptomatic swelling over the right zygomatic arch measuring approximately 3 cm in diameter. There were no recent changes in her ability to open her mouth, and no abnormalities were noted in either temporomandibular joint. CT scans confirmed the presence of a 3 cm pedunculated, well-circumscribed, radiopaque, lobulated structure along

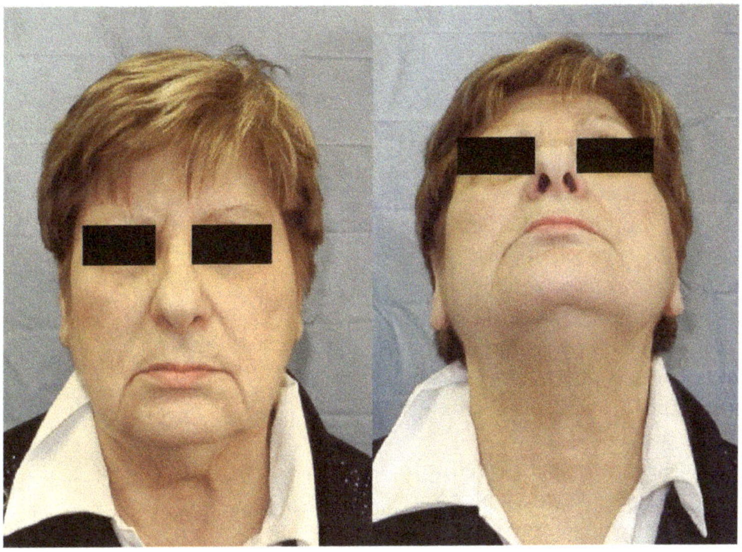

FIGURE 4: Clinical view 1 year after surgery.

TABLE 1: Summery of the published cases of peripheral osteomas of the zygomatic arch.

Case	Age/sex	Clinical symptoms	Size (cm)	Surgical approach	Follow-up	
1	55/F	None	Not reported	Preauricolar	Not reported	Furlaneto et al.
2	20/M	Local sensitivity	3 × 4	Direct facial approach	6 months	Akinmoladun et al.
3	61/M	None	8.5 × 6.7 × 9.85	None	Not reported	Durao et al.
4	35/M	Pain	2	Not reported	Not reported	Naikmasur et al.
5	32/F	Pain	3	Preauricolar	7 years	Quintans et al.
6	55/F	Pain	1.2 × 1.4	Preauricolar	1 year	Starch-Jensen
7	72/F	None	2.7 × 2 × 2.2	Preauricolar	5 years	Present case

the lateral border of the right zygomatic arch (Figure 2). Based on the clinical and radiographic findings, we diagnosed a peripheral osteoma of the zygomatic arch. Given the ongoing growth and cosmetic concerns, the decision was made to surgically remove the tumor.

Under general anaesthesia, the zygomatic arch was accessed via a preauricular incision with temporal extension (Al-Kayat and Bramley's modifications [16]). After incision, a complete view of the lesion was obtained and the tumor was easily excised. Histology revealed that the specimen was a normal cortical trabecular bone, confirming the diagnosis of an osteoma.

The patient's postoperative course was uneventful with only temporary dysesthesia along the V3 branch of the trigeminal nerve. The symptoms resolved spontaneously after 2 months. The patient was discharged home 5 days after surgery. CT scans 1 year after surgery showed normal bone architecture of the right zygoma, good symmetry, and no signs of relapse (Figures 3 and 4). No clinical evidence of recurrence was encountered at the 5-year follow-up.

3. Discussion

Peripheral osteomas of the maxillofacial region most frequently occur in the paranasal sinuses but can also be found in the jaw bones, external auditory canal, orbit, temporal bone, and pterygoid processes [3, 10, 13, 17]. Peripheral osteomas of the zygomatic arch are extremely uncommon. A literature review identified only six previously documented cases [18–23] (Table 1). According to Longo et al. [11] and Kashima et al. [14], the age of patients ranges from 20 to 72 years with a mean age of 47 years. In our study, despite the small number of cases, the prevalence of peripheral osteomas was slightly higher in women.

Several authors [1, 3, 10, 13] have reported that peripheral osteomas are usually asymptomatic. When present, the most common symptoms are pain, trismus, or limited mouth opening. In our review, we found that four of seven patients complained of pain or local dysesthesia, while the remainder of patients were asymptomatic. There did not appear to be any significant correlation between severity of the clinical symptoms and tumor size. Any clinical effects related to the growth of the osteoma were likely due to mass effects of the lesion and compression of adjacent anatomical structures [19, 20, 22, 23]. Surgery is indicated when a patient complains of symptoms or if a lesion presents as progressive growth, as was the case with our patient. An intraoral approach is preferable to avoid facial scarring and facial nerve damage. However, in our review, we found that all lesions were excised through an extraoral approach. A preauricolar approach was used in five cases, and one other report utilized a direct approach by "following the facial skin crease" [19].

Similar to Furlaneto et al. [18], we believe that a preauricular approach allows for adequate surgical exposure, a good view of the lesion, and complete tumor resection. Moreover, this approach has lower risks of facial injury and scarring than direct approaches. Akinmoladun et al. [19] reported a case in which the "tumor was excised under local anaesthesia by direct facial approach using an incision following the facial skin crease," but "caution was taken to avoid possible damage to the zygomatic arch." Furlaneto et al. [18] also described a case of osteoma recurrence in the zygomatic arch 10 years after surgical removal using a direct approach. In this case, it is likely that underexposure and poor visibility led to incomplete removal of the tumor.

Most cases of tumor excision have been performed with zygomatic arch preservation, with the exception of a case reported by Quintans et al. [22] , in which complete tumor excision required osteotomy of the zygomatic arch. In this case, positioning of a titanium plate was necessary to restore the normal bone architecture.

Acknowledgments

The English language in this document has been checked by at least two professional editors, both native speakers of English. For a certificate, please see http://www.textcheck.com/certificate/Am9xhA.

References

[1] N. Larrea-Oyarbide, E. Valmaseda-Castellón, L. Berini-Aytés, and C. Gay-Escoda, "Osteomas of the craniofacial region. Review of 106 cases," *Journal of Oral Pathology & Medicine*, vol. 37, no. 1, pp. 38–42, 2008.

[2] H. L. Jaffe, "Osteoid osteoma: a benign osteoblastic tumor composed of osteoid and atypical region," *Archives of Surgery*, vol. 31, no. 5, pp. 709–728, 1935.

[3] N. B. Sayan, C. Üçok, H. A. Karasu, and Ö. Günhan, "Peripheral osteoma of the oral and maxillofacial region: a study of 35 new cases," *Journal of Oral and Maxillofacial Surgery*, vol. 60, no. 11, pp. 1299–1301, 2002.

[4] P. Boffano, F. Roccia, P. Campisi, and C. Gallesio, "Review of 43 osteomas of the craniomaxillofacial region," *Journal of Oral and Maxillofacial Surgery*, vol. 70, no. 5, pp. 1093–1095, 2012.

[5] G. D. A. Orabona, G. Salzano, G. Iaconetta et al., "Facial osteomas: fourteen cases and a review of literature," *European Review for Medical and Pharmacological Sciences*, vol. 19, no. 10, pp. 1796–1802, 2015.

[6] E. J. GARDNER and H. P. PLENK, "Hereditary pattern for multiple osteomas in a family group," *American Journal of Human Genetics*, vol. 4, no. 1, pp. 31–36, 1952.

[7] L. Junquera-Gutierrez, J. S. Lopez-Arraz, J. M. Albertos-Castro, and J. C. De Vicente-Rodriguez, "Odontogenic tumors: classification, clinical features, diagnosis and treatment," *Medicina Oral*, vol. 2, no. 2, pp. 94–101, 1997.

[8] L. Bosshardt, R. C. Gordon, M. Westerberg, and A. Morgan, "Recurrent peripheral osteoma of mandible: report of a case," *Journal of Oral Surgery*, vol. 29, no. 6, pp. 446–450, 1971.

[9] K. Bessho, K. I. Murakami, T. Iizuka, and T. Ono, "Osteoma in mandibular condyle," *International Journal of Oral and Maxillofacial Surgery*, vol. 16, no. 3, pp. 372–375, 1987.

[10] L. Bodner, A. Gatot, N. Sion-Vardy, and D. M. Fliss, "Peripheral osteoma of the mandibular ascending ramus," *Journal of Oral and Maxillofacial Surgery*, vol. 56, no. 12, pp. 1446–1449, 1998.

[11] F. Longo, L. Califano, G. D. Maria, and R. Ciccarelli, "Solitary osteoma of the mandibular ramus: Report of a case," *Journal of Oral and Maxillofacial Surgery*, vol. 59, no. 6, pp. 698–700, 2001.

[12] F. K. Horikawa, R. R. de Freitas, F. A. Maciel, and A. J. Gonçalves, "Peripheral osteoma of the maxillofacial region: a study of 10 cases," *Brazilian Journal of Otorhinolaryngology*, vol. 78, no. 5, pp. 38–43, 2012.

[13] Y. Woldenberg, M. Nash, and L. Bodner, "Peripheral osteoma of the maxillofacial region. Diagnosis and management: A study of 14 cases," *Medicina Oral, Patología Oral y Cirugía Bucal*, vol. 10, Suppl2, pp. E139–E142, 2005.

[14] K. Kashima, O. I. F. Rahman, S. Sakoda, and R. Shiba, "Unusual peripheral osteoma of the mandible: Report of 2 cases," *Journal of Oral and Maxillofacial Surgery*, vol. 58, no. 8, pp. 911–913, 2000.

[15] S. C. White and M. J. Pharoah, "Oral radiology. Benign tumors of tha jaws," in *Oral Radiology: Principles and Interpretation*, pp. 392-393, Mosby Elsevier, 2009.

[16] A. Al-Kayat and P. Bramley, "A modified pre-auricular approach to the temporomandibular joint and malar arch," *The British Journal of Oral Surgery*, vol. 17, no. 2, pp. 91–103, 1979.

[17] T. Ishikawa, S. Yashima, H. Hasan, T. Shimosato, and S. Imada, "Osteoma of the lateral pterygoid plate of the sphenoid bone," *International Journal of Oral and Maxillofacial Surgery*, vol. 15, no. 6, pp. 786–789, 1986.

[18] E. C. Furlaneto, J. R. M. Rocha, and C. Heitz, "Osteoma of the zygomatic arch – report of a case," *International Journal of Oral and Maxillofacial Surgery*, vol. 33, no. 3, pp. 310-311, 2004.

[19] V. I. Akinmoladun, A. O. Akadiri, and A. A. Olusanya, "Peripheral osteoma of the zygoma: literature review and case presentation," *African Journal of Medicine and Medical Sciences*, vol. 36, no. 4, pp. 381–383, 2007.

[20] V. Naikmasur, A. Sattur, and A. Rai, "Osteoma of zygomatic arch and eminence: a case report," *Indian Journal of Stomatology*, vol. 2, no. 1, pp. 37-38, 2011.

[21] A. R. Durão, I. Chilvarquer, J. E. Hayek, M. Provenzano, and M. R. Kendall, "Osteoma of the zygomatic arch and mandible: report of two cases," *Revista Portuguesa de Estomatologia, Medicina Dentária e Cirurgia Maxilofacial*, vol. 53, no. 2, pp. 103–107, 2012.

[22] A. D. Quintans, J. A. D. Castro, P. E. M. Machado, and F. W. G. Costa, "Solitary osteoma in the zygomatic arch," *The Journal of Craniofacial Surgery*, vol. 24, no. 6, pp. 2209-2210, 2013.

[23] T. Starch-Jensen, "Peripheral solitary osteoma of the zygomatic arch: a case report and literature review," *The Open Dentistry Journal*, vol. 11, no. 1, pp. 120–125, 2017.

5

Treatment of Atypical Bifid Mandibular Condyle Associated with Ankylosis of the Temporomandibular Joint

Katheleen Miranda,[1] André Sander Carneiro,[1] Jennifer Tsi Gerber,[1] Suyany Gabriely Weiss,[1] Leandro Eduardo Klüppel,[1,2] and Rafaela Scariot[1,2]

[1]*School of Health Science, Positivo University, Curitiba, Brazil*
[2]*School of Health Science, Federal University of Paraná, Curitiba, Brazil*

Correspondence should be addressed to Rafaela Scariot; rafaela_scariot@yahoo.com.br

Academic Editor: Fabio Roccia

Introduction. The bifid mandibular condyle (BMC) is an unusual temporomandibular joint (TMJ) disorder with controversial etiology. The association of this entity with ankylosis is rare. *Objective.* The objective of the present study is to report a case of BMC with associated TMJ ankylosis in a patient with no history of trauma and/or infection. *Case Report.* A 17-year-old male patient sought care reporting pain on the right TMJ region and mastication difficulty due to a severe limitation of mouth opening. In the clinic and imaging examinations, a 15 mm mouth opening and BMC associated with ankylotic mass of the right TMJ were observed, besides a facial asymmetry with chin deviation to the right. The proposed treatment plan was condylectomy on the right side, bilateral coronectomy, and genioplasty, so the chin lateral deviation could be corrected, under general anesthesia. The patient remains under clinical and imaging follow-up of two years with functional stability and no signs of relapse of the ankylosis. *Conclusion.* The association of BMC with ankylosis is an atypical entity which must be diagnosed and treated early to prevent aesthetic and functional damages to the patient.

1. Introduction

Bifid mandibular condyle (BMC) is an anomaly characterized by a division of the mandibular head [1]. It was described for the first time by Hrdlicka in 1941, in 21 cases of a series of skull specimens. Sicher, in 1948, was the first researcher to report a case of BMC in a living person [2, 3]. Morphologically, a BMC may be restricted to a delicate notching on the condyle or extended as a complete lobulation of the condyles. Extensive division might result in two heads while in cases less completed, the heads are separated simply by a shallow groove [4].

The etiology of this entity is still controversial, even though two main theories have been discussed: traumatic origin and developmental anomaly [3]. Endocrine disorders, deficiency of some nutrients, irradiation, infection, ankylosis, and genetic factors are also cited as the potential cause for BMC induction [5, 6]. Its prevalence is still not clear [3]. The majority of studies sustains that there is no preference when it comes to sex or race and that it is usually unilateral [7]. It is often asymptomatic, being a radiological finding. However, when symptomatic, it may be associated with pain, limitation of mouth opening, ankylosis, facial asymmetry, and swelling in the affected region. Many types of temporomandibular joint (TMJ) imaging methods are adopted for different diagnostic purposes, including conventional radiography, computerized tomography (CT), MRI, ultrasonography, and cone beam CT scan [8].

The association of BMC with TMJ ankylosis is even more unusual, with very few cases reported in literature [9]. This change may cause a deformity of the articular fossa, compromising functions such as the speech, mastication, and limitation of mouth opening [10]. The BMC proper treatment depends on the symptomatology. Patients with

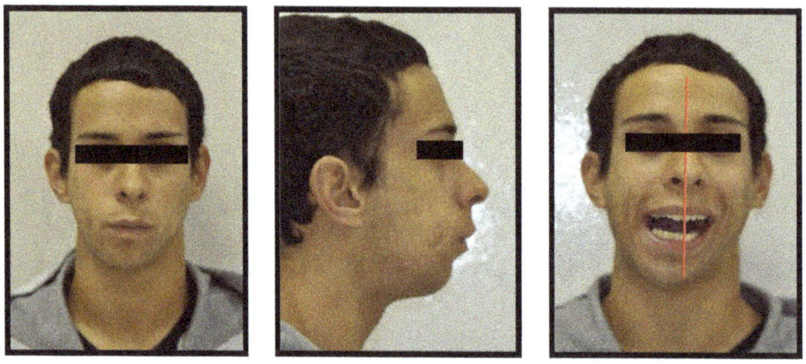

(a) (b) (c)

Figure 1: (a), (b), and (c) Preoperative pictures with front and lateral views emphasizing anteroposterior deficiency of the jaw and chin, mouth opening limitation, and chin deviation to the right.

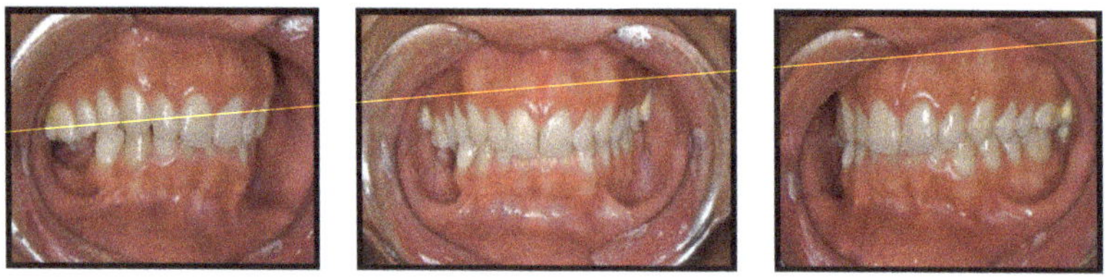

(a) (b) (c)

Figure 2: (a), (b), and (c) Preoperative intraoral pictures emphasizing deep bite and teeth absence on the right side.

associated articular ankylosis might need surgical condylectomy or arthroplasty [9].

Therefore, the objective of this study is to report a case of BMC with associated TMJ ankylosis in a patient with no history of trauma or previous ear infection, as well as its treatment alternatives.

2. Case Report

Written informed consent was obtained from the patient for publication of this case report and accompanying images. Patient D.G.B., a 17-year-old male, with no systemic changes, sought the services of Maxillofacial Surgery and Traumatology of Positivo University, Curitiba-PR, complaining of severe mouth opening limitation and pain on the right TMJ region. In the anamnesis, there was no record of trauma or ear infection during his childhood. At the clinical exam, the mouth opening limitation (15 mm) and a mandibular deviation to the right during the opening movement were verified. In addition, it was possible to observe a chin deviation to the right, associated with anteroposterior deficiency of the jaw and chin (Figure 1). The patient had a deep bite and teeth absence in the right posterior region of the mandible (Figure 2).

Imaging exams were requested—panoramic radiography and CT scan—in which could be observed altered condylar morphology on the right side, a characteristic of BMC, associated with TMJ ankylosis. Moreover, a chin deviation to the right and the impaction of the elements 47 and 48, in an unfavorable position and angulation, were observed (Figures 3 and 4).

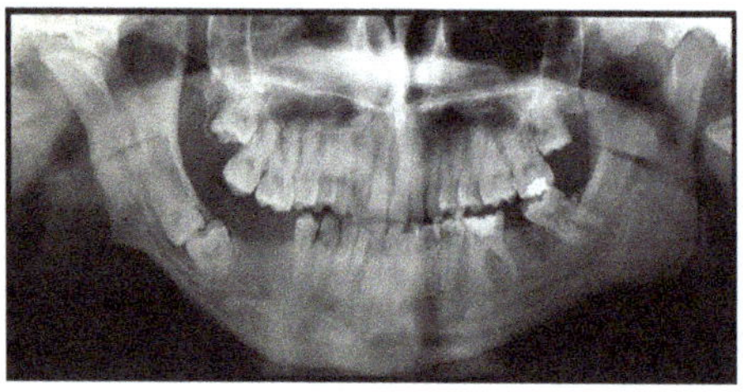

Figure 3: Preoperative panoramic radiography showing altered condylar morphology on the right side, mandibular asymmetry, and impaction of the teeth 47 and 48.

Based on this information, the proposed treatment plan was condylectomy on the right side and the removal of the bilateral coronoid process in order to detach the temporal muscle fibers and assist with the mouth opening. In addition, in the same surgical time, a genioplasty to the advancement of 10 mm and correction of the lateral chin deviation of 3 mm to the left was suggested. Due to the unfavorable position and absence of associated symptomatology to the impacted teeth 47 and 48, it was chosen not to remove these teeth at the time and have a clinic and radiographic follow-up.

The procedure was performed under general anesthesia through a nasotracheal intubation. An extraoral cleansing with iodine 10% with surfactant and intraoral cleansing with topical iodine 10% were conducted. The surgical access chosen was endaural, in order to leave the most imperceptible scar possible. A dissection of the tissues and exposure of the intra-articular spaces were performed with condylectomy

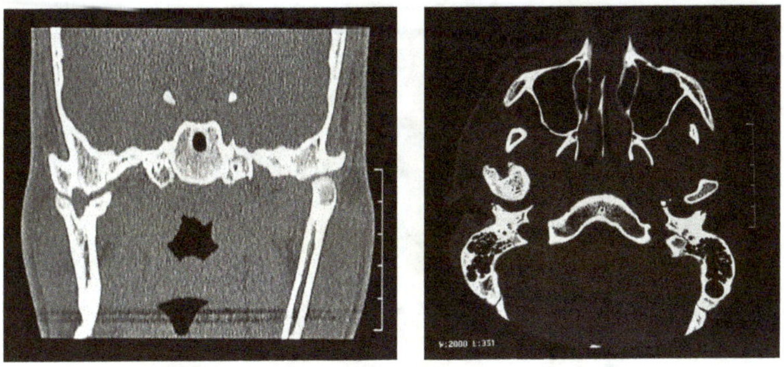

(a) (b)

FIGURE 4: (a) Coronal view of the CT scan emphasizing the bifid mandibular condyle in the laterolateral direction. (b) Axial view of the CT scan showing ankylosing mass.

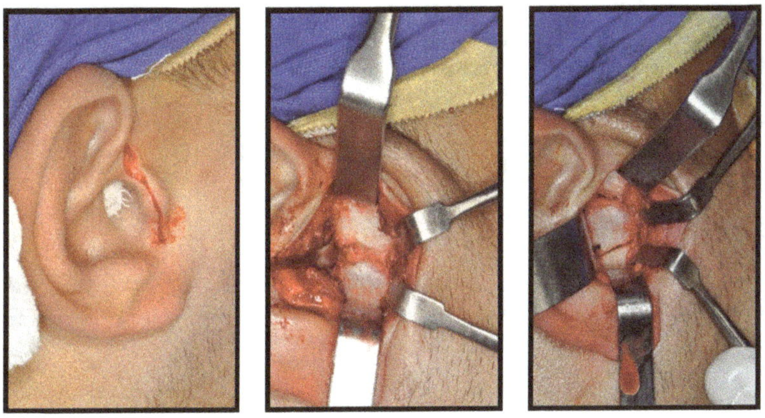

(a) (b) (c)

FIGURE 5: (a), (b), and (c) Transoperative pictures showing the endaural access and the exposure of the ankylosing mass.

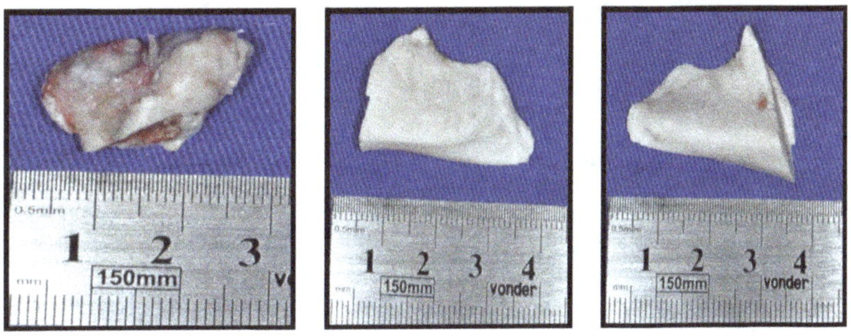

(a) (b) (c)

FIGURE 6: (a), (b), and (c) Surgical removal of the condylar process and bilateral coronoid process.

associated with the removal of the ankylosing mass with no interposition of tissue or material (Figure 5).

According to Sawhney's ankylosis classification, the mass found corresponds to type I, when the condyle is medially angled and associated with a deformed joint fossa along with a mild to moderate amount of new bone formation and fibrosis. This can be seen in the clinical picture (Figure 6(a)).

At the same time, a bilateral coronoidectomy and genioplasty were conducted. On the right side, the extraoral access was used to remove the coronoid process, while on the left side, an intraoral access was performed, at the bottom of the vestibule for the exposure and removal of the coronoid process. We chose to remove the right coronoid process to extraoral access only to use the same access used to perform the condylectomy. The stable internal fixation of the chin was conducted with a chin plate of 10 mm and four 2.0 screws (Figures 6 and 7).

At the transoperative, it was observed that the mouth opening was still not satisfactory. For that reason, besides the proposed treatment, an eminectomy on the left side in

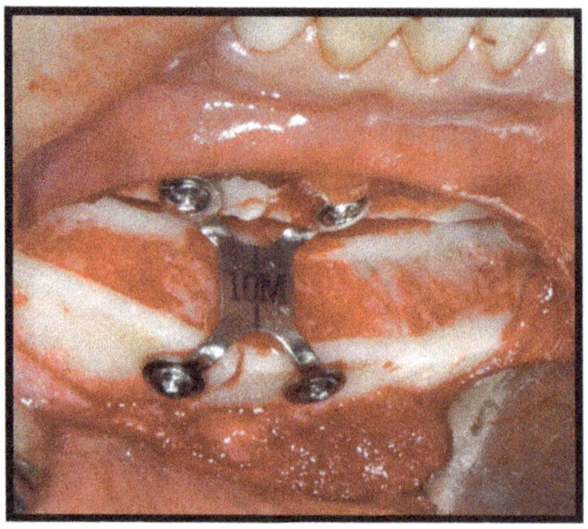

FIGURE 7: Stable internal fixation of the chin with a chin plate of 10 mm from the 2.0 mm system.

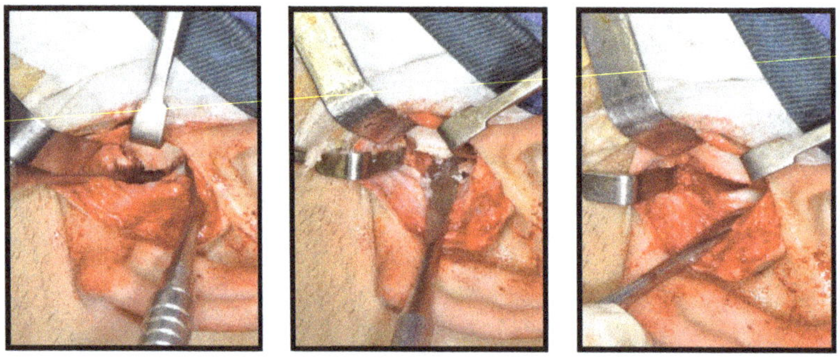

(a) (b) (c)

FIGURE 8: (a), (b), and (c) Transoperative pictures emphasizing the eminectomy on the left side.

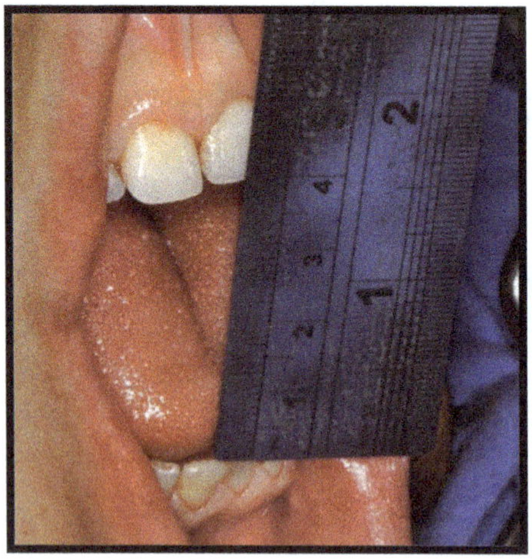

FIGURE 9: Mouth opening of 39 mm in the transoperative.

order to assist with the patient mouth opening was performed (Figure 8). After that, a 39 mm opening in the transoperative was achieved (Figure 9).

At the immediate postsurgery, the patient evolved with a slight anterior open bite, compatible with intra-articular swelling. Therefore, orthodontic brackets were installed so the occlusion could be guided with elastic bands. The patient continued with the follow-ups, with a mouth opening of 22 mm, no pain, and a satisfactory aesthetic and functional result (Figures 10 and 11). Seven days after the surgery, the patient performed a panoramic radiography, and the picture emphasized a good stability of the fixation and the bone gap on the right TMJ (Figures 12 and 13).

The patient was submitted to physiotherapy sessions with wooden spatulas, and after 30 days of postsurgery, he removed the orthodontic brackets, due to the stability of the occlusion (Figure 14). Since then, the patient remained in clinical and radiographic follow-up of two years, having no complaints and with a mouth opening of 35 mm (Figures 15, 16, 17, 18, and 19).

3. Discussion

Bifid mandibular condyle is an unusual condition, even though more cases are being reported as a result of enhanced imaging techniques [6, 7, 9, 11]. Its etiology is still contested. Most studies believe that this condition is associated with a trauma during childhood. However, there are theories about the persistency of fibrovascular septa during the formation of the mandibular condyle, teratogenic embryopathy, unusual insertion of muscle, endocrine disorders, and infection, which might explain the formation of BMC [5, 6, 9, 12]. In addition, the TMJ ankylosis may cause the development of BMC [2]. In a retrospective study, Rehman et al. [6] reported ten cases of BMC in 37 patients with TMJ ankylosis. Out of

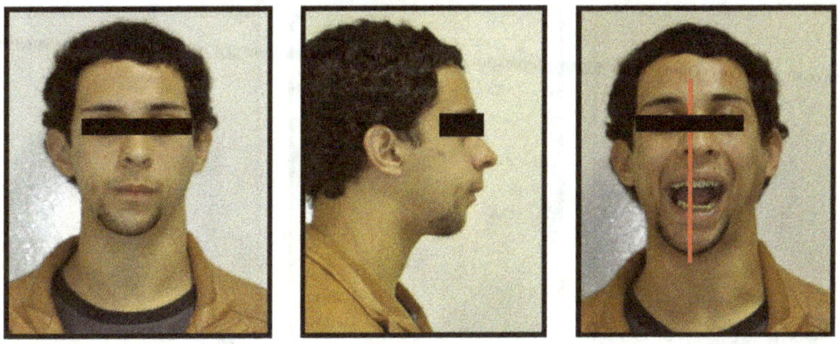

(a) (b) (c)

FIGURE 10: (a), (b), and (c) Postsurgery pictures after seven days emphasizing a more harmonic facial profile and improvement of the mouth opening and the mandibular deviation.

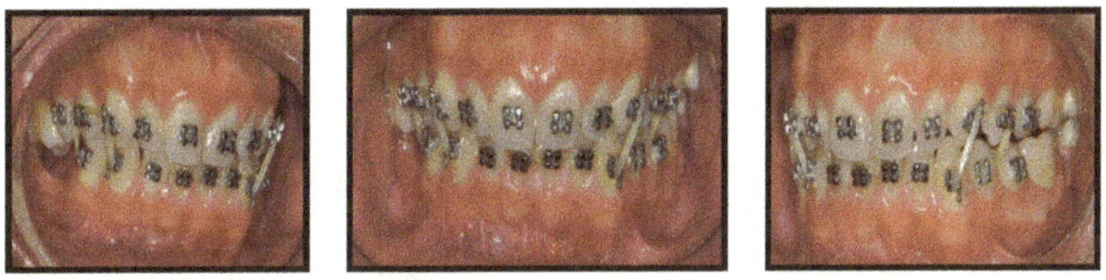

(a) (b) (c)

FIGURE 11: (a), (b), and (c) Intraoral pictures showing occlusion guided with elastic bands.

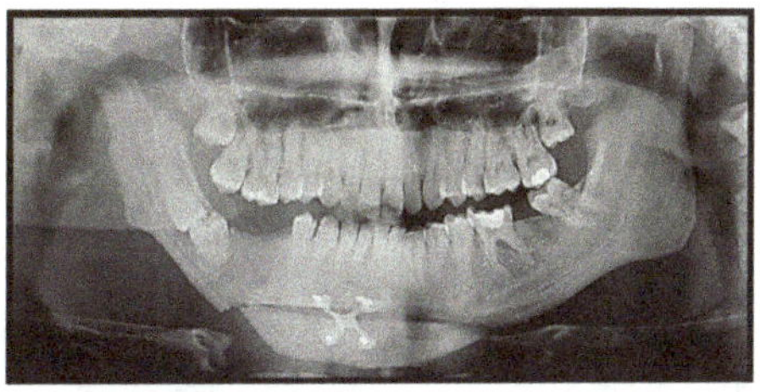

FIGURE 12: Panoramic radiography after seven days emphasizing the stable internal fixation of the chin and bone gap on the right side of the TMJ region.

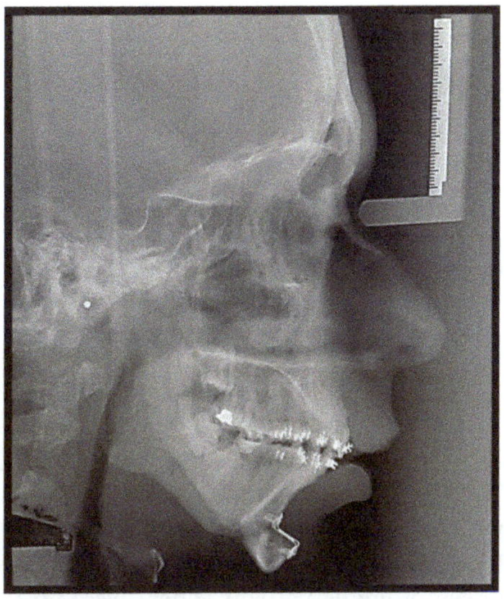

FIGURE 13: Profile teleradiograph after seven days showing a better facial profile with chin advancement.

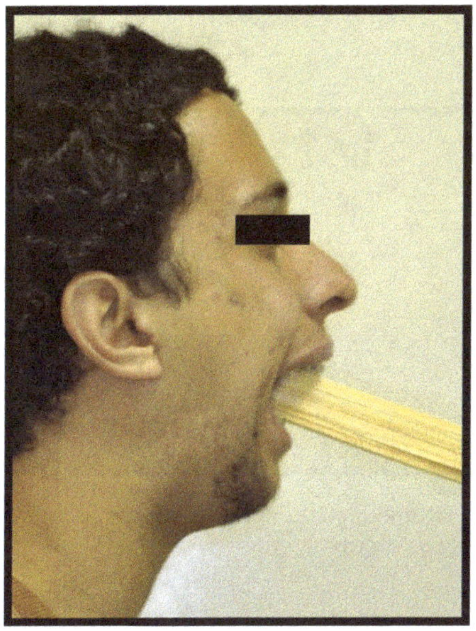

FIGURE 14: Physiotherapy with 15 wooden spatulas after 15 days of postsurgery.

these ten cases, nine were posttraumatic and one was postinfectious. In the present case, neither the patient nor his family remembered any trauma or infection during his childhood.

Bifid mandibular condyle is often unilateral, happening twice as much on the left side [7, 13]. In the literature, there is not a predilection when it comes to race or age. In a study reported by Loh and Yeo [14], most of the patients were over 20 years old. It is usually a radiographic finding. However, when symptomatic, it may be associated with pain, swelling,

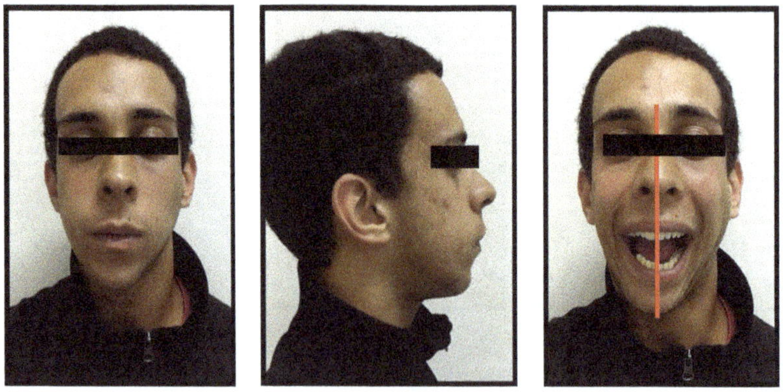

(a) (b) (c)

FIGURE 15: (a), (b), and (c) Postsurgery pictures after two years emphasizing the improvement in the facial harmony, mouth opening, and chin deviation.

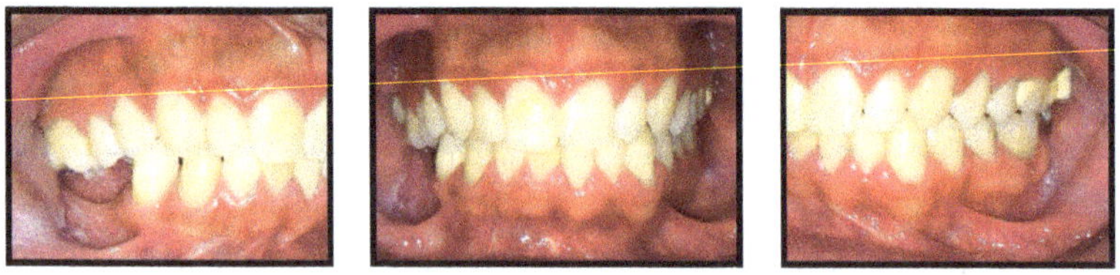

(a) (b) (c)

FIGURE 16: (a), (b), and (c) Intraoral pictures after two years showing stability in the occlusion.

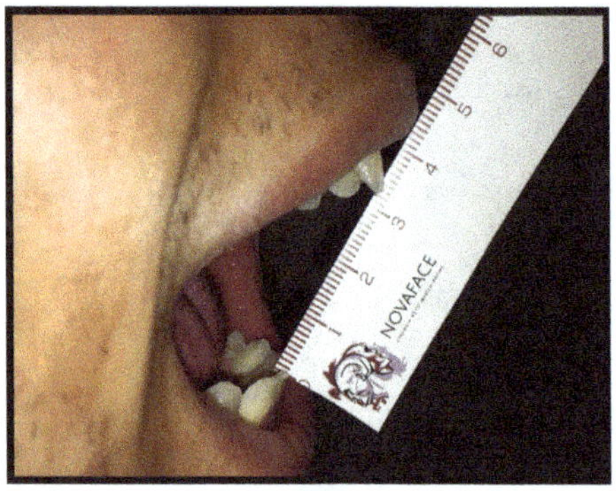

FIGURE 17: Picture emphasizing the mouth opening of 32 mm after two years of postsurgery.

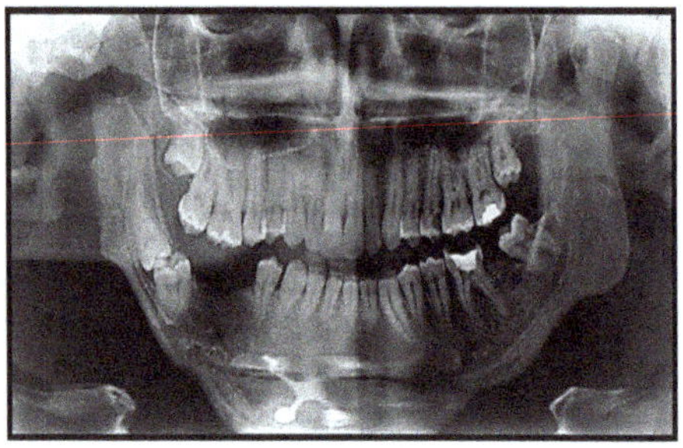

FIGURE 18: Panoramic radiography after two years emphasizing stability in the chin fixation and with no signs of ankylosis relapse.

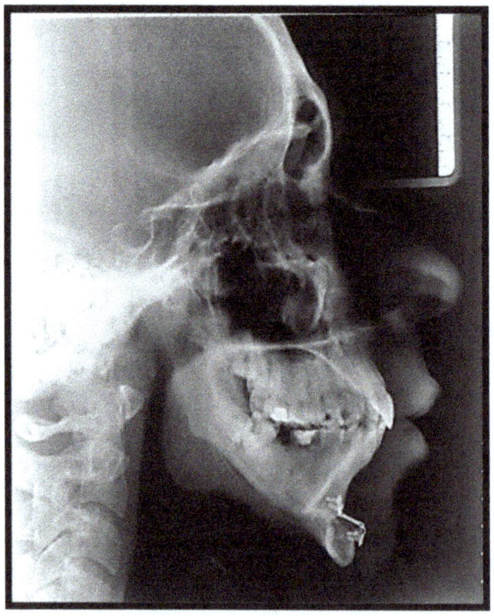

FIGURE 19: Profile teleradiograph after two years showing stability in the fixation and improvement of the facial profile.

asymmetries, and mouth opening limitation [6]. Cho and Jung [15] examined 3046 asymptomatic patients and 4378 patients with symptoms of TMJ dysfunction. They detected 15 (0.49%) cases of BMC in asymptomatic patients and 22 (0.50%) in symptomatic patients. There were no significant differences related to gender or to the affected side or any association with the symptoms in this study. Our report is about a 19-year-old male patient with BMC associated with TMJ ankylosis on the right side, with painful symptomatology and severe limitation of mouth opening, which is different from the usual cases, making this one atypical.

The most common radiographic image used in a diagnosis is the panoramic view, and it is used in most routine dental procedures [8]. However, it is known that the CT scan introduced a new image category, being increasingly used to evaluate the morphology of the mandibular condyle [16, 17]. The most usual imaging appearance is an anterior and a posterior head, separated by a shallow groove, although they can be oriented mediolaterally [3]. The TMJ ankylosis radiological aspect is more variable. There may be a deformity, with a complete loss of joint space and an unusual bone formation around the joint, or even a reduction of the joint space without complete obliteration, suggesting fibrous ankylosis [9, 18]. In this case report, the mandibular condyle was oriented mediolaterally.

The ideal treatment of these conditions depends on the clinical picture. Asymptomatic cases do not need any type of intervention [19]. When related to the ankylosis, the main objective of the treatment is to restore the function [11]. In these cases, Manganello-Souza and Mariani [10] described three basic techniques for the surgical correction of the temporomandibular ankylosis: gap arthroplasty (GA), interpositional arthroplasty (IA), and TMJ reconstruction.

Total joint replacement surgery is the most invasive treatment for TMJ disease. The goal of the procedure is to reduce pain, improve mouth opening, and correct occlusal changes and facial deformities [20]. Gold standard in treatment of this case is TMJ prosthesis, despite the young age of the patient, but this technique is expensive and not performed in all departments. Another option is to reconstruct the condyle with bone (rib) and interposition of fat, but the results are unpredictable.

In the present case, GA was the chosen technique. The GA has some advantages, such as the simple execution, less transoperative time, and low cost [21]. However, some authors have been associating it to a higher ankylosis recurrence rate [22]. A retrospective study designed by Danda et al. [23] could not find significant differences related to the mouth opening and the incidence of recurrence among the patients treated with GA and IA and concluded that the treatment's success depended on the patient's cooperation, active physiotherapy, and regular monitoring. Among the biological and nonbiological materials which can be used to the interposition after the GA are the remnant of the temporal muscle, skin, fat, cartilage, and silicon [22]. In this case report, the patient is in a two-year follow-up of gap arthroplasty, with no signs of recurrence of the ankylosis and with procedure stability. Any material since the patient presented an important gap was not lodged.

The GA is often combined with ipsilateral coronoidectomy because the prolonged immobility of the jaw, due to the ankylosis, usually results in coronoid hyperplasia. A contralateral coronoidectomy may be needed to facilitate the mouth opening [24], like it was performed in this case. Manganello-Souza and Mariani [10] reported 14 cases of TMJ ankylosis. Among the bilateral cases, five were submitted to bilateral coronoidectomy and one to unilateral coronoidectomy, while ipsilateral coronoidectomy was conducted in four of the eight unilateral cases. Moreover, the articular eminence has an important role in the TMJ's biomechanics, and it acts as an anterior barrier for the head of the mandible during the opening movement [25]. In this case report, after the gap arthroplasty and bilateral coronoidectomy, an eminectomy on the left side in order to increase the patient's mouth opening was performed.

It is known that the best treatment for the correction of the anteroposterior deficiency of the jaw is the mandibular advancement through orthognathic surgery. The most commonly performed technique for this condition is sagittal osteotomy of the mandibular ramus. However, some studies argue that the mandibular ramus in patients with ankylosis and with skeletal deformities usually has severe anatomic variations that may complicate or even prevent the sagittal split of the ramus [26]. For these cases, some authors suggest inverted L osteotomy to extend the mandibular ramus and body at the same time [26–28]. In this case report, despite the patient's anteroposterior deficiency, any type of osteotomy was not performed due to the inappropriate positioning of the teeth 47 and 48 and because that was not the patient's complaint. Therefore, it was chosen to work with advancement genioplasty to aesthetically soften the jaw and chin anteroposterior deficiency.

4. Conclusion

The association of BMC and ankylosis is an atypical condition that might compromise the patient's function and quality of life. The treatment variations must take into consideration the associated symptoms, the age, and the patient's cooperation.

References

[1] L. B. Artvinli and Ö. Kansu, "Trifid mandibular condyle: a case report," *Oral Surgery, Oral Medicine, Oral Pathology, Oral Radiology, and Endodontology*, vol. 95, no. 2, pp. 251–254, 2003.

[2] B. Kaur and S. Padda, "The prevalence, radiographic appearance and gender predilection of bifid mandibular condyles in Punjabi population of North India: a retrospective study," *Journal of Indian Academy of Oral Medicine and Radiology*, vol. 29, no. 3, pp. 180–185, 2017.

[3] F. M. de Moraes Ramos, J. O. de Vasconcelos Filho, F. R. Manzi, F. N. Bóscolo, and S. M. de Almeida, "Bifid mandibular condyle: a case report," *Journal of Oral Science*, vol. 48, no. 1, pp. 35–37, 2006.

[4] A. Haghnegahdar, P. Bronoosh, L. Khojastepour, and P. Tahmassebi, "Prevalence of bifid mandibular condyle in a selected population in south of Iran," *Journal of Dentistry, Shiraz University of Medical Sciences*, vol. 15, no. 4, pp. 156–160, 2014.

[5] S. Kamtane and A. Subramaniam, "Bifid mandibular condyle: a very rare entity," *Pakistan Oral & Dental Journal*, vol. 31, pp. 14–16, 2011.

[6] T. A. Rehman, S. Gibikote, N. Ilango, J. Thaj, R. Sarawagi, and A. Gupta, "Bifid mandibular condyle with associated temporomandibular joint ankylosis: a computed tomography study of the patterns and morphological variations," *Dento Maxillo Facial Radiology*, vol. 38, no. 4, pp. 239–244, 2009.

[7] M. A. O. Sales, J. X. Oliveira, and M. G. P. Cavalcanti, "Computed tomography imaging findings of simultaneous bifid mandibular condyle and temporomandibular joint ankylosis: case report," *Brazilian Dental Journal*, vol. 18, no. 1, pp. 74–77, 2007.

[8] H. Sahman, A. E. Sekerci, E. T. Ertas, M. Etoz, and Y. Sisman, "Prevalence of bifid mandibular condyle in a Turkish population," *Journal of Oral Science*, vol. 53, no. 4, pp. 433–437, 2011.

[9] A. Gulati, V. Virmani, S. Ramanathan, L. Verma, and N. Khandelwal, "Bifid mandibular condyle with temporomandibular joint ankylosis: report of two cases and review of literature," *Skeletal Radiology*, vol. 38, no. 10, pp. 1023–1025, 2009.

[10] L. C. Manganello-Souza and P. B. Mariani, "Temporomandibular joint ankylosis: report of 14 cases," *International Journal of Oral and Maxillofacial Surgery*, vol. 32, no. 1, pp. 24–29, 2003.

[11] J. S. M. Daniels and I. Ali, "Post-traumatic bifid condyle associated with temporomandibular joint ankylosis: report of a case and review of the literature," *Oral Surgery, Oral Medicine, Oral Pathology, Oral Radiology, and Endodontology*, vol. 99, no. 6, pp. 682–688, 2005.

[12] O. Güven, "A study on etiopathogenesis and clinical features of multi-headed (bifid and trifid) mandibular condyles and review of the literature," *Journal of Cranio-Maxillofacial Surgery*, vol. 46, no. 5, pp. 773–778, 2018.

[13] O. Miloglu, E. Yalcin, M. Buyukkurt, A. Yilmaz, and A. Harorli, "The frequency of bifid mandibular condyle in a Turkish patient population," *Dento Maxillo Facial Radiology*, vol. 39, no. 1, pp. 42–46, 2010.

[14] F. C. Loh and J. F. Yeo, "Bifid mandibular condyle," *Oral Surgery, Oral Medicine, and Oral Pathology*, vol. 69, no. 1, pp. 24–27, 1990.

[15] B.-H. Cho and Y.-H. Jung, "Nontraumatic bifid mandibular condyles in asymptomatic and symptomatic temporomandibular joint subjects," *Imaging Science in Dentistry*, vol. 43, no. 1, pp. 25–30, 2013.

[16] S. Shahidi, M. Vojdani, and M. Paknahad, "Correlation between articular eminence steepness measured with cone-beam computed tomography and clinical dysfunction index in patients with temporomandibular joint dysfunction," *Oral Surgery, Oral Medicine, Oral Pathology, Oral Radiology*, vol. 116, no. 1, pp. 91–97, 2013.

[17] J. Borras-Ferreres, A. Sanchez-Torres, and C. Gay-Escoda, "Bifid mandibular condyles: a systematic review," *Medicina Oral Patología Oral y Cirugia Bucal*, vol. 23, no. 6, pp. e672–e680, 2018.

[18] I. E. El-Hakim and S. A. Metwalli, "Imaging of temporomandibular joint ankylosis. A new radiographic classification," *Dentomaxillofacial Radiology*, vol. 31, no. 1, pp. 19–23, 2002.

[19] S. Phore, R. R. Singh, and M. Malhotra, "Bilateral double-headed condyles: a rare case report," *Saudi Journal of Oral Sciences*, vol. 5, no. 1, pp. 60–62, 2018.

[20] R. Sahdev, B. W. Wu, N. Anderson, S. N. Khawaja, S. Kim, and D. A. Keith, "A retrospective study of patient outcomes after temporomandibular joint replacement with alloplastic total joint prosthesis at Massachusetts General Hospital," *Journal of Oral and Maxillofacial Surgery*, 2018.

[21] O. Güven, "A clinical study on temporomandibular joint ankylosis," *Auris, Nasus, Larynx*, vol. 27, no. 1, pp. 27–33, 2000.

[22] J. Ma, H. Jiang, and L. Liang, "Interpositional arthroplasty versus reconstruction arthroplasty for temporomandibular joint ankylosis: a systematic review and meta-analysis," *Journal of Cranio-Maxillofacial Surgery*, vol. 43, no. 7, pp. 1202–1207, 2015.

[23] A. K. Danda, S. Ramkumar, and R. Chinnaswami, "Comparison of gap arthroplasty with and without a temporalis muscle flap for the treatment of ankylosis," *Journal of Oral and Maxillofacial Surgery*, vol. 67, no. 7, pp. 1425–1431, 2009.

[24] A. A. Heggie, "Concepts in the management of temporomandibular ankylosis," *Annals of the Royal Australasian College of Dental Surgeons*, vol. 13, pp. 132–135, 1996.

[25] F. H. Hirata, A. S. Guimarães, J. X. Oliveira, C. R. Moreira, E. T. T. Ferreira, and M. G. P. Cavalcanti, "Evaluation of TMJ articular eminence morphology and disc patterns in patients with disc displacement in MRI," *Brazilian Oral Research*, vol. 21, no. 3, pp. 265–271, 2007.

[26] S. Zhu, D. Wang, Q. Yin, and J. Hu, "Treatment guidelines for temporomandibular joint ankylosis with secondary dentofacial deformities in adults," *Journal of Cranio-Maxillofacial Surgery*, vol. 41, no. 7, pp. e117–e127, 2013.

[27] B. McMillan, R. Jones, P. Ward-Booth, and A. Goss, "Technique for intraoral inverted 'L' osteotomy," *British Journal of Oral and Maxillofacial Surgery*, vol. 37, no. 4, pp. 324–326, 1999.

[28] R. J. Naples, J. E. Van Sickels, and D. L. Jones, "Long-term neurosensory deficits associated with bilateral sagittal split osteotomy versus inverted 'L' osteotomy," *Oral Surgery, Oral Medicine, Oral Pathology*, vol. 77, no. 4, pp. 318–321, 1994.

6

Treatment of Complex Mandibular Body Fractures and Functional Reimplantation of the Maxillary Alveolar Fragment

Beatriz Sobrinho Sangalette,[1] **Rafaella Ferrari Pavoni**,[2] **Thayna da Silva Emídio**,[3] **Tiago Levatti**,[3] **Marcos Capelari**,[4] **Cláudio Maldonado Pastori**,[5] **and Gustavo Lopes Toledo**[6]

[1]*Department of Biological Sciences-Anatomy, Bauru School of Dentistry, University of São Paulo-FOB/USP Alameda Octávio Pinheiro Brisola, n° 9-75, Zip Code, 17012-901 Bauru-SP, Brazil*
[2]*State University of North Paraná-UENP. Av. Getúlio Vargas, no. 850, Zip Code, 86400-000 Jacarezinho, PR, Brazil*
[3]*Marília University-UNIMAR. Av. Higino Muzi Filho, n° 1001, Zip Code, 17525-902 Marília, SP, Brazil*
[4]*Oral Maxillofacial Surgery Department, Santa Casa da Misericórdia de Santa Cruz do Rio Pardo. Av. Dr. Ciro Melo Camarinha, n° 530, Zip Code, 18900-000 Santa Cruz do Rio Pardo, SP, Brazil*
[5]*Department of Bucomaxilofacial Surgery, University Center of Adamantina-UNIFAI. Av. Francisco Bellusci, n° 1000, CEP, 17800-000 Adamantina, SP, Brazil*
[6]*Oral Maxillofacial Surgery Department, State University of North Paraná-UENP. Av. Getúlio Vargas, no. 850, Zip code, 86400-000 Jacarezinho, PR, Brazil*

Correspondence should be addressed to Beatriz Sobrinho Sangalette; beatrizsangalett@gmail.com

Academic Editor: Christophoros Foroulis

Introduction. This report aims at demonstrating the treatment of complex mandibular fracture functional reimplantation of the maxillary alveolar fragment (FRAF), denoting the possibility and feasibility of this reduction with an excellent prognosis. *Case Report.* Patient E.M.S, 25 years old, male, leucoderma, referred to the Emergency Room of our institute. He reported being a victim of physical aggression, occlusal alteration, limitation of mouth opening, sensibility loss in the mentalis region, right infraorbital, and denied visual alteration. On physical examination, during the inspection and palpation, the crackling was observed in the right mandibular region and apical displacement of the maxillary alveolar process, corresponding to elements 13, 14, and 15. *Conclusion.* The rigid fixation of the complex jaw fracture and alveolar maxilla process, through functional reduction, indicated satisfactory applicability, and favorable prognosis.

1. Introduction

The bones of the face are part of the complex stomatognathic apparatus, of which the mandible occupies the second position among the most affected in craniofacial traumas [1]. Such prominence is related to the anatomy and projected anatomical disposition itself in relation to the other bones face, being preceded only by the nasal bones that occupy a prominent position when compared to the mandible [1, 2].

The etiology of mandibular fractures is concentrated in cases of physical aggression and automobile accidents, although sports accidents and pathological or mechanical fractures are present as predisposing factors, either in the involvement of neoplasms or during the extraction of lower third molars [1, 2]. Commonly, there are associated dentoalveolar fractures, varying with the direction and impact of the trauma, involving the alveolar process, adjacent teeth, and soft tissues [3].

For diagnosis, a thorough clinical and radiographic examination should be performed, taking into account factors such as impact energy, direction, and location, as well as the resilience of the structures involved [4]. The objective of this study was to report the treatment of complex mandibular fracture and block fracture of the alveolar process in the maxilla, involving dental elements, denoting singular technique of functional alveolar reimplantation of the respective alveolar bone fragment (FRAF), besides primary stabilization of the mandibular fracture before reconstruction plate placement, thus preserving the structure and restoring function.

2. Case Presentation

Patient E.M.S, 25 years old, male, leucoderma, was referred to the Emergency Room of our institute. During a medical-dental questionnaire, the patient mentioned having been a victim of physical aggression, reporting occlusal alteration, limitation of the amplitude of buccal opening, and loss of sensibility in the mental and infraorbital region. He denied visual and respiratory changes, although there were signs of subconjunctival ecchymosis and epistaxis. On physical examination, during the inspection and palpation, crepitation was observed in the body region and right mandibular angle and apical displacement of the bone fragment in the premaxilla, corresponding to elements 13, 14, and 15, with an evident sign of alveolar tooth fracture (Figure 1). In all maneuvers, the patient reported severe pain and great discomfort. Orthopantomographic radiography showed an image suggestive of loss of bone tissue continuity solution. However, the fragmentation of the alveolar process was obscure, with only sinus veining on the corresponding side, given the blood collection in the cavity.

After systemic stabilization, the patient was taken to the Buccomaxillofacial Surgery and Traumatology Service, after 10 days of the first care. In the surgical center, in HDD, under general anesthesia, antisepsis was started with topical PVP-i and placement of the sterile fields, followed by subperiosteal infiltrative terminal anesthesia in the right maxilla region, aiming at facilitating the detachment of the muco-suspicious flap and promoting hemostasis; through the Newman Modified incision, the detachment of the flap continued, evidencing the dentoalveolar fracture. In order to eliminate the granulation tissue at the interface of the fragment and maxilla, which would certainly prevent good bone repair, the fragment was removed (Figures 2–4). However, it was again juxtaposed through the FRAF technique, which consists of the removal of the bone fragment and subsequent repositioning of it in its pretraumatic place, being fixed by using guided plates and titanium screws, by steel wires positioned in Modified Kazagian ties (Figures 5 and 6). Note the absence of the element 15 in Figure 6, extracted due to loss of bone support, is understood as functional reduction when the occlusion prior to trauma is overcome through occlusal wear or even dental impression, which does not necessarily mean Angle Class I.

In the next step, through the Risdon incision in the mandible, the subcutaneous planes were approached, location and protection of the facial nerve and artery, and incision of the pterygomassetric band and detachment. With the separation of the fragments and evaluation of the lingual space, the reconstruction and anatomical repositioning of the fragments with transfixing screws and plates and screws of the 2.0 system (Figures 7 and 8) were started. To support the reduction, a plaque reconstruction was attempted, which promoted stability and the possibility of functional adaptation to occlusion (Figure 9).

The suture of the deep planes of the mandibular approach and oral cavity was performed with Vicryl 4.0 wire and on the skin was used Nylon 6.0.

The patient was preoperatively treated with Dexamethasone 8 mg, Cephalotin 1 g, and intravenous dipyrone 500 mg. All medications were maintained in trans and postoperative and were adapted for use in tablets. Postoperatively, N-acetylcysteine 500 mg was added to the bucosinusal communication.

2.1. Outcome and Follow-Up. The patient followed postoperative follow-up for 7, 14, 21, 35, and 64 days, presenting evolution within the norms of normality and cicatricial process compatible with the surgical procedure performed. There was an absence of secondary infections, occlusal restoration, and consolidation of the fragment in the maxilla. In respect to the regeneration of the nervous tissue, although it is known, by the literature, that the regeneration of the proximal stump occurs, in this specific case, it comes to an avulsion of fragment with involved teeth, which made the reasoning of this case to devolve in the same conditions and treatment of avulsioned teeth, that is, endodontic treatment after 14 days of the trauma. The patient was referred to the endodontic treatment of the elements 13 and 14, making it possible to maintain them in the oral cavity. A radiographic examination of the control was performed, in which titanium plates and screws were positioned, indicating a satisfactory reduction of the bone fragments (Figures 10 and 11).

3. Discussion

Facial fractures generate discussions among students ever since Hippocrates was alive, especially regarding the origin of the trauma, diagnosis, and treatment. In agreement with the findings found in the literature, this report presents a patient who suffered physical aggression of high intensity, generating maxillomandibular trauma. Such an etiology ranks first among the most common causes attended in emergency services [3, 4].

Among the anatomical subdivisions of the mandible, the body region corresponds to a significant percentage of the fractures, and the immediate reduction of the stumps is a determinant factor to obtain adequate occlusion [4, 5]. In the present case, the reduction was mediated due to the need for systemic stabilization of the victim, which has not been shown to cause significant harm to the resolution of the case. Literary scarcity is observed in cases where there is a fragmentation of the mandibular body with mediate reduction, demonstrating the relevance of this report to the scientific area.

The treatment choice was based on the analysis of complete clinical and radiographic examination, considering the possible sequels, both aesthetic and functional, that could be caused. According to most of the cases found in the literature, even in the other mandibular regions, the functional reduction was obtained through occlusal adjustment and

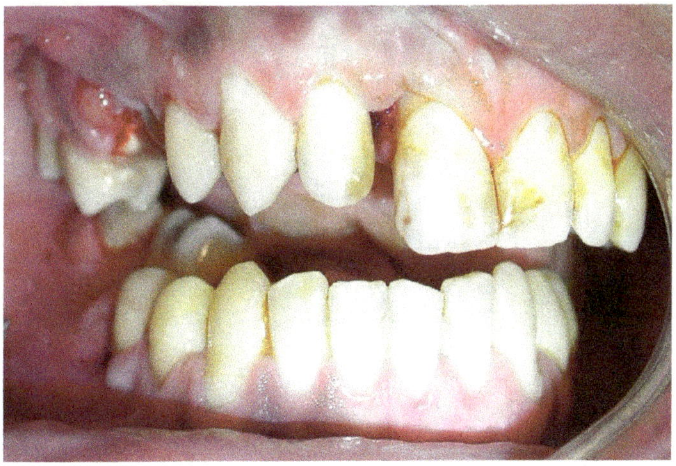

FIGURE 1: Initial appearance of the intraoperative showing apical fragment intrusion.

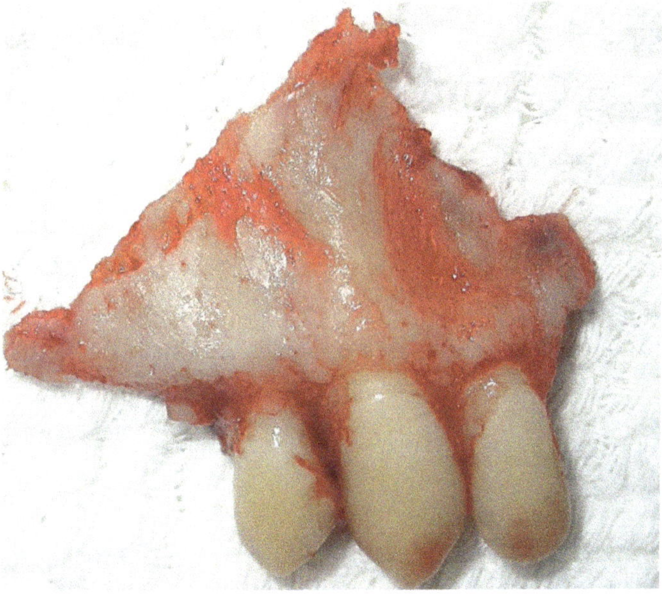

FIGURE 2: Alveolar fragment after removal of granulation tissue brought between it and the maxilla.

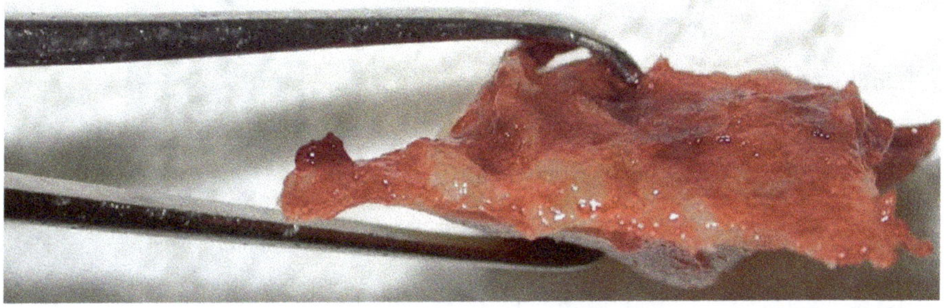

FIGURE 3: Super-inferior view of the premaxilla alveolar fragment.

rigid internal fixation, considering the complexity and biases of the reduction of complex fractures or maxillo-mandibular fractures [1, 5–7]. What has seemed a more viable solution in patients with great dental loss and inadequate occlusion.

According to a study carried out by Melo and Oleveira (2013), dentoalveolar trauma resulting from physical aggression accounts for about 35.8% of the cases, a study carried out on 1459 patients showed that in only 1% of the cases there

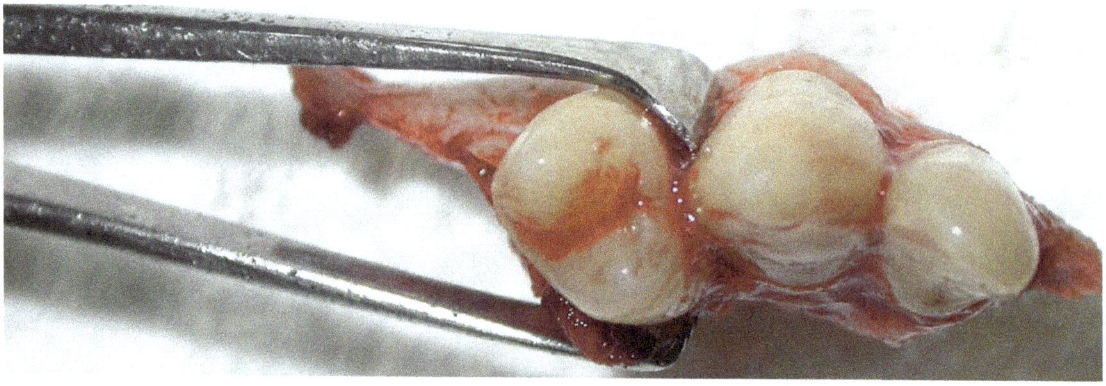

FIGURE 4: Occlusal view of the premaxilla alveolar fragment.

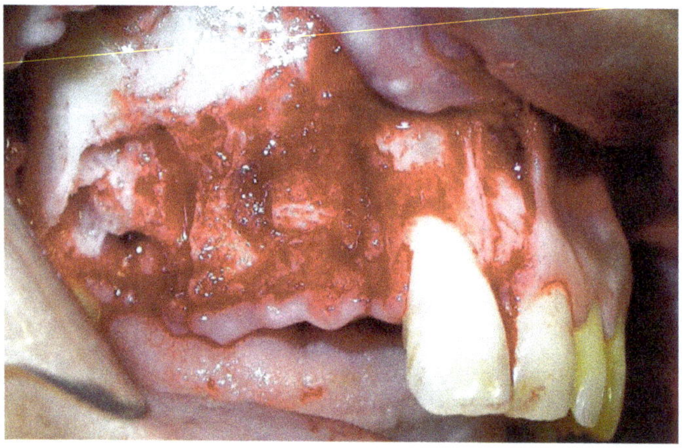

FIGURE 5: Curved surgical bed for functional reimplantation of the fragment.

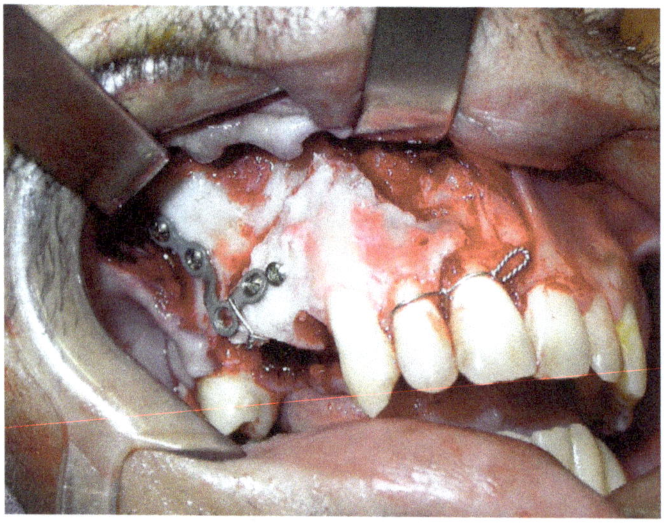

FIGURE 6: Functional reduction of the fragment with the aid of the "L" plate and 2.0 system titanium screws.

was an association of dentoalveolar trauma with mandible fracture [8]. Although there are few cases in the literature, the treatment of dentoalveolar trauma with bone fragment removal and repositioning should be performed, taking into consideration the adjacent structures and stage of dental development when there are elements involved [9]. However, the functional alveolar reimplantation technique advocated by the authors showed favorable results, indicating the viability and success of the technique provided that the reduction and fixation principles presented in the surgical steps have been obeyed.

It is important to observe that the removal of the fragment for removal of granulation tissue was indispensable; its nutrition was safeguarded by the periosteum itself

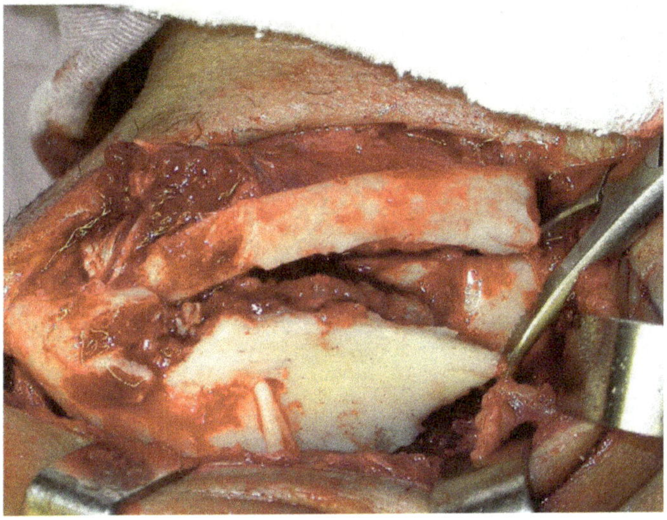

Figure 7: Exposure of complex mandible fracture.

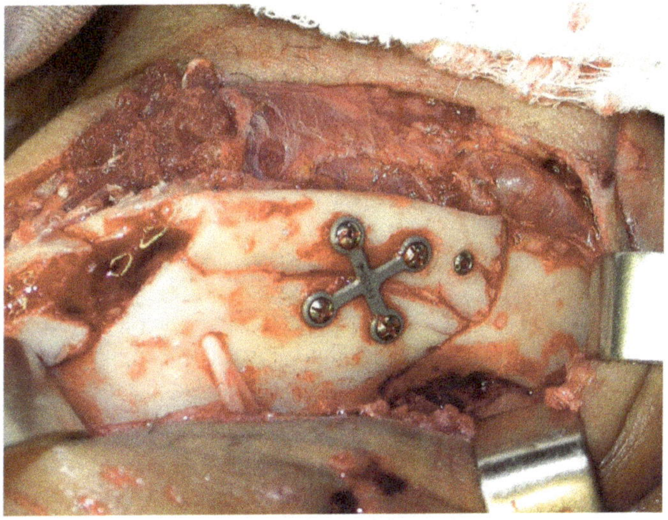

Figure 8: Reduction and stabilization of fractures with the lag screw, X-plate, and 2.0 system titanium screws.

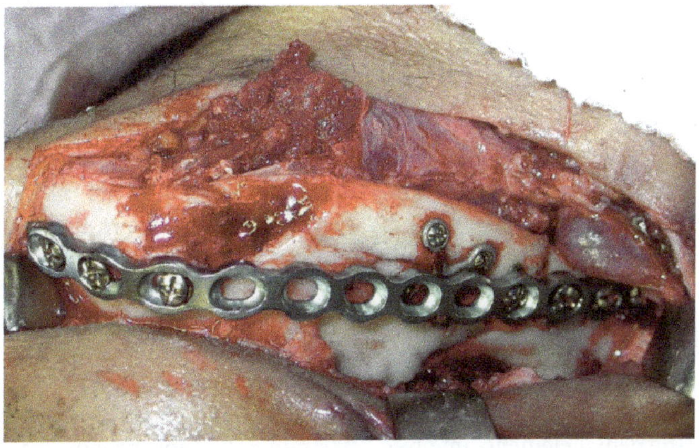

Figure 9: Rebuild plate installation overlapping stabilization material.

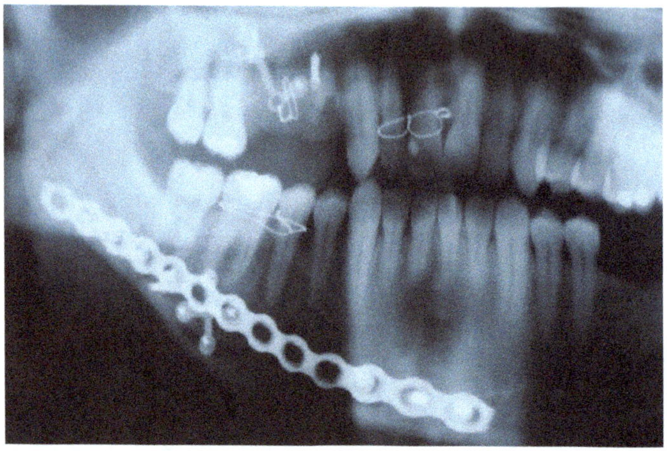

FIGURE 10: Orthopantomographic radiographic image of titanium plates and screws in position.

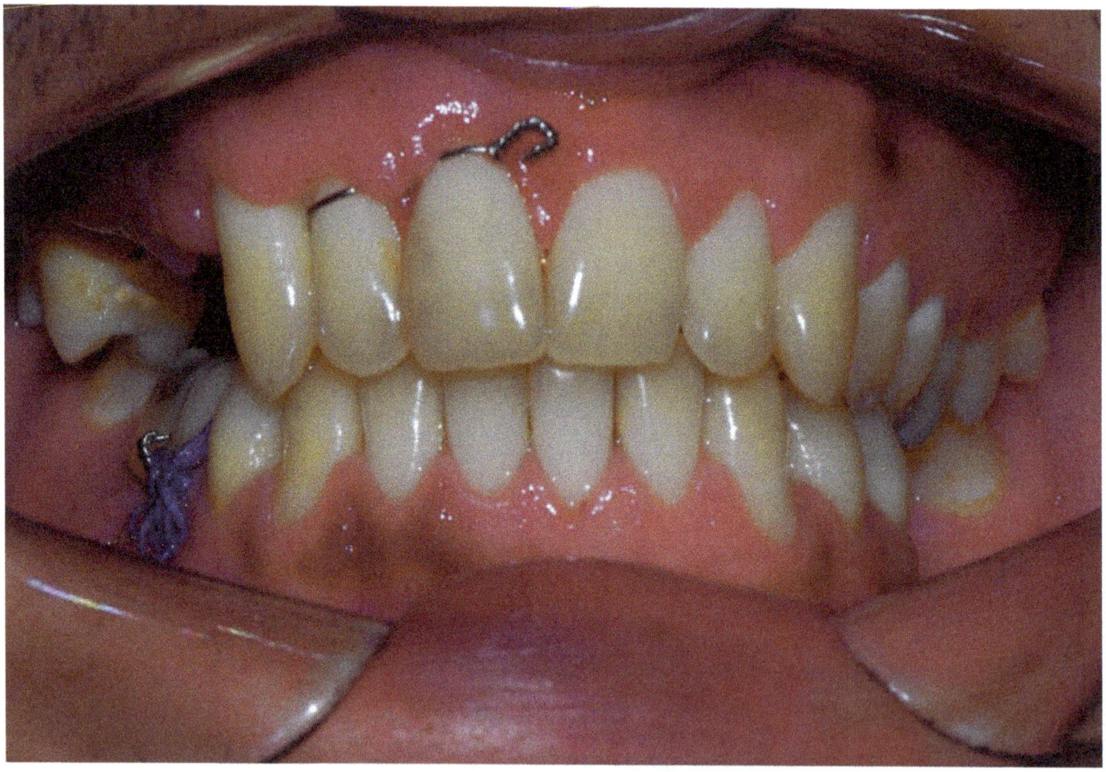

FIGURE 11: Postoperative appearance of 7 days, good healing aspect of the surgical approach, suture stitches in position, and reestablishment of functional occlusion.

carefully detached in the step of dieresis [10]. From its removal, it served as a free graft, a technique perfectly supported in the literature since it establishes a standard limit of up to 6 cm for its biological viability [11–13]. In addition, it is possible to verify the veracity of the postoperative orientation that did not show any signs of resorption or infectious processes. The fact that the noncoaptation of the fragment to the maxilla bone could be rejected could lead to osteomyelitis, a more damaging and unfavorable prognosis.

The nonrigid attachment of the dental elements involved should be indicated, when necessary, to stabilize them [14–16]. However, in this case, there was a fracture of the alveolar bone plates, where the technique recommended by the care team consisted of the use of rigid fixation of the fragment with titanium plates and screws, since there was enough room to use them.

With the evolution of the case, we can conclude that the proposed treatment proved to be effective, reestablishing the patient functionally. The FRAF technique process and primary stabilization of the anterior mandibular complex fracture and reconstruction plate are feasible and demonstrate a favorable prognosis when correctly indicated, following the basic principles of reduction, stabilization, and fixation even if mediated.

Consent

Written informed consent was obtained from the patient for publication of this case report and accompanying images. A copy of the written consent is available for review by the Editor-in-Chief of this journal on request.

Disclosure

This manuscript has not been submitted to, nor is under review at, another journal or other publishing venue.

Authors' Contributions

All authors have participated in (a) conception and design, or analysis and interpretation of the data; (b) drafting the article or revising it critically for important intellectual content; and (c) approval of the final version. All authors have participated in (a) conception and design, or analysis and interpretation of the data; (b) drafting the article or revising it critically for important intellectual content; and (c) approval of the final version.

Acknowledgments

For the contribution of translation and revision of the Portuguese language into the English language, we thank the language teacher Bruno Oliver and the native Michael Zeigler.

References

[1] J. C. G. Mendonça, L. A. Bento, and G. P. Freitas, "Tratamento das fraturas de côndilo mandibular: revisão da literatura," *Revista Brasileira de Cirurgia Craniomaxilofacial*, vol. 13, no. 2, 2010.

[2] L. J. Peterson et al., *Cirurgia oral e maxilofacial contemporânea*, Guanabara Koogan, Rio de Janeiro, 3 edition, 2000.

[3] C. B. Xavier, G. D. Faria, B. F. Vigi, K. F. Collares, and R. Dickel, "Estudo dos traumatismos alvéolo-dentários em pacientes atendidos em um Setor de Cirurgia e Traumatologia Buco-Maxilo Facial," *RGO. Revista Gaúcha de Odontologia*, vol. 59, no. 4, pp. 565–570, 2011.

[4] L. F. Simoneti, J. L. Toledo Filho, C. Marzola et al., "Estudo da parestesia do nervo lingual em pacientes submetidos à expansão rápida da maxila cirurgicamente assistida - Revista da literatura e relato de dois casos clínicos cirúrgicos," *Revista de Odontologia (Academia Tiradentes de Odontologia - ATO) Bauru*, vol. 15, no. 2, pp. 106–116, 2015.

[5] M. F. Carvalho Neto, "Tratamento das Fraturas Mandibulares com Fixação Interna Rígida: Estudo Comparativo entre Via de Acesso ExtraOral e Intra-Oral com Uso de Trocarte Percutâneo," *Revista Brasileira de Cirurgia Craniomaxilofacial*, vol. 11, no. 4, pp. 132–141, 2008.

[6] E. C. Gaetti-Jardim, L. P. Faverani, and J. L. Gullineli, "Facial injuries: a retrospective study of 1190 cases in the region of Araçatuba," *Revista Brasileira de Cirurgia da Cabeça e Pescoço*, vol. 38, no. 3, pp. 163–165, 2009.

[7] M. E. Muller, M. Allgöwer, R. Schneider, and R. Willenegger, *Manual of internal fixation: techniques recommended by the AO/ASIF*, SpringerVerlog, Berlin, 1991.

[8] R. E. V. A. Melo and M. G. Oliveira, "Rizólize / reabsorção dentária," *Revista Odonto Ciência, Porto Alegre*, vol. 12, no. 23, pp. 87–97, 1997.

[9] T. von Arx, A. Filippi, and D. Buser, "Splinting of traumatized teeth with a new device: TTS (Titanium Trauma Splint)," *Dental Traumatology*, vol. 17, no. 4, pp. 180–184, 2001.

[10] J. J. Barros and L. C. M. Souza, *Traumatismo Buco-maxilo-facial*, Roca, São Paulo, 2 edition, 2000.

[11] R. D. Foster, J. P. Anthony, A. Sharma, and M. A. Pogrel, "Vascularized bone flaps versus nonvascularized bone grafts for mandibular reconstruction: an outcome analysis of primary bony union and endosseous implant success," *Head & Neck*, vol. 21, no. 1, pp. 66–71, 1999.

[12] J. C. Dinato and W. D. Polido, *Implantes osseointegrados: cirurgia e prótese*, Artes Médicas, São Paulo, 2001.

[13] H. Schliephake, R. Schmelzeisen, H. Husstedt, and L. U. Schmidt-Wondera, "Comparison of the late results of mandibular reconstruction using nonvascularized or vascularized grafts and dental implants," *Journal of Oral and Maxillofacial Surgery*, vol. 57, no. 8, pp. 944–950, 1999.

[14] A. M. B. Santos, C. F. R. Cardoso, E. Azoubel, E. S. Cardoso, P. H. C. Souza, and R. B. D. Oliveira, "Métodos de contenção em traumatismo dentoalveolar," *Revista Odonto Ciencia*, vol. 13, no. 25, pp. 143–149, 1998.

[15] R. A. Dale, "Dentoalveolar trauma," *Emergency Medicine Clinics of North America*, vol. 18, no. 3, pp. 521–538, 2000.

[16] E. H. Vieira, M. A. C. Gabrielli, R. D. Rêgo, and R. Q. Ramos, "Fixação interna rígida em fratura alvéolo-dentária na maxila," *Revista da Associacao Paulista de Cirurgioes Dentistas*, vol. 52, no. 6, pp. 471–473, 1998.

7

Customized Titanium Mesh for Guided Bone Regeneration in the Posterior Mandible in a Patient Previously Treated with Bisphosphonates

Johannes Müller[1,2] **and Rüdiger Junker**[1]

[1]*Department of Prosthodontics and Biomaterials, Danube Private University, Krems, Austria*
[2]*Deputy Medical Director, Danube Private University, Krems, Austria*

Correspondence should be addressed to Rüdiger Junker; ruediger.junker@dp-uni.ac.at

Academic Editor: Asja Celebic

We describe the restorative treatment of an 86-year-old female patient who was referred to our specialist prosthodontics clinic. Due to secondary osteoporosis, she underwent oral antiresorptive therapy with ibandronic acid for 10 years. Although she was classified as a patient at increased risk of drug-induced osteonecrosis of the jaw, she eventually signed a consent form for fixed implant-supported prosthetic rehabilitation in her 4th sextant. However, after tooth extraction, the bone ridge was too small at the intended implant positions. Therefore, guided bone regeneration was performed with a computer-aided design/computer-aided manufacturing three-dimensional printed titanium mesh. Finally, a continuous augmented hard tissue ridge above 7 mm was found, and three implants were inserted. Eventually, after four months of submerged healing, the implants were loaded with single crowns. Now, the patient is seen regularly for supportive peri-implant therapy.

1. Introduction

In our time, prosthetic rehabilitation of missing teeth with dental implants has become a predictable treatment option [1, 2]. However, a common clinical problem in implant dentistry is the lack of sufficient bone width and bone height to allow for prosthetically driven implant position and placement [3]. In view of this, scientific evidence supports lateral [3, 4] and vertical [3, 5] bone augmentation prior to implant placement as effective procedures to achieve sufficient ridge width and height for implant placement. In this context, guided bone regeneration (GBR)—in principle, the application of a barrier membrane to exclude cells from the soft tissue to allow protected migration of osteoblasts and eventually bone formation [6]—with resorbable, collagenous barrier membranes in combination with space maintaining xenografts is considered useful and predictable [3–5, 7]. However, such a combination might lack mechanical stability, which ultimately leads to a smaller increase in bone volume [4, 9]. To overcome this, individualized computer-aided design/computer-aided manufacturing (CAD/CAM) three-dimensional printed titanium meshes have been successfully introduced into GBR [10].

Here, we present the rehabilitation of the posterior mandible—in an elderly patient previously under bone resorptive therapy—with implants and implant-supported single crowns after guided bone augmentation supported by a printed titanium mesh.

2. Patient Information

An 86-year-old female patient was referred to our specialist prosthodontic clinic in August 2018 for comprehensive therapy due to a vertical root fracture on tooth 35 (Figure 1) and the patient's desire for fixed rehabilitation. She presented with fixed, tooth- and implant-supported prosthetic restorations that were fitted about 17 years ago. But in recent years, she has not seen a dental hygienist or a general dentist regularly. She has also never smoked and is mentally and physically fit. However, due to secondary osteoporosis, she underwent oral antiresorptive therapy with ibandronic acid (i.e., one

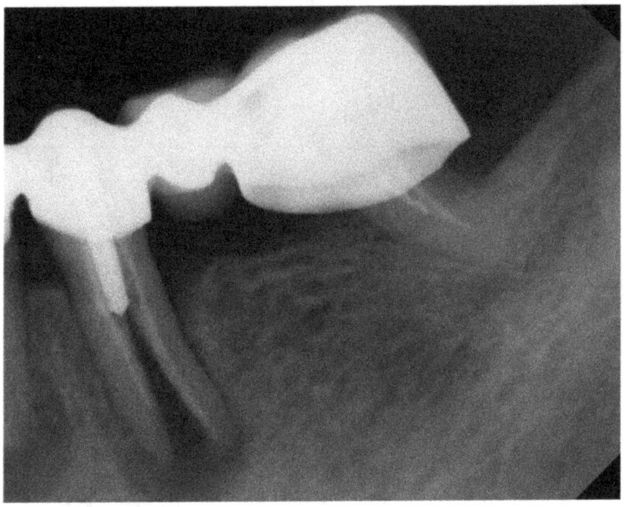

FIGURE 1: Radiograph tooth 35 at intake August 2018.

150 mg tablet once a month; Bonviva®, Future Health Pharma GmbH, Wetzikon, Switzerland) from 2005 to 2015. For the treatment of osteoporosis, she continues to take Calciduran® vitamin D3 tablets (calcium carbonate; Recipharm Stockholm AB, Jordbro, Sweden) once a day and Oleovit® D3 drops (colecalciferol; Fresenius Kabi Austria GmbH, Graz, Austria) once a week. The patient is otherwise healthy. Her chief complaint was bite pain in the lower left posterior mandible. In addition, she insisted on fixed prosthodontic rehabilitation.

3. Clinical and Radiographic Findings

In brief, at intake, teeth 13, 12, 11, 21, 22, 23, 24, 25, and 27 as well as implants in regions 15 and 16 were present with corresponding fixed prostheses (Figure 2). Due to insufficient crown margins, caries, tooth mobility, and peri-implant bone loss, it was decided to extract all teeth in the maxilla and rehabilitate it with a one-piece fixed dental prosthesis (FDP) on seven implants (Table 1 and Figure 3). This treatment will not be presented and discussed in detail in this case report. In the mandible, teeth 37, 35, 34, 33, 32, 31, 41, 42, 43, 44, and 48 were present with corresponding fixed prostheses (Figure 2). Here, extractions of 37 (insufficient root canal treatment), 35 (vertical root fracture), and 34 (insufficient root canal treatment associated with peri-apical radiolucency), and replacement with three implant-borne single crowns were planned. No intervention was planned for the 6th sextant (Table 1). In addition, the patient had acceptable oral hygiene (Approximal Plaque Index 28%) but is prone to periodontitis (could be classified as stage III, grade B [11]).

4. Timeline

The timeline for the treatment of the left posterior mandible is shown in Table 2.

5. Therapeutic Intervention

As mentioned above, in the 4th sextant, the extractions of teeth 34 due to insufficient root canal treatment associated

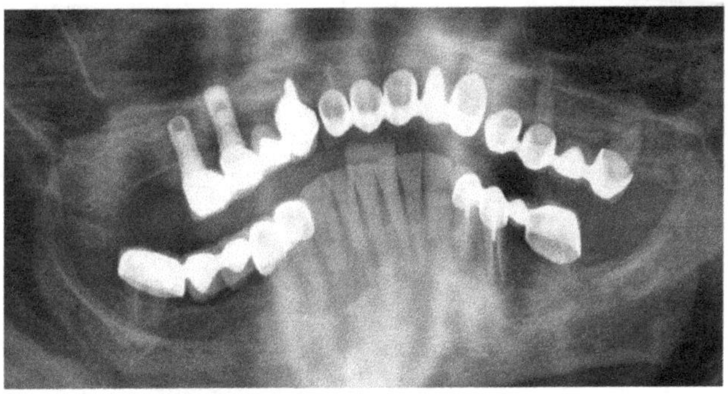

FIGURE 2: DPT section at intake August 2018.

with peri-apical radiolucency, 35 due to a vertical root fracture, and 37 due to insufficient root canal treatment (as well as assuming that it would be unreasonable to treat and retain this tooth under the concept of prosthetic rehabilitation with implant-supported single crowns), and subsequent rehabilitation with three implant-supported single crowns were planned.

6. Risk Assessment for Medication-Related Osteonecrosis of the Jaw

Due to secondary osteoporosis, the patient had been taking oral antiresorptive medication (i.e., the bisphosphonate ibandronic acid, one 150 mg tablet once per month; Bonviva®, Future Health Pharma GmbH) from 2005 to 2015. Unfortunately, drug-induced osteonecrosis of the jaw (medication-related osteonecrosis of the jaw [MRONJ]) has been reported as a rare side effect of bisphosphonates. It is defined as exposed bone or bone that can be probed through an intraoral or extraoral fistula in the jaw region that has been present for more than eight weeks in patients who have been treated with anti-resorptive drugs in the past, without radiotherapy to the jaw or obvious metastatic disease of the jaw [12]. In this context, it should be understood that dentoalveolar surgery (e.g., GBR or placement of dental implants) is considered a risk factor for MRONJ [13]. However, the risk of MRONJ, for example, after the placement of dental implants, is unknown [14, 15]. However, as bisphosphonates are known to remain in the body for a considerable time after cessation of use, it is recommended that patients who have taken the drug for more than five years should be assigned to a risk group as if they were still taking the drug. [13]. Therefore, the patient was classified as a higher risk patient [13]. This risk assessment was discussed between the treating dentists and, of course, with the patient. Finally, the patient gave informed consent to the treatment (i.e., GBR and dental implants).

7. GBR—Planning

After the extraction of teeth 34, 35, and 37 and thirteen months of bone healing, a digital volume tomography (DVT) of the jaws was made in June 2020 for final treatment planning. Tapered Screw Vent TSVT MTX Zimmer Biomet™ implants (Zimmer Biomet Holdings Inc., Warsaw, IN, USA) were considered. The minimum diameter of this type of

Table 1: DPT, dental status at intake, and treatment planning.

								FDP								
Treatment plan			I		I	I		I		I	I			I		
			X	X		X	X	X	X	X	X	X	X		X	
				FDP					FDP					FDP		
Dental status	M	M	I	I	M									M		M
	8	7	6	5	4	3	2	1	1	2	3	4	5	6	7	8

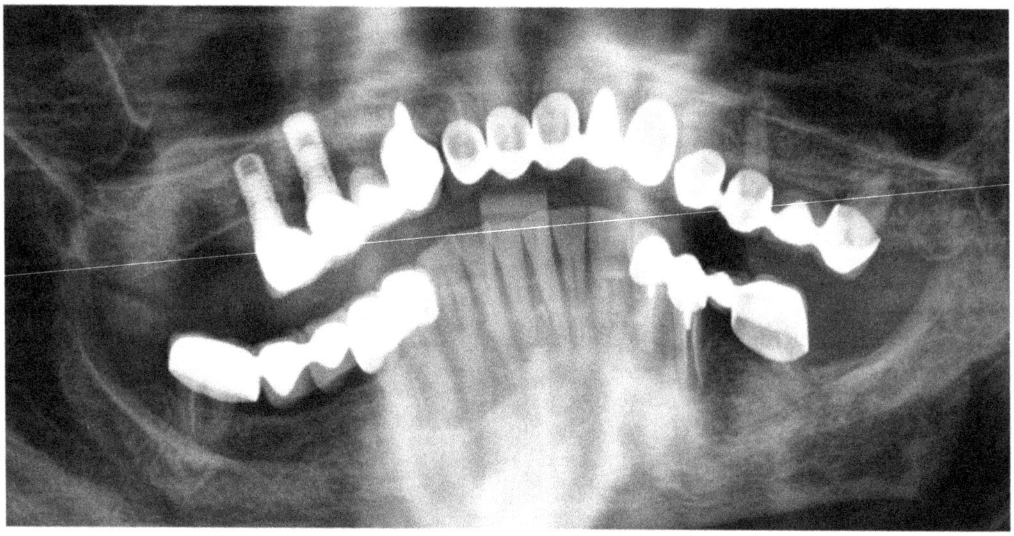

	8	7	6	5	4	3	2	1	1	2	3	4	5	6	7	8
Dental status		M	M											M		M
			FDP											FDP		
Treatment plan												I	I	I		
												SC	SC	SC		

M: Missing tooth. I: Implant. X: To be extracted or explanted. SC: Single crown. FDP: Fixed dental prosthesis.

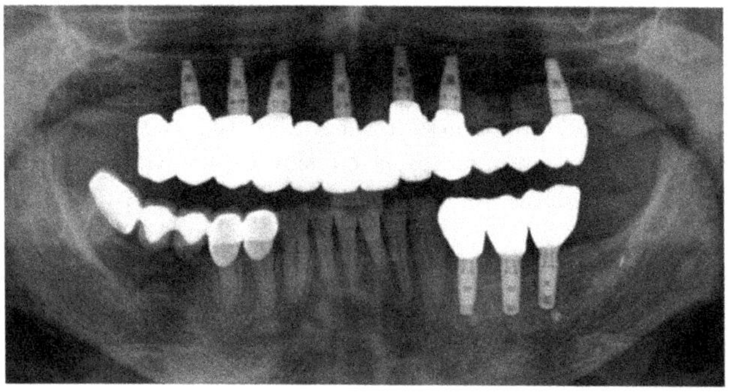

Figure 3: Section of a DPT immediately after cementation of the single crowns.

implants used for the replacement of premolars and molars is 3.7 mm, and the minimum length is 8 mm. When measuring the intended implant positions in regions 34, 35, and 36, the bone crest was found to be too narrow (<5 mm; Figures 4–6). Therefore, a GBR with a CAD/CAM-printed three-dimensional titanium mesh (YxOss CBR®; ReOss®, Filderstadt, Germany) in combination with autogenous bone (AB) and xenografts (Bio-Oss®/Bio-Gide®; Geistlich, Baden-Baden, Germany) was planned and prepared.

To create the conditions for successful implant placement and osteointegration, the first step was to simulate a primary horizontal augmentation to 8 mm in the 34–37 regions on the patient's DVT (Orthophos SL 3D, Dentsply Sirona Deutschland GmbH, Bensheim, Germany) from June 2020. The data were uploaded to and discussed with experienced clinical consultants (ReOss®, Filderstadt, Germany). Based on this, an individual YxOss CBR® titanium mesh was designed and visualized by ReOss® (Figure 7). After evaluation of the three-dimensional design and position by the treating specialist dentist, it was manufactured and delivered.

7.1. GBR—First Surgical Intervention. On July 9, 2020, the corresponding surgical procedure was performed. As premedication, the patient received 40 mg Urbason® (methylprednisolone; Sanofi-Aventis Deutschland GmbH, Frankfurt, Germany), 1 g Augmentin® (amoxicillin + clavulanic acid; GlaxoSmithKline Pharma GmbH, Vienna, Austria), and 600 mg Ibuprofen® (nonsteroidal anti-inflammatory painkiller; BASF, Ludwigshafen, Germany) one hour before the surgery. Furthermore, regions 38–33 were anaesthetized with a total of 5.1 ml Ultracain® D-S forte (Sanofi-Aventis Deutschland GmbH, Frankfurt am Main, Germany). Then, after a mid-crestal incision form region 38 into the gingival sulcus of 33 and a realising incision into the vestibulum distal to 33, a muco-periosteal flap was prepared (Figure 8).

TABLE 2: Chronological order of the treatment.

Timeline—left posterior mandible	
Intake	August 2018
Clinical examination	
DPT	
Articulated models of maxilla and mandible	
Preliminary treatment plan and initial treatment	Up to June 2020
Oral hygiene improvement	
Non-surgical periodontal therapy	
Extraction of teeth 34, 35, and 37	
Supportive therapy 4 times per year	
DVT	June 2020
Definitive treatment plan	
Implant positions	
CAD-titanium mesh for guided bone regeneration	
First surgical approach (i.e., GBR)	July 2020
CAM-printed titanium mesh (YxOss®; ReOss, Filderstadt, Germany)	
Xenografts (Bio-Oss®/Bio-Gide®; Geistlich, Baden-Baden, Germany)	
Submerged healing	
Second surgical approach	May 2021
Removal of the titanium mesh	
Implant placement (Tapered Screw Vent Zimmer Biomet™; Zimmer Biomet Holdings Inc., IN, USA)	
Submerged healing	
Third surgical approach	August 2021
Uncovering of the implants	
Healing abutments	
Prosthodontics (i.e., loading the implants)	
Individualized titanium abutments	
Monolithic, coloured SCs (Zirkon GEN-X®; Amman Girrbach™, Koblach, Austria)	
Cemented (KetacCem®; 3M; Vienna, Austria)	

DPT: digital panoramic tomography. DVT: digital volume tomography. GBR: guided bone regeneration. CAD: computer assisted design. CAM: computer assisted manufacturing. SC: single crown.

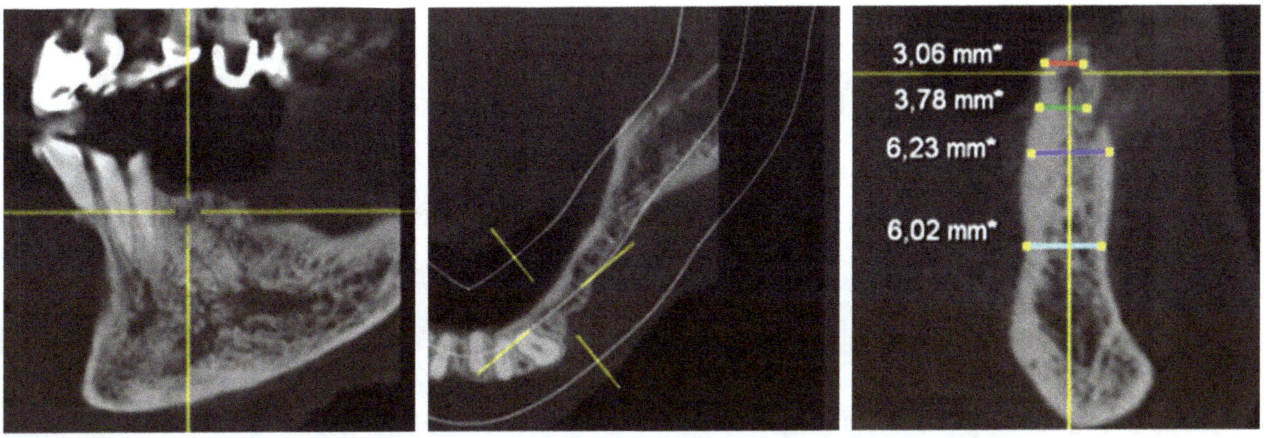

FIGURE 4: DVT—section region 34.

Next, the sterilized YxOss CBR® titanium mesh was tried on and checked for accuracy of fit. Buccal cortical bone was then harvested apically and distally to the final mesh position for mixing with a xenograft (Safescraper™ Twist Cortical Bone Collector; Zimmer Biomet Austria GmbH, Vienna, Austria). Subsequently, to support adequate healing of the bone graft, the crestal and buccal cortical bone of the bed to be augmented was perforated with a drill (alveolar process

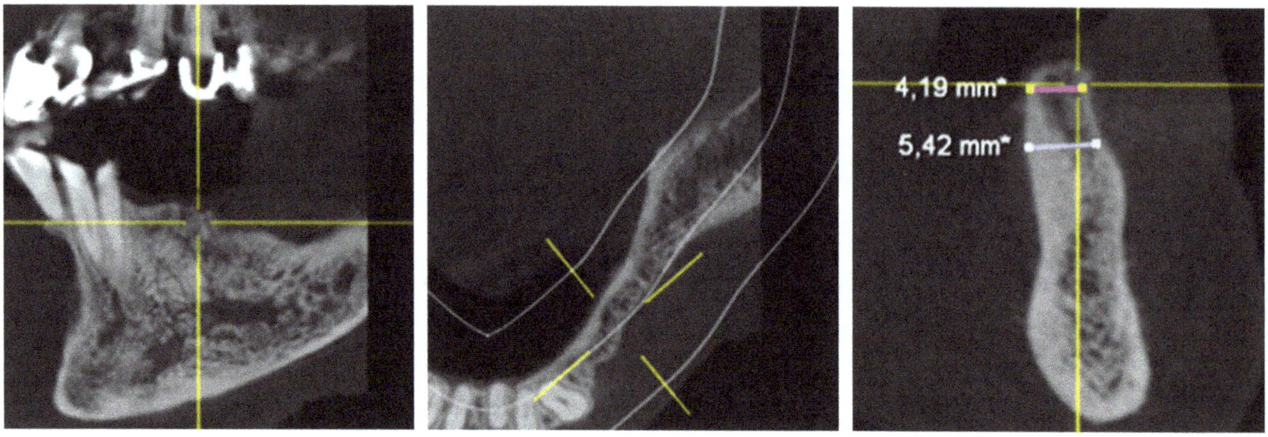

Figure 5: DVT—section region 35.

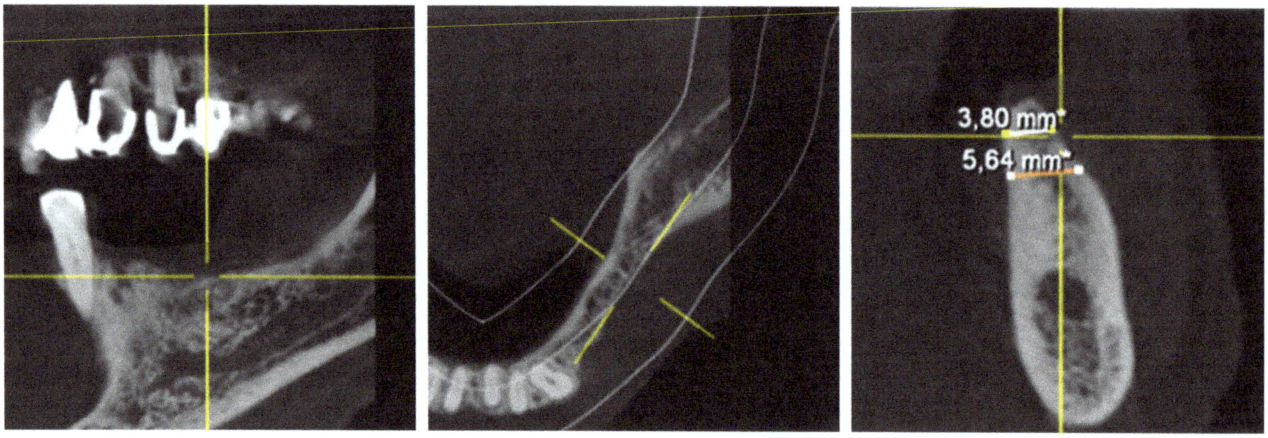

Figure 6: DVT—section region 36.

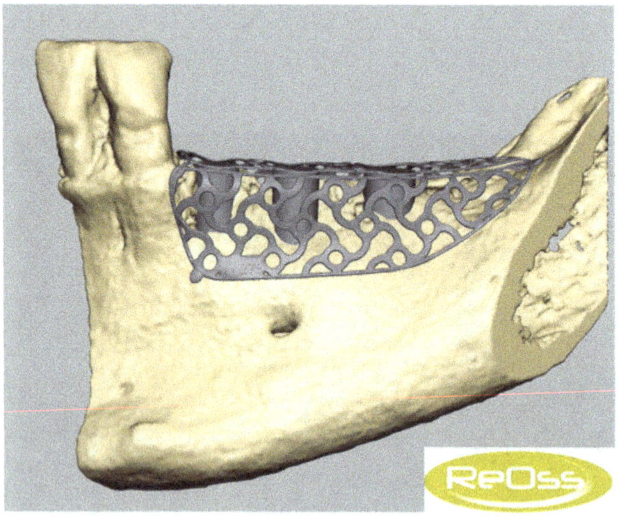

Figure 7: Individualized YxOss CBR® titanium mesh designed and visualized by ReOss®.

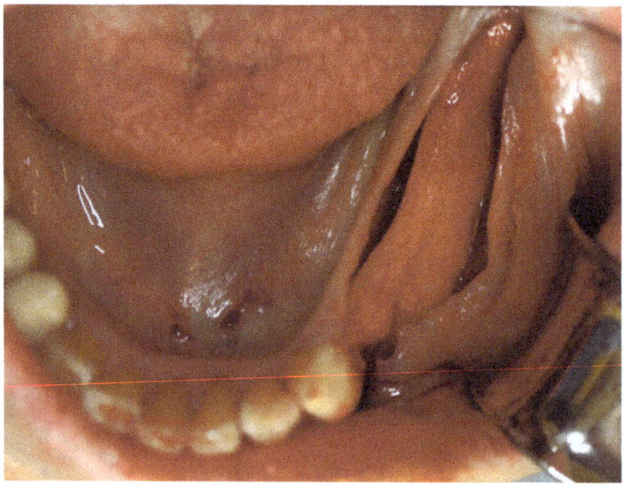

Figure 8: Muco-periosteal flap in the 4th sextant.

drill: diameter 1.2 mm and length 8 mm; Straumann Holding AG, Basel, Switzerland). After repositioning the YxOss CBR® titanium mesh, holes were drilled through the corresponding mesh openings (alveolar process drill; Straumann Holding AG), and the mesh was screwed onto the bone with four titanium screws (titanium osteosynthesis screws: diameter 1.5 mm and length 8 mm; Straumann Holding AG; Figure 9). Then, 0.5 g Bio-Oss® small granules (0.25–1 mm) and 2 g Bio-Oss® large granules (1–2 mm) were mixed with autologous bone and blood from the surgical site and placed

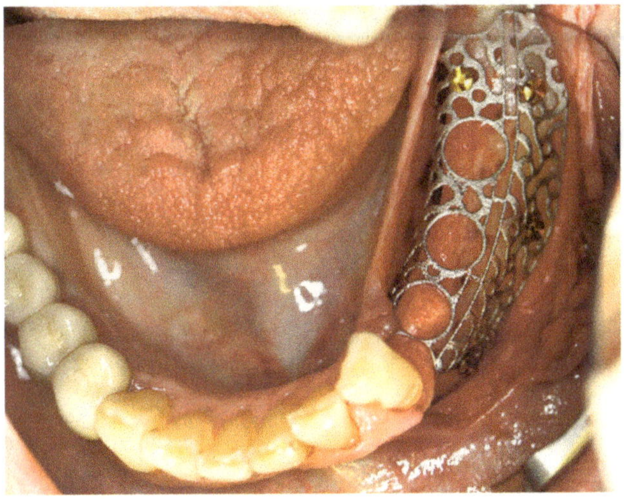

Figure 9: YxOss CBR® titanium mesh screwed onto the bone.

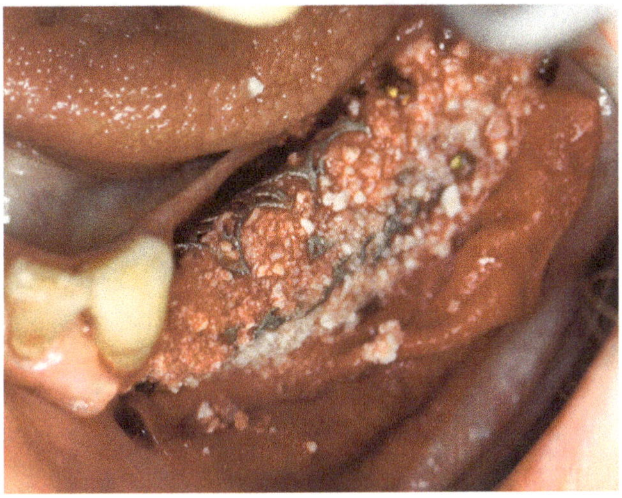

Figure 10: YxOss CBR® titanium mesh filled with the bone replacement graft.

in the titanium mesh (Figure 10). Thereafter, a Bio-Gide® membrane (30mm × 40mm) was cut to cover the YxOss CBR® titanium mesh and about 3 mm of the surrounding bone in a single layer. The membrane was stabilized in position with three titanium pins (Straumann Holding AG; Figure 11). To ensure tension-free wound closure, underlying vertical mattress sutures with absorbable suture material (Vicryl 4-0; Ethicon, Johnson & Johnson Medical GmbH, Norderstedt, Germany) were placed. Primary wound closure was achieved with a continuous suture (GORE-TEX® Suture CV5; W.L Gore & Associates, Phoenix, AZ, USA). In addition, a sling suture was applied to 33 for coronal positioning and stabilisation of the mucoperiosteal flap (Figure 12). A digital pantomogram (DPT) was obtained immediately after suturing (Figure 13). Augmentin® (2 g × 1 g daily, for 7 days) and Ibuprofen® (3 mg × 600 mg daily, for 3 days, then as needed) were prescribed, and the patient was again informed about postoperative behaviour (e.g., cooling). An absence of at least three weeks from her interim prosthesis was agreed with the patient. In addition, the patient was asked not to

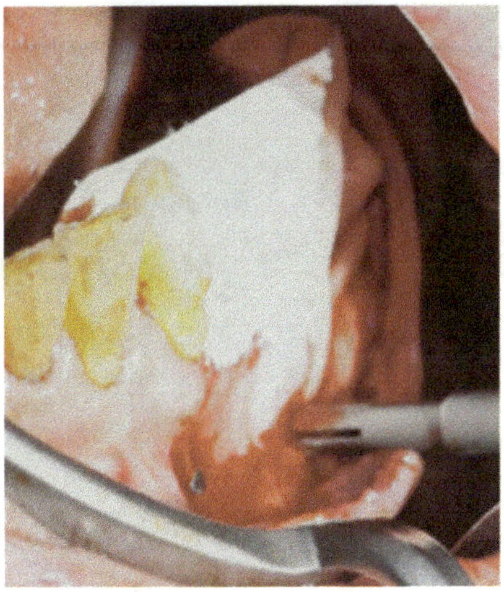

Figure 11: Bio-Gide® membrane stabilized in its position with titanium pins.

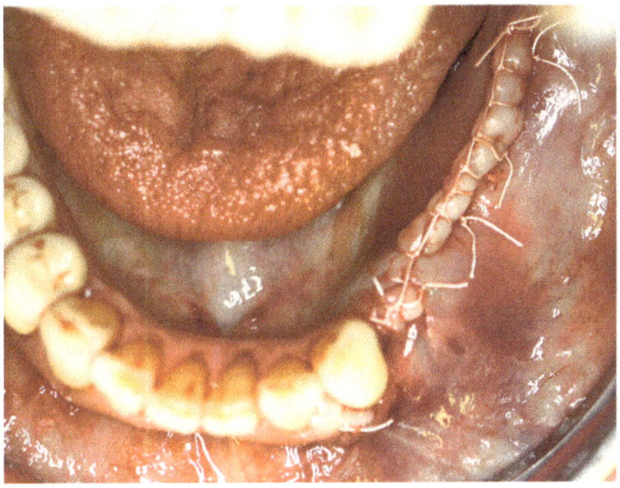

Figure 12: GORE-TEX® suture in place.

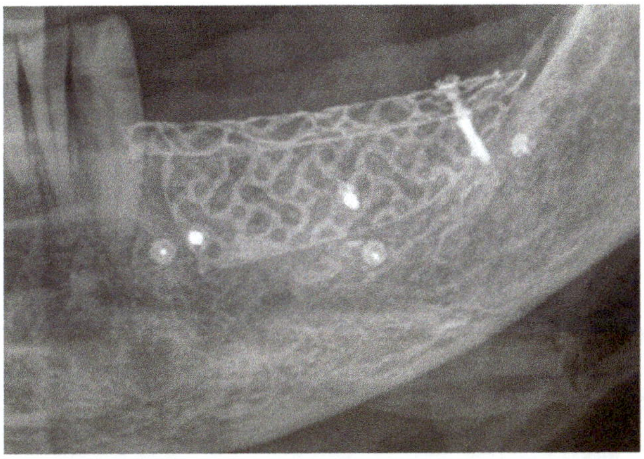

Figure 13: DPT section after GBR surgery was completed.

brush the surgical area until the suture was removed, but to rinse regularly (at least twice a day) with Chlorhexamed® (0.1%; GlaxoSmithKline Consumer Healthcare GmbH,

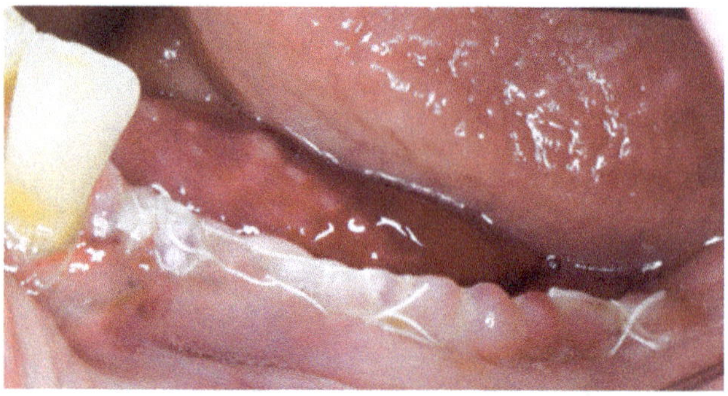

Figure 14: Day 1 after surgery.

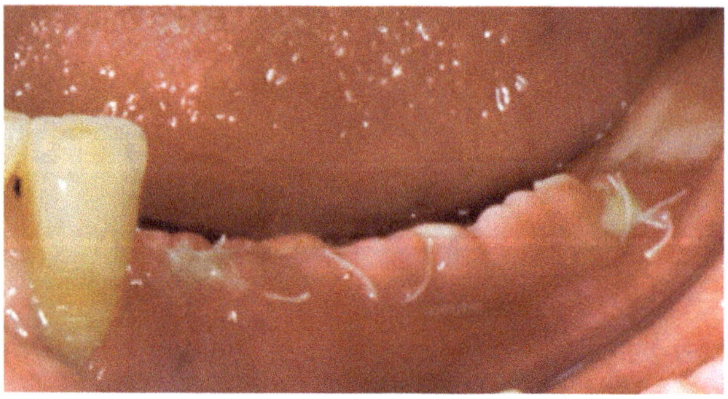

Figure 15: Day 7 after surgery.

Munich, Germany) according to the instructions for use. From the first postoperative day until the removal of the sutures, the surgical area was checked and cleaned (cotton swabs soaked with Chlorhexamed® 0.1%) every other day (Figures 14 and 15). In addition, plaque on adjacent teeth was removed with curettes (Hu-Friedy Mfg. Co., LLC., Frankfurt, Germany). Until suture removal, twelve days after surgery, the wound healing was uneventful.

7.2. GBR—YxOss CBR® Titanium Mesh Removal. After an uneventful—completely submerged—healing period of ten months, the titanium mesh was surgically removed on April 20, 2021 (delay due to COVID-19; usually 6 months according to Geistlich for BioOss®). As premedication, the patient received 1 g Augmentin® and 600 mg Ibuprofen® one hour before the surgery. In addition, regions 38–33 were anaesthetized with a total of 6.8 ml Ultracain® D-S forte. Then, after a mid-crestal incision from region 38 into the gingival sulcus of 33 (to keep the surgical area as small as possible without releasing incision), a muco-periosteal flap was prepared (Figure 16), and the YxOss CBR® titanium mesh, the four associated titanium screws, and one titanium pin were removed. Due to the decision to keep the surgical area as small as possible, the disto-apical and distal titanium pins were left in situ. Obviously, the graft was ossified (Figure 17).

7.3. Implant Placement. To plan the implant position, the bone edges were smoothed, and a DVT was taken immediately after removal of the YxOss CBR® titanium mesh. A continuous augmented hard tissue ridge, at the coronal margin above 7 mm, was found. Furthermore, the augmented

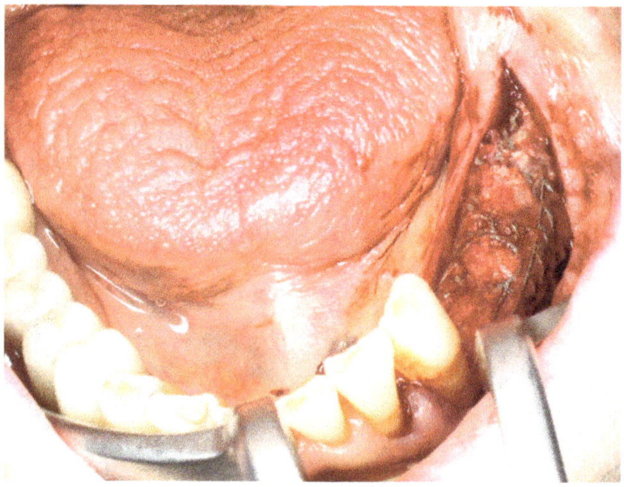

Figure 16: Exposed YxOss CBR® titanium mesh.

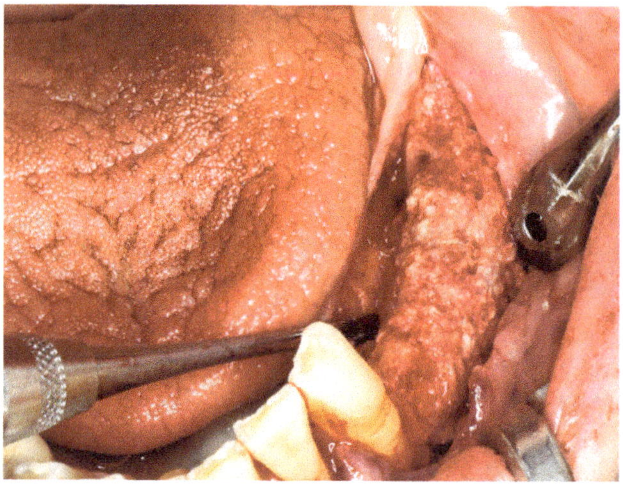

Figure 17: Ossified graft after YxOss CBR® titanium mesh removal.

hard tissue volume could be clearly distinguished from the native bone. As mentioned above, Tapered Screw Vent TSVT MTX Zimmer Biomet™ implants with a minimum coronal diameter of 3.7 mm and a minimum length of 8 mm had to be considered for the replacement of premolars and molars. When measuring the intended implant positions in regions 34, 35, and 36, the bone ridge was found to be sufficient in width and height (width: >7 mm, height (distance from coronal edge to upper edge of mandibular canal: >14 mm; Figures 18–20). Figures 21–23 show the approximate comparison of the hard tissue volume in the different regions where the implants were to be placed before and after GBR.

Immediately after planning the implant position, three Tapered Screw Vent TSVT MTX Zimmer Biomet™ implants (region 34: diameter 3.7 mm and length 10 mm; region 35: diameter 3.7 mm and length 10 mm; region 36: diameter 4.1 mm and length 10 mm) were implanted slightly subcrestal with an insertion torque of 35 Ncm each (Figure 24). Primary wound closure for healing of the submerged implants

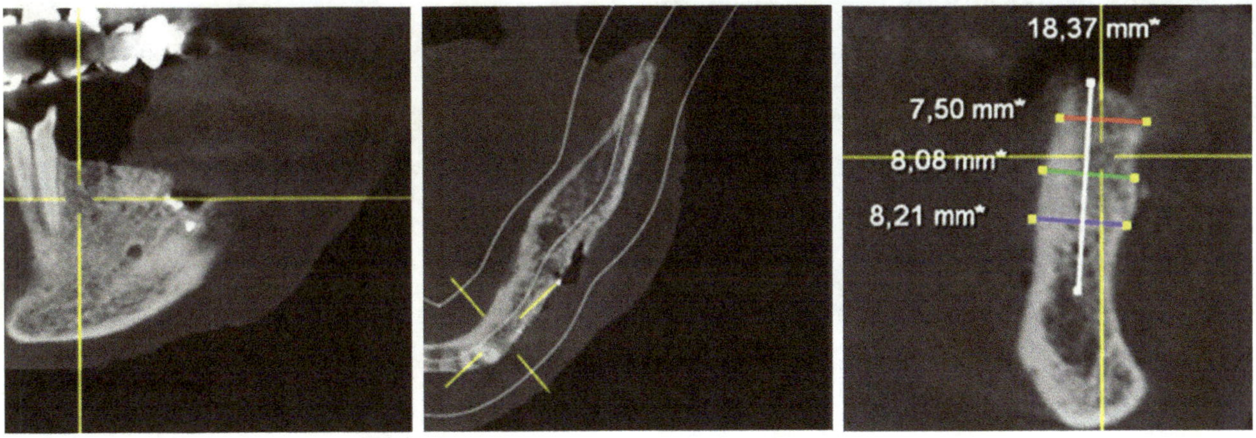

Figure 18: DVT—section; implant position region 34.

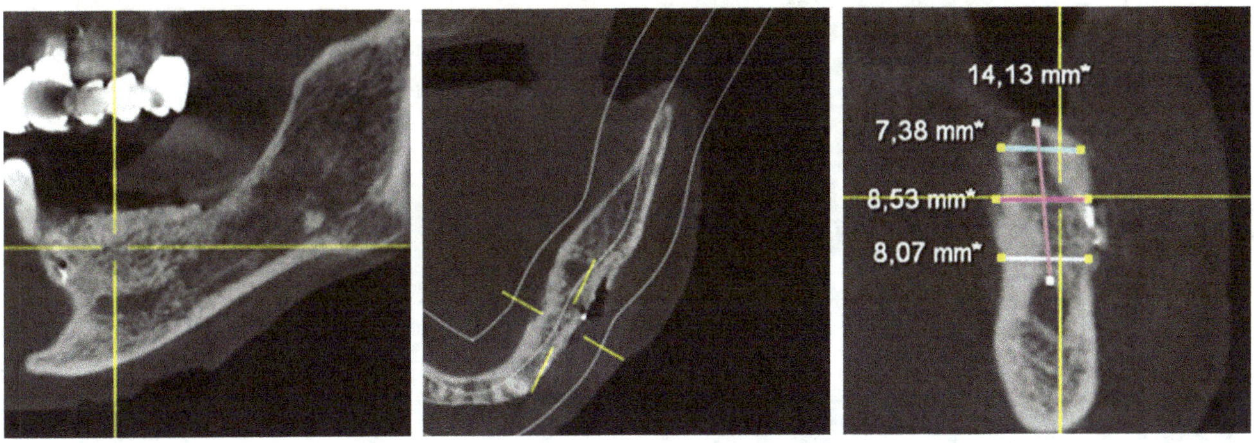

Figure 19: DVT—section; implant position region 35.

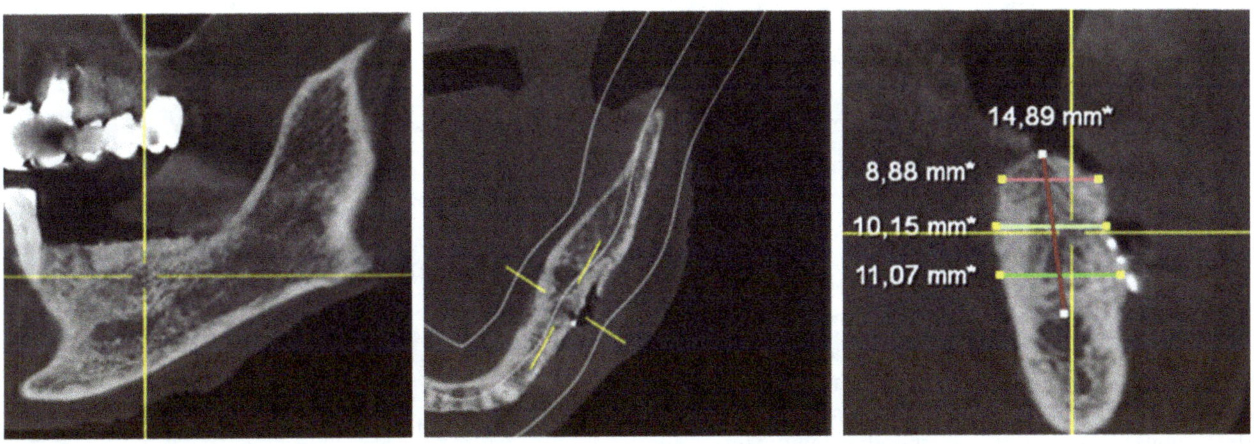

Figure 20: DVT—section; implant position region 36.

was achieved with interrupted single sutures (GORE-TEX® suture CV5). A DPT was taken immediately after suturing (Figure 25). Again, Augmentin® ($2\,g \times 1\,g$ daily, for 7 days) and Ibuprofen® ($3\,g \times 600\,mg$ daily, for 3 days, then as required) were prescribed, and the patient was asked not to brush the surgical area until the suture was removed, but to rinse regularly (at least twice a day) with 0.1% Chlorhexamed®. From the first postoperative day until the removal of the suture, the surgical area was checked and cleaned (cotton swabs soaked with Chlorhexamed® 0.1%) every fourth day. Plaque on the adjacent teeth was also removed with curettes. Until the suture was removed, thirteen days after surgery, wound healing was uneventful.

7.4. Prosthodontics and Supportive Therapy. In August 2021, after four months of submerged healing, the prosthetic

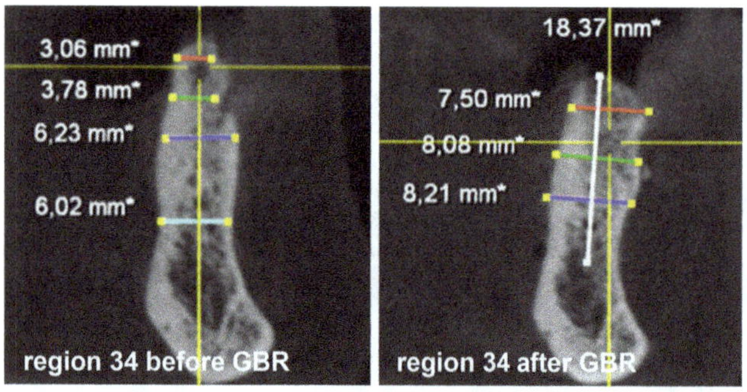

Figure 21: DVT—sections; implant position region 34 before and after GBR.

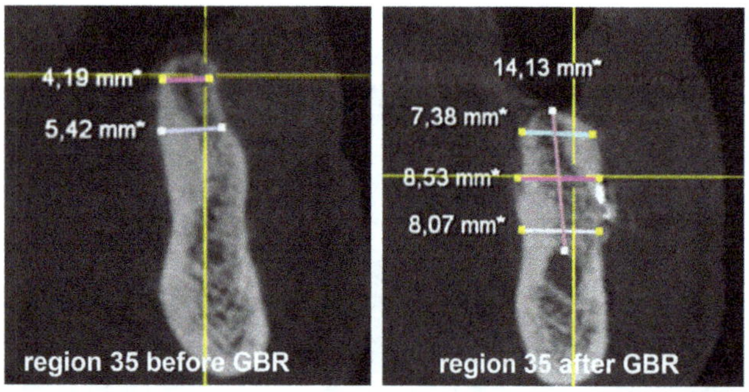

Figure 22: DVT—sections; implant position region 35 before and after GBR.

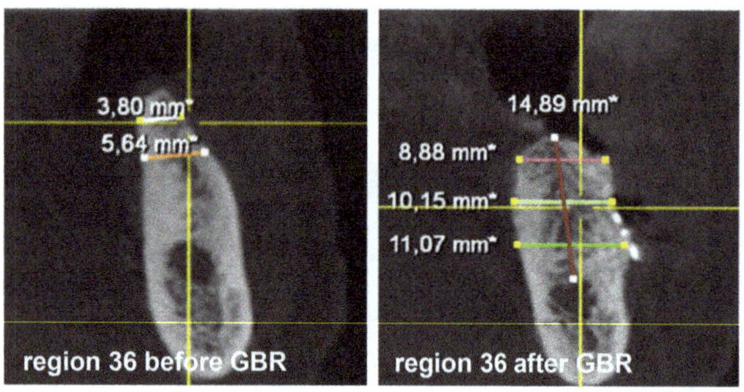

Figure 23: DVT—sections; implant position region 36 before and after GBR.

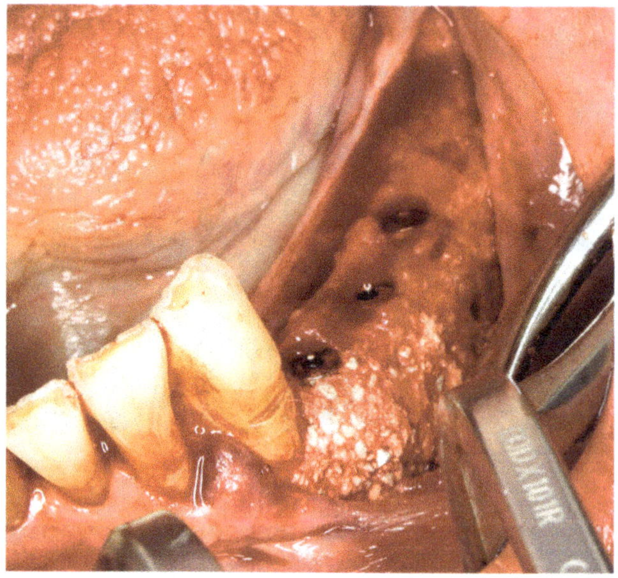

Figure 24: Tapered Screw Vent TSVT MTX Zimmer Biomet™ implants inserted in region 34, 35, and 36.

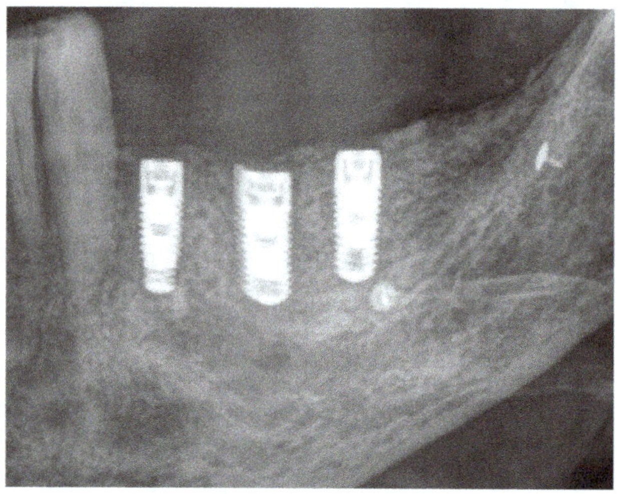

Figure 25: DPT—section; Tapered Screw Vent TSVT MTX Zimmer Biomet™ implants inserted in region 34, 35, and 36.

phase was initiated. In detail, after surgical exposure of the implants and open impression technique (ImpregumTM PentaTM; 3 M Deutschland GmbH, Neuss, Germany), individual single crowns and corresponding abutments were finally designed (ExocadTM GmbH, Darmstadt, Germany). The individual abutments were milled from Zimmer Biomet™ pre-milled abutment blanks (Zfx™ GenTek™ Titanium Pre-milled Abutment Blank, 4.5 mm diameter). In addition, the matching single crowns were monolithically milled from a zirconia oxide blank (zircon GEN-X®; Amman Girrbach™, Koblach, Austria) and shaded according to the patient needs. Finally, the crowns were cemented onto the titanium abutments with KetacCem® (3MTM; Vienna, Austria). Immediately after cementation, a DPT was taken to check the exact fit and to exclude cement residues (Figure 3).

Thereafter, the patient received two further appointments, each two weeks apart, to (1) check and, if necessary, correct static and dynamic occlusion and (2) check and, if necessary, support oral hygiene. In the further course, the patient was enrolled in a supportive therapy programme, and visits were arranged every three months.

7.5. GBR—Calculated Hard Tissue Gain. Figure 26 shows an overlay of DVTs before (2019) and after guided bone augmentation (2021). For this purpose, the corresponding 3D data sets were converted into 3D STL files using CoDiagnostiX® software (Dental Wings™, Montreal, QC, Canada) and then overlaid using Autodesk Netfabb 2020.0® software (Autodesk™, San Rafael, CA, USA). Furthermore, a

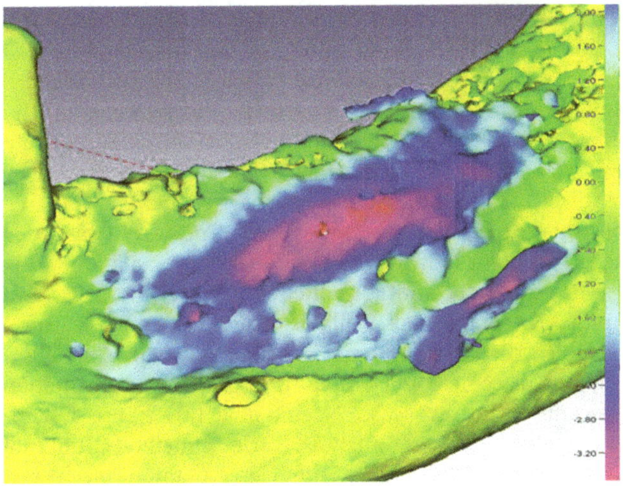

Figure 26: Graphical representation of the volume gain. The colour coding divides the gain from 0.0 mm (yellow) to 4.0 mm (red) at the respective positions of the third quadrant.

matching was performed with the software Final Surface® (Gesellschaft zur Förderung angewandter Informatik e.V., GFaI, Berlin, Germany; modified best-fit method), and a volume gain of 1.3–1.4 cm^3 was calculated. However, it should be clearly stated that this calculation method is not validated and that some referencing error (i.e., inaccuracies due to, e.g., artefact reduction during digital processing of the datasets used or conversion into STL files) remains in the 3D composite image.

8. Discussion

Here, we describe the restorative treatment of an 86-year-old patient who was referred to our specialist prosthodontics clinic in August 2018. Due to secondary osteoporosis, she received oral antiresorptive therapy with ibandronic acid from 2005 to 2015. Despite being classified as a patient at higher risk of MRONJ [13], she insisted on fixed implant-supported prosthetic rehabilitation in her 4th sextant and eventually signed the informed consent form. However, after extraction of teeth 34, 35, and 37 and thirteen months of bone healing, it was found that the coronal aspect of the bone ridge was too small (<5 mm horizontally) at the planned implant sites in regions 34, 35, and 36. Therefore, GBR was performed with a CAD/CAM-printed three-dimensional titanium mesh in combination with AB and a xenographic bone replacement graft. To create the conditions for successful implant placement and osseointegration, a horizontal augmentation of 8 mm ridge width in regions 34–37 was planned and performed. After ten months of submerged healing, a new DVT was taken, and a hard tissue ridge was found at the coronal margin, which was consistently above 7 mm. This allowed three implants (region 34: diameter 3.7 mm and length 10 mm; region 35: diameter 3.7 mm and length 10 mm; region 36: diameter 4.1 mm and length 10 mm) to be placed slightly subcrestal with an insertion torque of 35 Ncm each. After a four-month healing phase, the implants were finally restored with single crowns. Now the patient is seen regularly—every three months—for supportive peri-implant therapy.

During treatment planning, the previous antiresorptive therapy with Bonviva® (i.e., orally administered, 150 mg tablets once monthly; therapeutic indication: treatment of osteoporosis in postmenopausal women [16]) was critically reviewed. Each tablet of Bonviva® contains 150 mg ibandronic acid (molecular formula: $C_9H_{23}NO_7P_2$; structural formula: [1-hydroxy-3-(methylpentylamino)propylidene]diphosphonic acid), a medicine from the group of bisphosphonates for the treatment of, for example, osteoporosis. Hence, Bonviva® belongs to the pharmacological group of medicinal products for the treatment of bone diseases, bisphosphonates, and its Anatomical Therapeutic Chemical Classification System code is M05-BA06. Thereby, ibandronic acid is a highly effective bisphosphonate that belongs to the group of nitrogen-containing bisphosphonates (N-BPs; group of so called powerful antiresorptives [pARs]) that act selectively on bone tissue and specifically inhibit osteoclast activity without directly affecting bone formation. It does not interfere with osteoclast recruitment. Consequently, it leads to a progressive net increase in bone mass due to the reduction in increased bone turnover to premenopausal levels in postmenopausal women [16]. The principle molecular mechanisms underlying the inhibition of bone resorption by osteoclasts mediated by ibandronic acid are known. In brief, since bisphosphonates target bone mineral and osteoclasts are capable of releasing bone-bound bisphosphonate, a direct effect on mature osteoclasts appears to be the most important route of action. Ibandronic acid seems to act as analogues of isoprenoid diphosphate lipids, thereby inhibiting farnesyl diphosphate synthase. Inhibition of this enzyme in osteoclasts prevents the biosynthesis of isoprenoid lipids (farnesyl pyrophosphate and geranylgeranyl pyrophosphate), which are essential for posttranslational farnesylation and geranylgeranylation of small GTPase signalling proteins. Then, the loss of bone resorptive activity and osteoclast apoptosis is primarily a consequence of the loss of these geranylgeranylated small GTPases [17].

Unfavourably, MRONJ is a potentially severe adverse event affecting patients with osteoporosis (this applies also to patients with cancer, of course) who have been treated with, for example, N-BPs, pARs [18] as ibandronic acid. Thus, the European Public Assessment Report of the European Medicines Agency for Bonviva® lists osteonecrosis of the jaw (ONJ; i.e., MRNOJ) as a very rare adverse reaction (<1/10,000) reported in post-marketing settings in postmenopausal women receiving Bonviva 150 mg once monthly [16]. However, it should not be left unmentioned that this is generalized in a footnote to "Cases of osteonecrosis of the jaw have been reported, predominantly in cancer patients treated with medicinal products that inhibit bone resorption, such as ibandronic acid. Cases of ONJ have been reported in the post-marketing setting for ibandronic acid." [16] And thus, also for Bonviva®, indicating, and consistent with published data, that pAR-related MRONJ has similar general MRONJ pathophysiology in cancer and osteoporosis patients [12, 19, 20], but that pAR-related MRONJ occurs less frequently in patients treated for osteoporosis (incidence of 0.01–0.03%) than in cancer patients (incidence of 1.8–5%)

[12, 19, 21, 22]. Accordingly, that pAR-treated patients are at risk for MRONJ is reflected in guidelines [13, 23]. On this basis, we primarily classified our patient as being at higher risk of developing MRONJ. However, preclinical and clinical data suggest that most MRONJ cases require systemic risk factors (e.g., pARs) in combination with local oral risk factors, including inflammatory dental disease (e.g., periodontitis), tooth extractions, trauma from removable dentures, and possibly placement of dental implants [12, 19, 20, 24–39]. Be that as it may, even when looking very cautiously at scientific papers published to date, there seems to be convincing evidence that placing dental implants in patients receiving oral bisphosphonate therapy (as opposed to intravenous bisphosphonate therapy) has no significant negative impact on the development of MRONJ, implant survival, and implant success rate alone [15, 39–44]. Furthermore, since the teeth 34–37 would have had to be extracted anyway and periodontitis was successfully treated in advance and, moreover, as the general pathophysiology of MRONJ associated with pAR is at least similar in cancer and osteoporosis patients, and therefore trauma from removable dentures could be a theoretical risk factor for the development of MRONJ in patients with oral pAR therapy [35, 38], and since the patient presented here was otherwise healthy (i.e., beside an age of more than 60 years and female sex, no other non-dental risk factors for developing MRONJ; for review see Wan et al. [24]), we finally categorised her as a patient at lower risk for the development of MRONJ and were willing to realize the patient's request for a fixed—implant-supported—prosthetic restoration. However, the actual statistical or even individual risk of developing MRONJ (during or) after oral therapy for postmenopausal osteoporosis with Bonviva® following GBR and dental implantation remains unknown. All this was discussed with the patient in detail. Finally, the patient agreed to the therapy and signed the corresponding consent form. It should not go unmentioned that the treatment outcome confirms our assessment regarding not developing MRONJ.

Since oral surgical procedures should generally be considered risk factors for the development of MRONJ also in patients on oral pAR therapy (e.g., tooth extraction, bone augmentation, and implant placement), we chose a multistage approach. First, although the evidence especially for oral pAR therapy should be regarded as low, the teeth 34, 35, and 37 were extracted under a preventive protocol [28, 45–48]. In brief, before extraction, care was taken (especially in the 3rd quadrant) to ensure that plaque was reduced as much as possible and that there were no clinical signs of gingivitis [28]. As premedication, the patient received 1 g Augmentin® and 600 mg Ibuprofen® one hour before the intervention. In addition, immediately before tooth extraction, the oral cavity was thoroughly rinsed with Chlorhexamed® FORTE 0.2% for one minute. Furthermore, tension-relieving incisions were made for tooth extraction, bone edges were removed after the extraction, and the entire wound was completely closed in a passive manner (i.e., tension-free) [28, 46, 47]. In addition, Augmentin® (2 g × 1 g daily, for 7 days) and Ibuprofen® (3 mg × 600 mg daily, for 3 days, then as required) were prescribed. Furthermore, the patient was asked not to brush the surgical area until suture removal, but to rinse regularly (at least twice a day) with Chlorhexamed® 0.1%. Starting on the first post-surgical day until suture removal, the surgical area was checked and cleaned (cotton swabs soaked in Chlorhexamed® 0.1%) every second day. In addition, plaque on adjacent teeth was removed with curettes (Hu-Friedy Mfg. Co., LLC.). Until suture removal, wound healing was uneventful. Based on this experience, this prevention protocol was used accordingly for bone augmentation and implantation.

In general (i.e., not for patients with previous or current oral pAR therapy), the available evidence suggests that predictable correction of horizontal bone deficits that allow implant placement is possible through bone augmentation procedures (for review, see Naenni et al. [4]). In this systematic review and meta-analysis, various methods (but not graft-stabilising techniques with, e.g., a titanium mesh) and materials for lateral bone augmentation were analysed. The mean horizontal hard tissue gain was calculated to be 3.30 mm (95% confidence interval (CI): 2.81–3.79 mm; prediction interval (PI): 0.96–5.65 mm) for all available studies (i.e., twenty studies) and to 3.43 mm (95% CI: 2.83–4.03 mm; PI: 1.31–5.55 mm) for only seven studies that presented data for all three time points investigated (pre-augmentation, post-augmentation, and re-entry). Furthermore, the mean decrease of the augmented horizontal hard tissue was calculated as −1.33 mm (95% CI: −1.78 to −0.88 mm; PI: −2.98 to 0.32 mm (all studies) and −1.54 mm (95% CI: −2.17 to −0.91 mm; PI: −3.77 to 0.69 mm (seven studies with data for all three time points). This means, however, that due to the high variability of hard tissue augmentation achieved, predictability for actual treatment (for not graft-stabilising techniques with, e.g., a titanium mesh) is certainly difficult.

Moreover, for Bonviva® in particular, there was (and still is to our knowledge) no published evidence regarding bone augmentation procedures. For that reason, during treatment planning, it was assumed that since Bonviva® does not interfere with osteoclast recruitment and leads to an increase in bone mass [16], new bone formation should not be compromised during bone augmentation (i.e., GBR), and therefore, correction of the horizontal bone deficit should be predictably possible in the current patient to allow implant placement. Since, as mentioned above, any oral surgery should be considered a risk factor for the development of MRONJ, even in patients receiving oral pAR therapy, defect augmentation was not performed with bone harvested intraorally from a second surgical site (chin, ramus mandibulae), but for mixing with a xenograft, buccal cortical bone was collected apical and distal to the final mesh position with a Safescraper™.

For the augmentation method in the present case (i.e., Bio-Oss® mixed with AB, and Bio-Gide®; but not stabilized with a titanium mesh), there is some evidence regarding lateral hard tissue gain, graft reduction during wound healing, and predictability of implant placement [49]. In brief, in a randomized clinical trial (RCT) Bio-Oss®, particles were mixed by weight with AB particles either in a ratio of 90 : 10 (mean; 1.2 g Bio-Oss® : 0.14 g AB) or in a ratio of 60 : 40 (mean; 1.1 g Bio-Oss® : 0.7 g AB) together with autogenous blood from the surgical site. However, in contrast to the present case, 0.25 ml of fibrin glue was added to each of the graft mixtures to make the graft moldable and prevent the particles from migrating from the augmented area. Finally, all grafts were covered by Bio-Gide® membranes without further fixation. The width of the alveolar ridge ranged preoperatively from 1.6 to 6.1 mm and 1.4 to 6.5 mm, 3 and 6 mm from the top of the alveolar ridge, respectively. After a submerged healing period of approximately 7.5 months, the hard tissue gain was 0.4–6.3 mm (graft reduction: 0–94.9%) and 0.4–6.3 mm (graft reduction: −8.6% to 89.7%), 3 and 6 mm from the upper edge of the alveolar ridge, respectively. Finally, all the implants could be placed in all the planned locations, except for one, where the ridge was still too narrow, and the graft was very soft at this point. As noted for the review and meta-analysis by Naenni et al. [4], this again means that due to the high variability of hard tissue gain and graft reduction, predictable treatment planning (i.e., predictable implant placement) with the method and material used may indeed be difficult. In addition, Meijndert et al. [50–52] studied Bio-Oss® in combination with Bio-Gide® in one group (five patients) of a parallel-group RCT. In brief, all patients had a single-tooth diastema in the anterior region of the maxilla. Bio-Oss® was mixed with blood from the surgical site (but, unlike the present case, not mixed with AB, and no graft stabilising titanium mesh was used) and covered with a Bio-Gide® membrane. After six months of submerged healing, ridge enlargement of 2–3 mm was reported [50]. Two implants inserted in a Bio-Oss®/Bio-Gide® graft failed to osseointegrate and were lost within six months of placement [52]. In addition, the marginal peri-implant bone loss between 1 and 120 months after prosthetic loading (i.e., crown placement) was calculated to be −0.64 mm (SD: 1.46 mm) at mesial and −0.37 mm (SD: 1.47 mm) at distal sites in the Bio-Oss®/Bio-Gide® group. During this 10-year period, no further implant in the Bio-Oss®/Bio-Gide® group was lost [52]. But again, predictable treatment planning for long-term implant success may be difficult with the method and material used.

Therefore, to augment the region 34–37 predictably for successful implantation and osseointegration, a graft-stabilising three-dimensional printed titanium mesh for horizontal bone augmentation of up to 8 mm was planned and used in the present case. The graft biomaterials used were Bio-Oss® (mixed with AB and blood from the surgical site) and a Bio-Gide® membrane (to prevent ingrowth of connective tissue and to ensure osteogenic potential in the marginal area of the graft), stabilized with titanium pins. After a submerged healing period of ten months, a continuous augmented hard tissue ridge, at the coronal margin above 7 mm, was found, and all three implants could be placed in a prosthodontically driven position with an insertion torque of 35 Ncm each. Furthermore, after four months of submerged implant healing, the implants were clinically stable (i.e., osseointegrated) and restored with single crowns. Thus, the lateral bone width gain in the entire augmentation area in the 4th sextant was approximately between more than 3 mm and more than 5 mm. This is within the 95% prediction interval of bone width gain of the systematic review and meta-analysis on lateral bone augmentation before implant placement without graft stabilising techniques (e.g., a titanium mesh) published by Naenni et al. [4] and within the range of bone width gain (without graft stabilising technique) in the study by Mordenfeld et al. [49]. Moreover, such a continuous increase in hard tissue was never observed in our hands in similar GBRs without titanium mesh and might be attributed to the positional stability of the augmentation, which allows undisturbed bone healing free from compressive loads and other physical influences. Furthermore, compared to the data of Naenni et al. [4] and Mordenfeld et al. [49], the associated graft reduction was minimal in the current case.

Besides, there is a limited evidence for lateral bone augmentation with a graft-stabilising titanium mesh in general (for review see [53, 54]) and for the YxOss titanium mesh in combination with Bio-Oss® mixed with AB and Bio-Gide® in particular [55, 56] for lateral hard tissue gain, wound healing, and predictability of implant placement. In brief, Sagheb et al. [55] retrospectively analysed GBR (i.e., Bio-Oss® mixed with AB (AB form different intraoral donor sites and from the iliac crest or AB alone/YxOss titanium mesh/Bio-Gide® plus platelet-rich fibrin (PRF) membrane or Bio-Gide® alone) in 17 patients with 21 principally three-dimensional bone defects (i.e., vertical and horizontal bone augmentation). The postoperative healing was uneventful in 14 GBR sites (67%) during the follow-up time of six months until re-entry. However, at seven GBR sites (33%), exposure of the YxOss titanium mesh was observed after periods of five to twelve weeks after the first-stage surgery. Re-entry with explantation of the YxOss titanium mesh and simultaneous implantation of 44 implants was performed after six months. Cone beam computed tomography was performed preoperatively and six months postoperatively to measure bone height and width. A mean vertical bone gain of 6.5 mm (SD: 1.7 mm) and a mean horizontal bone gain of 5.5 mm (SD: 1.9 mm) were observed. Furthermore, after a mean follow-up time of 12 months (SD: 6 months) after second-stage surgery, none of the 44 inserted implants were lost, which corresponds to a survival rate of 100%. In the end, the authors only very generally concluded that individualized CAD-CAM fabricated titanium meshes are a safe and predictable procedure for large vertical and horizontal ridge augmentations. Similar results are reported by Hartmann and Seiler [56]. They also retrospectively analysed GBR (i.e., Bio-Oss® mixed with AB (in one patient, only Bio-Oss®; AB from different intraoral donor sites and from the iliac crest; ratio 1 : 1/YxOss titanium mesh/Bio-Gide® or Bio-Gide® plus an Advanced- (A-PRF®) membrane) in 55 patients with 68 three-dimensional bone defects (i.e., vertical and horizontal bone augmentation). Overall (i.e., Bio-Gide® or Bio-Gide® plus A-PRF® membrane), exposure of the YxOss titanium mesh was observed in 25% of treated defect sites ($n = 17$) in association with partial (11.8%, $n = 8$) and complete (15%, $n = 1$) loss of graft material. The YxOss titanium meshes were removed after a mean healing time of 6.5 months (SD: 2.7 months). A total of 98 implants were placed as planned. These authors also very generally concluded that the surgical protocol of individual bone regeneration has proven to be a promising technique for complex bone reconstructions. But the variability of GBR treatment performed in the studies of Sagheb et al. [55] and Hartmann and Seiler [56] (vertical and horizontal bone augmentation/different biomaterials) makes an actual evidence-based, meaningful comparison with the case presented here difficult.

Nevertheless, this case shows that GBR with a CAD/CAM-printed three-dimensional titanium mesh can predictably fulfil the desire for fixed, implant-supported single crowns, and a corresponding quality of life even in an older, medically compromised patient.

However, this result should not be generalized (predictable horizontal bone augmentation width, minimum reduction of the graft) as such a statement would require clinical trials with appropriate patient numbers.

9. Patient Perspective

To be able to describe an objective assessment of patient satisfaction, the Oral Health Quality questionnaire with 53 questions was used for the evaluation. There was a clear increase in the quality of life, and in particular, the patient did not describe any problems or complaints with chewing functionality or phonetics.

Consent

The patient gave informed consent on 20th July 2020.

Acknowledgments

This case report was not funded by third parties and was performed as a part of the employment of the authors (Danube Private University).

References

[1] D. Buser, L. LSennerby, and H. De Bruyn, "Modern implant dentistry based on osseointegration: 50 years of progress, current trends and open questions," *Periodontology 2000*, vol. 73, no. 1, pp. 7–21, 2017.

[2] N. P. Lang, "Oral implants: the paradigm shift in restorative dentistry," *Journal of Dental Research*, vol. 98, no. 12, pp. 1287–1293, 2019.

[3] S. Jepsen et al., "Regeneration of alveolar ridge defects. Consensus report of group 4 of the 15th European workshop on periodontology on bone regeneration," *Journal of Clinical Periodontology*, vol. 46, no. S21, pp. 277–286, 2019.

[4] N. Naenni, H. C. Lim, S. N. Papageorgiou, and C. H. F. Hämmerle, "Efficacy of lateral bone augmentation prior to implant placement: a systematic review and meta-analysis," *Journal of Clinical Periodontology*, vol. 46, Suppl 21, pp. 287–306, 2019.

[5] I. A. Urban, E. Montero, A. Monje, and I. Sanz-Sánchez, "Effectiveness of vertical ridge augmentation interventions: a systematic review and meta-analysis," *Journal of Clinical Periodontology*, vol. 46, Suppl 21, pp. 319–339, 2019.

[6] A. H. Melcher, "On the repair potential of periodontal tissues," *Journal of Periodontology*, vol. 47, no. 5, pp. 256–260, 1976.

[7] M. Sanz, C. Dahlin, D. Apatzidou et al., "Biomaterials and regenerative technologies used in bone regeneration in the craniomaxillofacial region: consensus report of group 2 of the 15th European workshop on periodontology on bone regeneration," *Journal of Clinical Periodontology*, vol. 46, Suppl 21, pp. 82–91, 2019.

[8] H. J. Haugen, S. P. Lyngstadaas, F. Rossi, and G. Perale, "Bone grafts: which is the ideal biomaterial?," *Journal of Clinical Periodontology*, vol. 46, Suppl 21, pp. 92–102, 2019.

[9] C. H. F. Hämmerle and R. E. Jung, "Bone augmentation by means of barrier membranes," *Periodontology*, vol. 2003, no. 33, pp. 36–53, 2000.

[10] A. Hartmann, M. Peetz, B. al-Nawas, and M. Seiler, "Patient-specific titanium meshes: future trend or current technology?," *Clinical Implant Dentistry and Related Research*, vol. 23, no. 1, pp. 3–4, 2021.

[11] P. N. Papapanou, M. Sanz, N. Buduneli et al., "Periodontitis: consensus report of workgroup 2 of the 2017 world workshop on the classification of periodontal and peri-implant diseases and conditions," *Journal of Clinical Periodontology*, vol. 45, Suppl 20, pp. S162–S170, 2018.

[12] S. L. Ruggiero, T. B. Dodson, J. Fantasia et al., "American Association of Oral and Maxillofacial Surgeons position paper on medication-related osteonecrosis of the jaw–2014 update," *Journal of Oral and Maxillofacial Surgery*, vol. 72, no. 10, pp. 1938–1956, 2014.

[13] (SDCEP), S.D.C.E.P. Oral Health Management of Patients at Risk of Medication-related Osteonecrosis of the Jaw—Dental Clinical Guidance, 2017, http://www.sdcep.org.uk.

[14] B. Owen and H. Bradley, "Is it safe to place implants in patients at risk of MRONJ?," *Evidence-Based Dentistry*, vol. 22, no. 3, pp. 108–109, 2021.

[15] V. Mendes, G. O. dos Santos, M. D. Calasans-Maia, J. M. Granjeiro, and V. Moraschini, "Impact of bisphosphonate therapy on dental implant outcomes: an overview of systematic review evidence," *International Journal of Oral and Maxillofacial Surgery*, vol. 48, no. 3, pp. 373–381, 2019.

[16] EMAEPAR-BONOVIA-INFORMATION_EN. Annex I Summary of Product characteristics, 2022.

[17] M. J. Rogers, "New insights into the molecular mechanisms of action of bisphosphonates," *Current Pharmaceutical Design*, vol. 9, no. 32, pp. 2643–2658, 2003.

[18] J. I. Aguirre, E. J. Castillo, and D. B. Kimmel, "Preclinical models of medication-related osteonecrosis of the jaw (MRONJ)," *Bone*, vol. 153, pp. 116184–116184, 2021.

[19] A. A. Khan, A. Morrison, D. A. Hanley et al., "Diagnosis and management of osteonecrosis of the jaw: a systematic review and international consensus," *Journal of Bone and Mineral Research*, vol. 30, no. 1, pp. 3–23, 2015.

[20] T. Kikuiri, I. Kim, T. Yamaza et al., "Cell-based immunotherapy with mesenchymal stem cells cures bisphosphonate-related osteonecrosis of the jaw–like disease in mice," *Journal of Bone and Mineral Research*, vol. 25, no. 7, pp. 1668–1679, 2010.

[21] P. Rugani et al., "Prevalence of medication-related osteonecrosis of the jaw in patients with breast cancer, prostate cancer, and multiple myeloma," *Dentistry Journal*, vol. 4, no. 4, p. 32, 2016.

[22] R. E. Coleman, M. Collinson, W. Gregory et al., "Benefits and risks of adjuvant treatment with zoledronic acid in stage II/III breast cancer. 10 years follow-up of the AZURE randomized clinical trial (BIG 01/04)," *Journal of Bone Oncology*, vol. 13, pp. 123–135, 2018.

[23] S. Ruggiero, E. R. Carlson, and L. A. Assael, "Comprehensive review of bisphosphonate therapy: implications for the oral and maxillofacial surgery patient," *Journal of Oral and Maxillofacial Surgery*, vol. 67, no. s1, pp. 1–12, 2009.

[24] J. T. Wan, D. M. Sheeley, M. J. Somerman, and J. S. Lee, "Mitigating osteonecrosis of the jaw (ONJ) through preventive dental care and understanding of risk factors," *Bone Research*, vol. 8, no. 1, p. 14, 2020.

[25] A. Soundia, D. Hadaya, N. Esfandi et al., "Osteonecrosis of the jaws (ONJ) in mice after extraction of teeth with periradicular disease," *Bone*, vol. 90, pp. 133–141, 2016.

[26] M. Song, A. Alshaikh, T. Kim et al., "Preexisting periapical inflammatory condition exacerbates tooth extraction-induced bisphosphonate-related osteonecrosis of the jaw lesions in mice," *Journal of Endodontia*, vol. 42, no. 11, pp. 1641–1646, 2016.

[27] H. Katsarelis, N. P. Shah, D. K. Dhariwal, and M. Pazianas, "Infection and medication-related osteonecrosis of the jaw," *Journal of Dental Research*, vol. 94, no. 4, pp. 534–539, 2015.

[28] T. Hasegawa, S. Hayashida, E. Kondo et al., "Medication-related osteonecrosis of the jaw after tooth extraction in cancer patients: a multicenter retrospective study," *Osteoporosis International*, vol. 30, no. 1, pp. 231–239, 2019.

[29] T. L. Aghaloo, B. Kang, E. C. Sung et al., "Periodontal disease and bisphosphonates induce osteonecrosis of the jaws in the rat," *Journal of Bone and Mineral Research*, vol. 26, no. 8, pp. 1871–1882, 2011.

[30] J. I. Aguirre, M. P. Akhter, D. B. Kimmel et al., "Oncologic doses of zoledronic acid induce osteonecrosis of the jaw-like lesions in rice rats (Oryzomys palustris) with periodontitis," *Journal of Bone and Mineral Research*, vol. 27, no. 10, pp. 2130–2143, 2012.

[31] R. S. de Molon, S. Cheong, O. Bezouglaia et al., "Spontaneous osteonecrosis of the jaws in the maxilla of mice on antiresorptive treatment: a novel ONJ mouse model," *Bone*, vol. 68, pp. 11–19, 2014.

[32] J. G. Messer, J. M. Jiron, J. L. Mendieta Calle et al., "Zoledronate treatment duration is linked to bisphosphonate-related osteonecrosis of the jaw prevalence in rice rats with generalized periodontitis," *Oral Diseases*, vol. 25, no. 4, pp. 1116–1135, 2019.

[33] J. G. Messer, J. L. Mendieta Calle, J. M. Jiron et al., "Zoledronic acid increases the prevalence of medication-related osteonecrosis of the jaw in a dose dependent manner in rice rats (Oryzomys palustris) with localized periodontitis," *Bone*, vol. 108, pp. 79–88, 2018.

[34] B. Kang, S. Cheong, T. Chaichanasakul et al., "Periapical disease and bisphosphonates induce osteonecrosis of the jaws in mice," *Journal of Bone and Mineral Research*, vol. 28, no. 7, pp. 1631–1640, 2013.

[35] K. Vahtsevanos, A. Kyrgidis, E. Verrou et al., "Longitudinal cohort study of risk factors in cancer patients of bisphosphonate-related osteonecrosis of the jaw," *Journal of Clinical Oncology*, vol. 27, no. 32, pp. 5356–5362, 2009.

[36] L. Levin, A. Laviv, and D. Schwartz-Arad, "Denture-related osteonecrosis of the maxilla associated with oral bisphosphonate treatment," *Journal of the American Dental Association (1939)*, vol. 138, no. 9, pp. 1218–1220, 2007.

[37] L. M. Hess, J. M. Jeter, M. Benham-Hutchins, and D. S. Alberts, "Factors associated with osteonecrosis of the jaw among bisphosphonate users," *The American Journal of Medicine*, vol. 121, no. 6, pp. 475–483.e3, 2008.

[38] A. Kyrgidis, K. Vahtsevanos, G. Koloutsos et al., "Bisphosphonate-related osteonecrosis of the jaws: a case-control study of risk factors in breast cancer patients," *Journal of Clinical Oncology*, vol. 26, no. 28, pp. 4634–4638, 2008.

[39] C. Walter, B. al-Nawas, T. Wolff, E. Schiegnitz, and K. A. Grötz, "Dental implants in patients treated with antiresorptive medication – a systematic literature review," *International Journal of Implant Dentistry*, vol. 2, no. 1, p. 9, 2016.

[40] R. Gelazius, L. Poskevicius, D. Sakavicius, V. Grimuta, and G. Juodzbalys, "Dental implant placement in patients on bisphosphonate therapy: a systematic review," *Journal of Oral & Maxillofacial Research*, vol. 9, no. 3, article e2, 2018.

[41] A. Stavropoulos, K. Bertl, P. Pietschmann, N. Pandis, M. Schiødt, and B. Klinge, "The effect of antiresorptive drugs on implant therapy: systematic review and meta-analysis," *Clinical Oral Implants Research*, vol. 29, Suppl 18, pp. 54–92, 2018.

[42] M. Nisi, F. la Ferla, D. Karapetsa et al., "Risk factors influencing BRONJ staging in patients receiving intravenous bisphosphonates: a multivariate analysis," *International Journal of Oral and Maxillofacial Surgery*, vol. 44, no. 5, pp. 586–591, 2015.

[43] M. Tallarico, L. Canullo, E. Xhanari, and S. M. Meloni, "Dental implants treatment outcomes in patient under active therapy with alendronate: 3-year follow-up results of a multicenter prospective observational study," *Clinical Oral Implants Research*, vol. 27, no. 8, pp. 943–949, 2016.

[44] V. Chappuis, G. Avila-Ortiz, M. G. Araújo, and A. Monje, "Medication-related dental implant failure: systematic review and meta-analysis," *Clinical Oral Implants Research*, vol. 29, Suppl 16, pp. 55–68, 2018.

[45] S. Ferlito, C. Liardo, and S. Puzzo, "Dental extractions in patient treated with intravenous bisphosphonates and risk of osteonecrosis of jaws: presentation of a preventive protocol and case series," *Minerva Stomatologica*, vol. 59, no. 11–12, pp. 593–601, 2010.

[46] S. Ferlito, S. Puzzo, and C. Liardo, "Preventive protocol for tooth extractions in patients treated with zoledronate: a case series," *Journal of Oral and Maxillofacial Surgery*, vol. 69, no. 6, pp. e1–e4, 2011.

[47] M. J. Heufelder, J. Hendricks, T. Remmerbach, B. Frerich, A. Hemprich, and F. Wilde, "Principles of oral surgery for prevention of bisphosphonate-related osteonecrosis of the jaw," *Oral Surgery, Oral Medicine, Oral Pathology, Oral Radiology*, vol. 117, no. 6, pp. e429–e435, 2014.

[48] E. Gaudin, L. Seidel, M. Bacevic, E. Rompen, and F. Lambert, "Occurrence and risk indicators of medication-related osteonecrosis of the jaw after dental extraction: a systematic review and meta-analysis," *Journal of Clinical Periodontology*, vol. 42, no. 10, pp. 922–932, 2015.

[49] A. Mordenfeld, C. B. Johansson, T. Albrektsson, and M. Hallman, "A randomized and controlled clinical trial of two different compositions of deproteinized bovine bone and

autogenous bone used for lateral ridge augmentation," *Clinical Oral Implants Research*, vol. 25, no. 3, pp. 310–320, 2014.

[50] L. Meijndert, G. M. Raghoebar, P. Schüpbach, H. J. A. Meijer, and A. Vissink, "Bone quality at the implant site after reconstruction of a local defect of the maxillary anterior ridge with chin bone or deproteinised cancellous bovine bone," *International Journal of Oral and Maxillofacial Surgery*, vol. 34, no. 8, pp. 877–884, 2005.

[51] L. Meijndert, G. M. Raghoebar, H. J. A. Meijer, and A. Vissink, "Clinical and radiographic characteristics of single-tooth replacements preceded by local ridge augmentation: a prospective randomized clinical trial," *Clinical Oral Implants Research*, vol. 19, no. 12, pp. 1295–1303, 2008.

[52] C. M. Meijndert, G. M. Raghoebar, L. Meijndert, K. Stellingsma, A. Vissink, and H. J. A. Meijer, "Single implants in the aesthetic region preceded by local ridge augmentation; a 10-year randomized controlled trial," *Clinical Oral Implants Research*, vol. 28, no. 4, pp. 388–395, 2017.

[53] Y. Xie, S. Li, T. Zhang, C. Wang, and X. Cai, "Titanium mesh for bone augmentation in oral implantology: current application and progress," *International Journal of Oral Science*, vol. 12, no. 1, p. 37, 2020.

[54] F. Briguglio, D. Falcomatà, S. Marconcini, L. Fiorillo, R. Briguglio, and D. Farronato, "The use of titanium mesh in guided bone regeneration: a systematic review," *International Journal of Dentistry*, vol. 2019, 2019.

[55] K. Sagheb, E. Schiegnitz, M. Moergel, C. Walter, B. al-Nawas, and W. Wagner, "Clinical outcome of alveolar ridge augmentation with individualized CAD-CAM-produced titanium mesh," *International Journal of Implant Dentistry*, vol. 3, no. 1, p. 36, 2017.

[56] A. Hartmann and M. Seiler, "Minimizing risk of customized titanium mesh exposures – a retrospective analysis," *BMC Oral Health*, vol. 20, no. 1, p. 36, 2020.

8

Customized Polymethyl Methacrylate Implants for the Reconstruction of Craniofacial Osseous Defects

André Luis Fernandes da Silva,[1] Alexandre Meireles Borba,[1,2,3] Niverso Rodrigues Simão,[1] Fábio Luis Miranda Pedro,[1] Alvaro Henrique Borges,[1] and Michael Miloro[2]

[1] *Post-Graduation Department, Faculty of Dentistry, University of Cuiaba (UNIC), 3100 Manoel Jose de Arruda Street, 78065-480 Cuiaba, MT, Brazil*

[2] *Department of Oral and Maxillofacial Surgery, College of Dentistry, University of Illinois (UIC), 801 South Paulina Street, Chicago, IL 60612-7211, USA*

[3] *Division of Dentistry, University General Hospital, 2101 Treze de Junho Street, 78025-000 Cuiaba, MT, Brazil*

Correspondence should be addressed to Alexandre Meireles Borba; alex80@terra.com.br

Academic Editor: Fabio Roccia

Craniofacial defects represent alterations in the anatomy and morphology of the cranial vault and the facial bones that potentially affect an individual's psychological and social well-being. Although a variety of techniques and restorative procedures have been described for the reconstruction of the affected area, polymethyl methacrylate (PMMA), a biocompatible and nondegradable acrylic resin-based implant, is the most widely used alloplastic material for such craniomaxillofacial reconstruction. The aim of this study was to describe a technique for aesthetic and functional preoperative customized reconstruction of craniofacial bone defects from a small series of patients offered by the Brazilian public health system. Three adult male patients attended consultation with chief complaints directly related to their individual craniofacial bone defects. With the aid of multislice computed tomography scans and subsequent fabrication of the three-dimensional craniofacial prototype, custom-made PMMA implants were fabricated preoperatively. Under general anesthesia, with access to the craniofacial defects with a coronal approach, the PMMA implants were adapted and fixated to the facial skeleton with titanium plates and screws. Postoperative evaluation demonstrated uneventful recovery and an excellent aesthetic result. Customized prefabricated PMMA implants manufactured over the rapid prototyping models proved to be effective and feasible.

1. Introduction

Craniofacial defects represent alterations in the anatomy and morphology of the cranial vault and the facial bones as a result of trauma, tissue necrosis associated with infections, or sequel following surgical procedures [1]. Craniofacial traumas from sport-related accidents, falls, physical assault, or, in particular, automobile accidents are associated with a high incidence of craniofacial defects by maxillofacial bone fracture caused by the trauma itself or bone loss caused by a neurosurgical craniotomy performed for intracranial decompression [2]. Such defects are not always corrected immediately due to the patient's compromised systemic condition(s) that may contraindicate immediate repair; this creates aesthetic and functional impairments of the facial skeleton that will need to be corrected at a later period of time [3]. Regardless of the etiology, these defects potentially affect an individual's psychological and social well-being [4].

Reconstruction of craniofacial defects requires a combination of function and aesthetic repair principles [3]. A variety of techniques and restorative procedures have been described for this purpose, including autogenous or allogeneic bone grafting, as well as the use of alloplastic materials that can be molded during, or prior to, surgical reconstruction [3, 4]. Each of the possible options has advantages and disadvantages in its use [5]. Autogenous bone grafting remains the first choice for reconstruction of bone defects, but often the patient refuses a second surgical site with resultant morbidity to obtain bone or the amount of bone available is insufficient; for such cases, alloplastic implant materials are used [3, 6]. Currently, the most widely used alloplastic material for these craniomaxillofacial reconstructions is polymethyl methacrylate (PMMA), a biocompatible and nondegradable acrylic resin-based implant, which can be fabricated prior to surgery, with the advantages of reduced surgical time, the use of a simple technique, and excellent long-term aesthetic results [3, 5, 7].

The construction of the PMMA implant can be performed during surgery, or even preoperatively, with the aid of three-dimensional (3D) reconstruction [1, 2, 4]. However, such technology is not always available depending upon the specific location, or the high cost of design and materials might preclude its use. Considering the cost-free availability of 3D reconstruction of the craniofacial skeleton for patients of the Brazilian public health system by the *Centro de Tecnologia da Informação Renato Archer* (CTI), the aim of this study was to describe a technique for aesthetic and functional preoperative customized reconstruction of craniofacial bone defects from a small series of patients.

2. Cases Report

Three adult male patients attended consultation at the Department of Oral and Maxillofacial Surgery at the General Hospital of Cuiaba, which is affiliated with the University of Cuiaba, MT, Brazil, with chief complaints directly related to their individual craniofacial bone defects.

2.1. Case 1. A 25-year-old male patient reported a work-related accident 18 months ago. At the time, he underwent decompressive craniectomy and remained hospitalized at an intensive care unit for a period of two months. Following hospital discharge, due to cosmetic and functional concerns about his craniofacial defect, the patient sought consultation and evaluation from our department. Physical examination showed a significant bony depression at the right frontoorbital region associated with right eye enophthalmos, orbital vertical dystopia, and right eyelid ptosis (Figures 1(a)–1(d)).

2.2. Case 2. A 30-year-old male patient was the victim of an altercation involving a large animal about five years ago. At the time of the accident, he was primarily treated at his hometown and referred to our department for evaluation and treatment of complex facial bone fractures. Several weeks later, the patient underwent reconstructive surgery for open reduction and internal fixation of the comminuted fractures of the frontal bone. At a late postoperative evaluation, it became evident that the patient presented with resorption of the anterior wall of the frontal sinus where titanium plates had been used for fixation of the fractures. During the next four years, the patient was noncompliant with regular follow-up visits and appeared in our clinic with a chief complaint of a significant frontal bone defect (Figures 1(e)–1(h)).

2.3. Case 3. A 33-year-old male patient was the victim of a motor vehicle accident when he was 18 years of age. At that time, he underwent decompressive craniectomy, exenteration of the right eyeball due to extensive injury, and tracheotomy while being hospitalized in the intensive care unit for a period of two months. The patient remained untreated due to the extensive distance from his hometown to the nearest health services facility until he was referred to our department for evaluation and management. Physical examination revealed a significant depression involving the right frontonasoorbital region (Figures 1(i)–1(l)).

2.4. Preoperative Planning. In order to obtain a precise diagnosis and perform surgical planning for reconstruction of the craniofacial defects, all patients underwent multislice computed tomography scan (CT) according to the protocol of the CTI (Figures 2(a)–2(c)). Then, these images were sent to the CTI for subsequent fabrication of the 3D craniofacial prototype.

With the aid of the prototype, custom-made PMMA implants were fabricated preoperatively. Since none of the patients presented with functional defects of the frontal sinus, the proposed reconstructive surgeries were intended primarily to recreate the premorbid anatomical and morphological craniofacial contours.

The prototypes were reconstructed with modeling wax at the defective regions of the skull to accurately simulate the morphology of the PMMA implants. Then, the thickness of the wax was reduced by approximately three millimeters, which allowed all involved areas to receive insulating liquid. This liquid allowed the PMMA material to be poured over these areas during its plastic phase, in accordance with the desired anatomical contour, with lateral small edge-shaped extensions, to provide support over healthy bone. After polymerization of the PMMA, the implant was polished and underwent ethylene oxide sterilization (Figures 3(a)–3(i)).

2.5. Surgical Technique. All surgical procedures were performed under general anesthesia, with access to the craniofacial defect(s) with a coronal approach, providing adequate exposure of the affected region(s). After careful debridement of the osseous defects, with removal of soft tissue fibrous ingrowth and small bone irregularities, the PMMA implants were adapted and fixated to the facial skeleton with titanium plates and screws. In all cases, the PMMA implants fit precisely and passively at the craniofacial defects, requiring only minor corrections to provide better adaptation (Figures 4(a)–4(f)). None of the patients had their frontal sinus approached, since no preoperative sinus complaints were reported or observed.

Postoperative objective and subjective patient evaluation demonstrated uneventful recovery and an excellent aesthetic result (Figures 5(a)–5(l)).

3. Discussion

Frontal bone fractures comprise about 2% to 15% of all facial fractures. The goals of craniofacial fracture treatment are isolation of the intracranial contents, treatment of any associated cerebrospinal fluid leak, and functional, as well

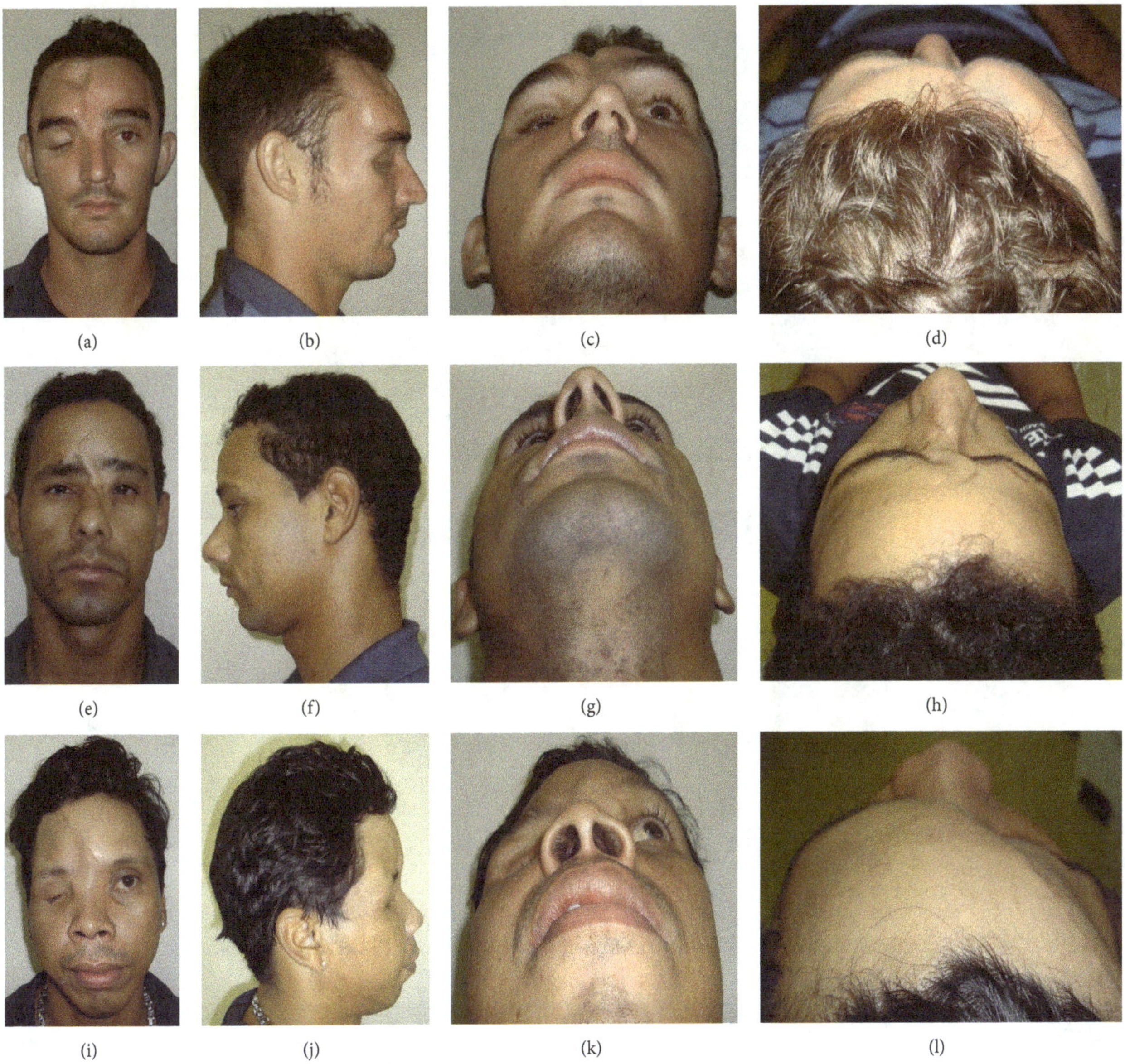

(a) (b) (c) (d)
(e) (f) (g) (h)
(i) (j) (k) (l)

FIGURE 1: Clinical preoperative evaluation.

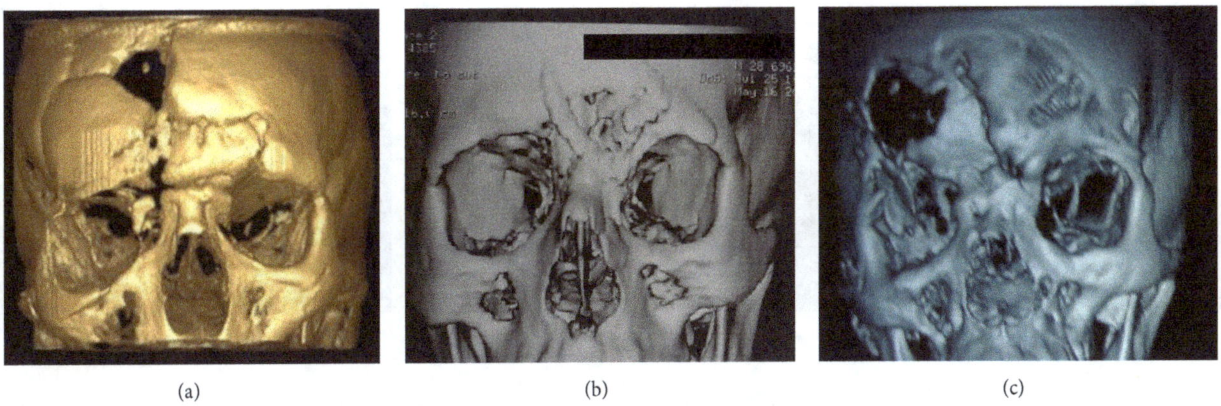

(a) (b) (c)

FIGURE 2: Preoperative 3D CT scans for Cases 1, 2, and 3 ((a), (b), and (c), resp.).

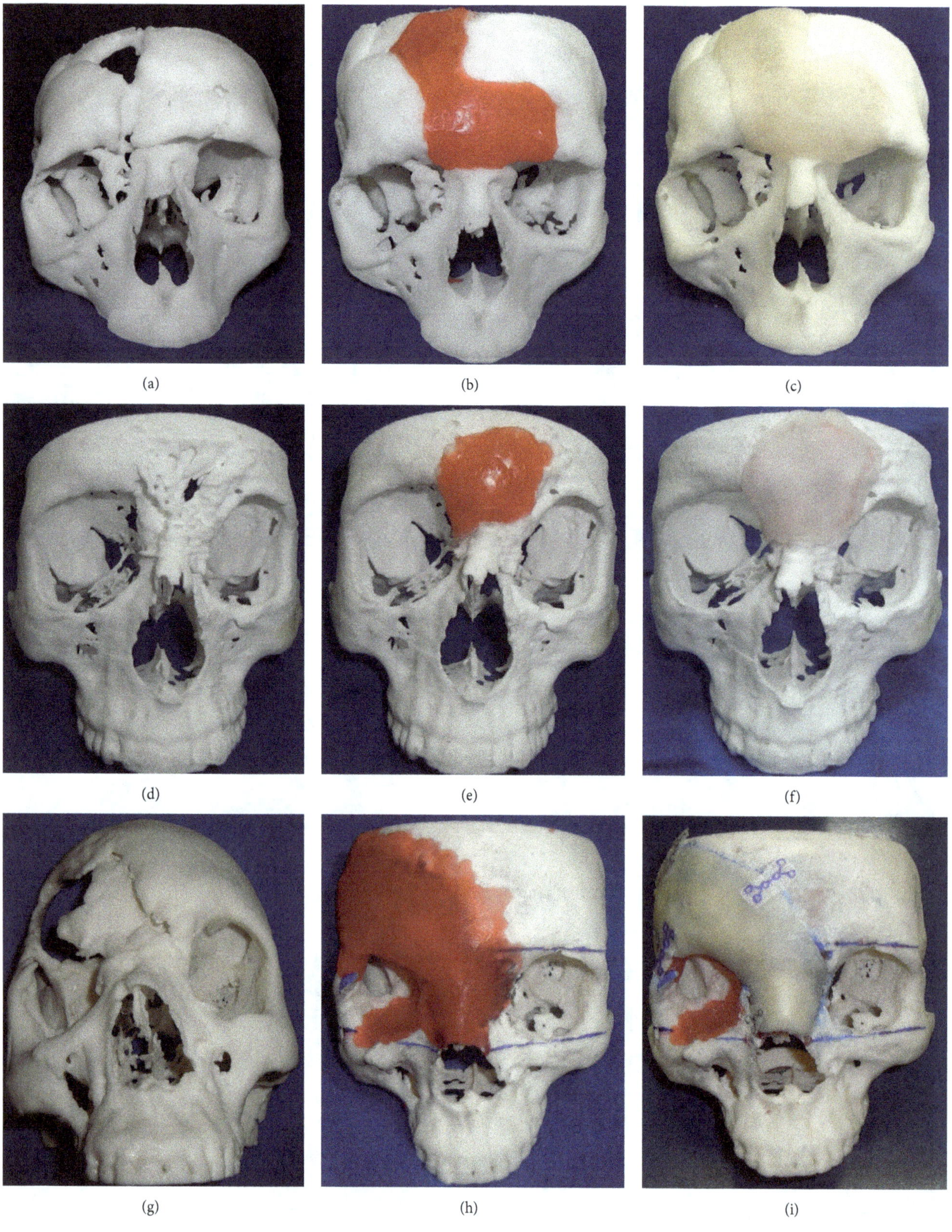

FIGURE 3: Preoperative customization of PMMA implants: initial aspect of the defect, wax covering the defects with a thickness-reduced wax, and PMMA reconstruction of the defect according to the desired anatomical contour (Case 1 ((a)–(c)), Case 2 ((d)–(f)), and Case 3 ((g)–(i))).

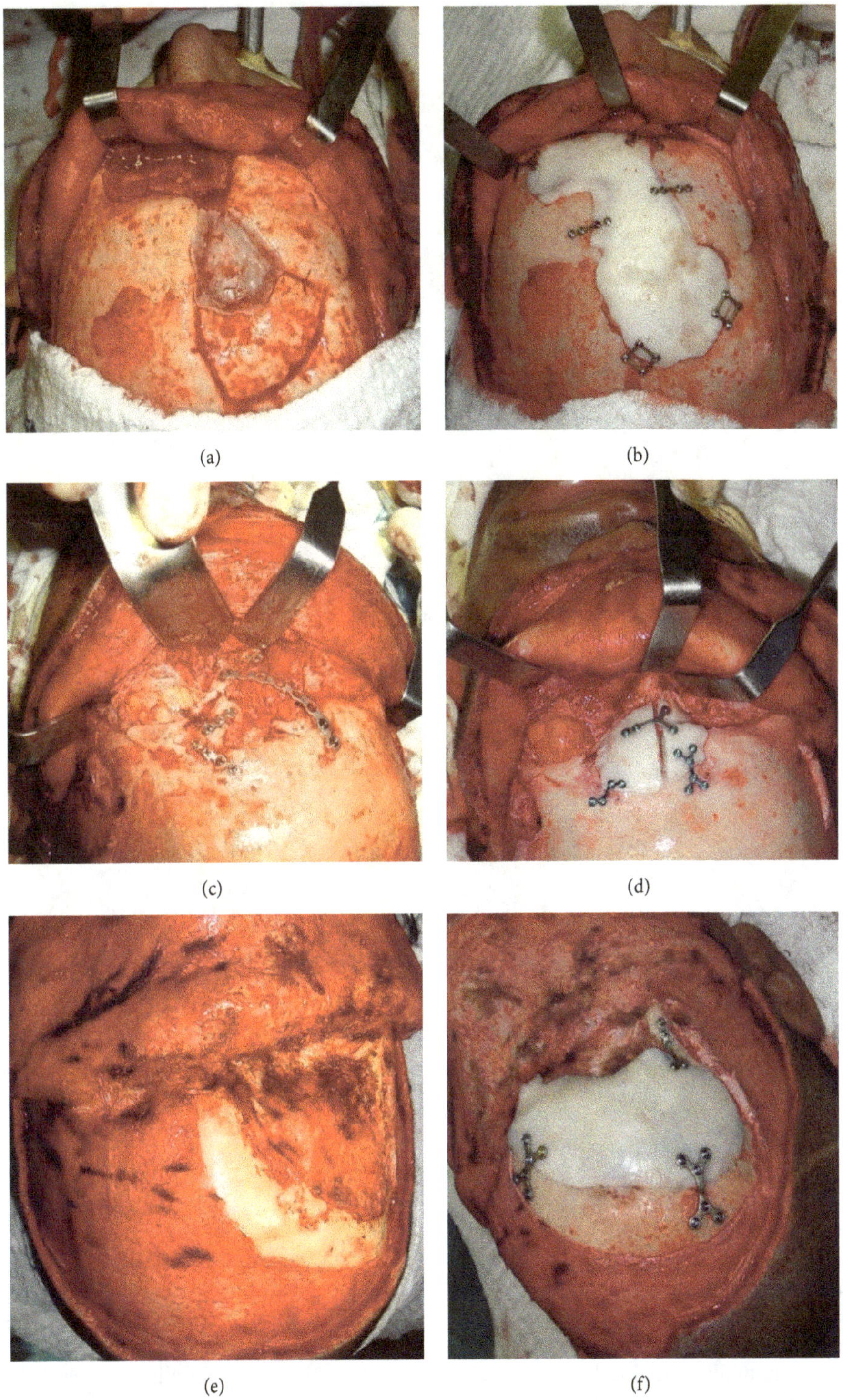

Figure 4: Intraoperative view of the defect and reconstruction with the PMMA implant (Case 1 ((a)-(b)), Case 2 ((c)-(d)), and Case 3 ((e)-(f))).

as aesthetic, restoration of the original bone anatomy and contour [2]. Although it is not the purpose of this paper, it is important to note that upper facial reconstruction may involve management of the frontal sinus since the frontonasal duct might be impaired as a result of the craniofacial defect. Also, management of frontal sinus posterior wall fractures might indicate the need for frontal sinus obliteration or cranialization [2]. When a decompressive craniotomy is performed, the bone fragment removed from the skull may be banked and used to reconstruct the defect later. For this,

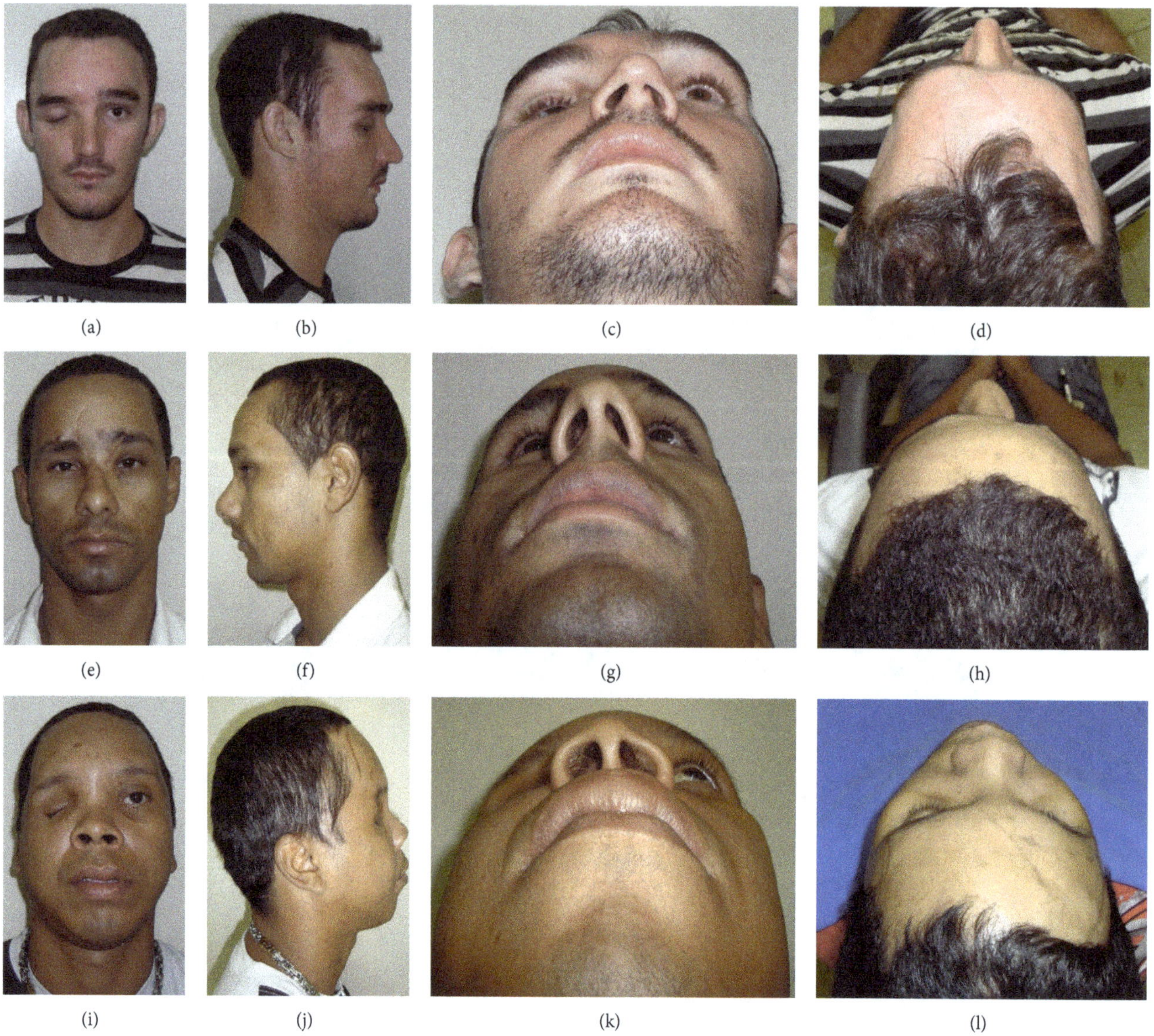

FIGURE 5: Clinical postoperative evaluation.

the fragment might be stored in the abdominal wall and then frozen in storage [1]. However, such techniques may have the disadvantages such as resorption of the bone graft or infection [4, 7]. Patients undergoing decompressive craniotomy can develop the "syndrome of the trephined," with symptoms such as dizziness, anxiety, irritability, and intolerance to noise or vibration. The reconstruction of cranial bone defects has proven to be effective in the treatment of this syndrome [4, 8]. This reinforces the concept that reconstructive procedures are intended for not only aesthetic restoration but also functional rehabilitation.

The use of autogenous bone remains the first choice for reconstruction of bone defects, and this may include corticocancellous bone or vascularized bone flaps that may also provide a soft tissue pedicle for reconstruction of significant soft tissue defects. However, disadvantages include the risk of bone graft resorption, insufficient availability of the required quantity of bone, or the refusal of the patient to approach another surgical site for harvest of the bone graft due to the associated morbidity. These factors would tend to favor the use of an alloplastic material [2, 3, 5–7, 9]. Advantages of alloplastic materials include ready availability, resistance to resorption, easy handling and workability during surgical procedures, and long-term stable and satisfactory cosmetic results [3, 5, 7]. The materials used most commonly are hydroxyapatite cement, hydroxyapatite block, hydroxyapatite granules, carbonated calcium phosphate bone cement, calcium phosphate paste of calcium carbonate, carbonated calcium phosphate plate, titanium mesh, high-density porous polyethylene implants, bioactive glass ceramic implants, polyetheretherketone, and acrylic materials (PMMA) [2, 3, 5].

The use of titanium mesh is limited due to its high cost and the difficulty to contour and model the material, and it is also time consuming to perform these adjustments at the time of reconstructive surgery [5, 9]. The use of demineralized bone allograft material is promising but still carries the risk of resorption, immunologic reactions, and transmission of infectious disease, thus limiting its widespread use. Although hydroxyapatite is becoming increasingly popular due to its biocompatibility and possible osteoconductive and osteoinductive properties, when compared to PMMA, the latter is less expensive, more readily accessible, and easier to handle and contour for specific craniofacial defects [9].

Currently, the alloplastic material mostly used by surgeons for these craniomaxillofacial reconstructions is PMMA, which is composed of fine particles of prepolymerized resin mixed with methyl methacrylate [1–4]. The polymerization process is initiated by the reaction between the benzoyl peroxide and N-dimethyl-p-toluidine. A radiopaque material such as barium sulfite or zirconium dioxide is also added as a component of the powder. The polymerization reaction is highly exothermic, and the PMMA material may exceed 80°C. It is currently well tolerated and supports bone formation on its surface (osteoconductive). After polymerization, typically within five minutes, the PMMA releases about 3 to 5% of monomer residues and decreases to 1.2% over time. The monomer toxicity should disappear completely within four hours [3]. No monomer fragments are released after PMMA implantation, and no PMMA toxicity occurs after 48 and 78 months following surgical reconstruction [10].

Infection, foreign body reaction, and growth restriction (in skeletally immature individuals) are a few major disadvantages of the use of alloplastic materials. The risk of infection can be reduced by adding gentamicin to the acrylic mixture, using it in a sterile environment, covering the alloplast with vascularized tissues, and maintaining systemic broad-spectrum antibiotic for a period of five days after implantation [5]. To reduce the risk of foreign body reaction, the implant must be stabilized well with immobility with the use of titanium plates and screws [9]. Growth restriction in the growing patient can be prevented by avoiding the use of PMMA placed directly over craniofacial sutures in children [5]. Of course, the initial injury and subsequent scarring may be an independent risk factor for growth restriction irrespective of the use of PMMA in the reconstruction.

PMMA can be used directly during surgery, by applying it over the bony defect, while the material is in the plastic phase of polymerization. When the implant begins to polymerize, an exothermic reaction takes place, generating heat that should be controlled by cold saline irrigation. In cases of total thickness cranial reconstruction, a titanium mesh is indicated to be placed over the PMMA implant in order to protect the implant from direct trauma [9]. After polymerization occurs, the implant is removed for trimming and then replaced and fixated. Increased operative time, the exothermic reaction, contact of PMMA resin fluid with blood, and material toxicity are all disadvantages of the use of this PMMA technique [1, 2, 4]. The allergic reaction to PMMA is rare and occurs due to a reaction against a component of the PMMA, N-dimethyl-p-toluidine, which is used as an accelerator (MMA monomer). A small amount of the population is allergic to MMA, which may manifest with symptoms of stomatitis, burning mouth syndrome, or chronic hives [3].

An alternative to intraoperative placement and polymerization is prefabrication of the PMMA implant, thereby avoiding the intraoperative disadvantages and still providing excellent aesthetic results [3, 8]. With the aid of computer-planning technology, many emerging techniques provide 3D design and construction of implants using the information provided by high-definition CT images, known as computer-aided design and computer-aided manufacturing (CAD-CAM) [1, 2, 4, 6, 7]. Undoubtedly, there are many advantages with such a technique, but it should be noted that there is a higher cost when employing additional technology in the planning process.

The rapid prototyping techniques include stereolithography, fused deposition modeling, and selective laser sintering. The prototyping technology has been widely used in the industrial area but still has been used less extensively in medical and dental healthcare, mainly due to the limited number of companies providing prototyping services, the cost of this technology, and also the lack of knowledge from health professionals regarding the application of this technology, although this is improving internationally [11]. For the construction of the prefabricated PMMA implant according to the technique presented here, a rapid prototyping model, produced by stereolithography, was used to customize a structure directly from a 3D model. Rapid prototyping has been presented as a technology that favors the direct relationship between the model and the actual anatomy. This allows for surgical simulation and planning as well as preoperative customization of implants, thus reducing surgical time and allowing better communication between the surgical team and the patient [11]. Healthcare specialty areas such as orthopedic surgery, neurosurgery, maxillofacial surgery, and implantology might benefit from this technology when planning treatment of cases of trauma, pathology, and congenital or acquired craniomaxillofacial deformities.

The technique described here combines favorable factors supported by the current literature. Besides using PMMA which is widely accepted for this reconstructive purpose, the use of a rapid prototyping technique to customize a prefabricated implant without additional financial cost to patients within the Brazilian public health system was only available through a partnership with the CTI, a governmental research unit. This might not reflect public healthcare systems in other countries, which might limit their ability to provide adequate treatment for such complex cases due to financial constraints.

In large craniofacial reconstruction procedures, PMMA implants have proven to be effective, easy to handle, and biocompatible, providing excellent aesthetic and functional results. 3D reconstruction of the defect greatly assists in the diagnosis and surgical planning, allowing surgical time to be decreased. Customized prefabricated PMMA implants manufactured over the rapid prototyping models, such as those described in this study, proved to be effective and feasible. In addition to features inherent to PMMA implants, the

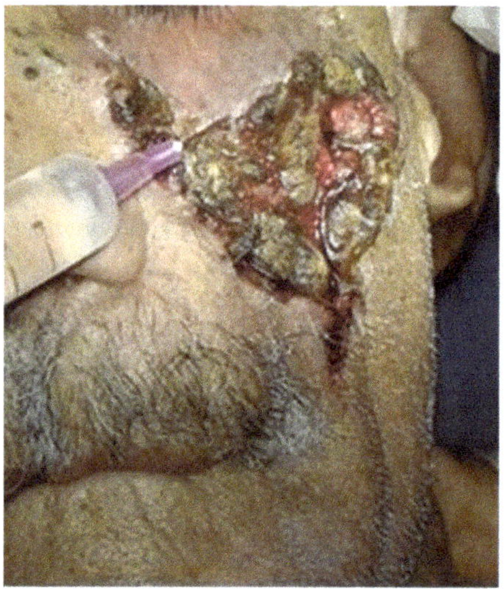

FIGURE 1: Ulcerated lesion involving the left cheek.

cervicofacial flap. The entire procedure was performed under local anesthesia as the patient was a high risk category for general anesthesia.

3. Procedure

Wide excision of the lesion with a 5 mm margin was done (Figure 2). The incision for the flap started directly posterior from the superior most extent of the resection and carried straight till the preauricular crease for improved cosmetics. Medially, the incision was made without disturbing the anatomic boundary of the nose. The entire flap was elevated in a subcutaneous plane till along the lateral aspect of the mandible to enhance the reach and rotation of the flap (Figure 3). The entire defect could be reconstructed with good esthetic and functional results (Figure 4). This technique reduced the operating and recovery time without compromising the results. The postop period was uneventful with no observation of flap necrosis or significant facial nerve deficits. There was no other unanticipated outcome when the patient followed up for suture removal (Figure 5).

The flap design was straightforward with slight modification to a conventional cervicofacial flap. Even though deep plane dissection has been advocated by some to improve vascularity and reduce complications, it has been shown that the subcutaneous flap is much easier to raise with comparable and even lower complication rates than deep plane flaps [5, 6]. Also, performing a deep plane dissection needs more surgical expertise and experience. The reconstruction was one stage and did not require any later refinements.

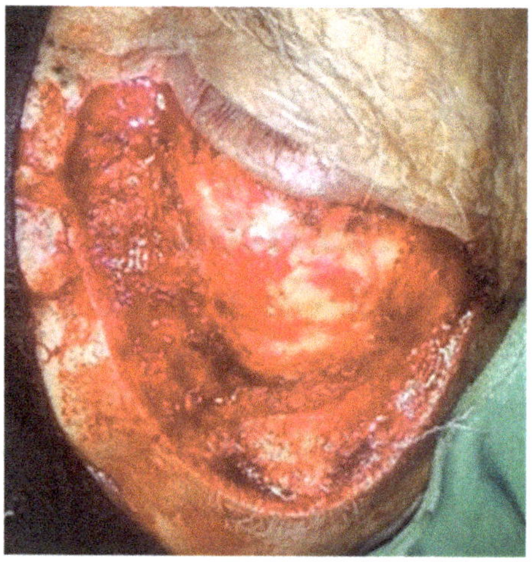

FIGURE 2: Defect following tumor resection.

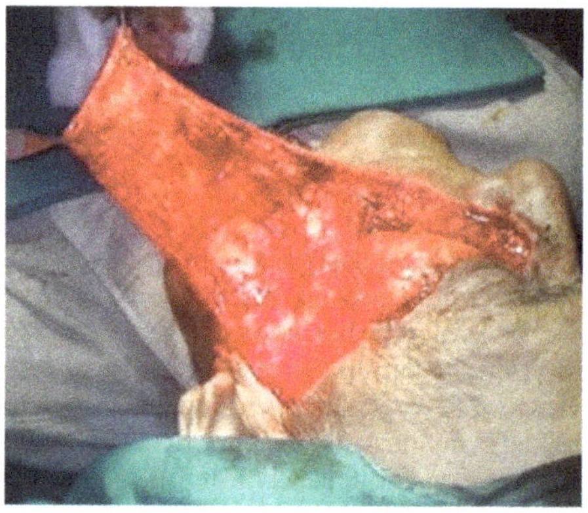

FIGURE 3: Elevated flap.

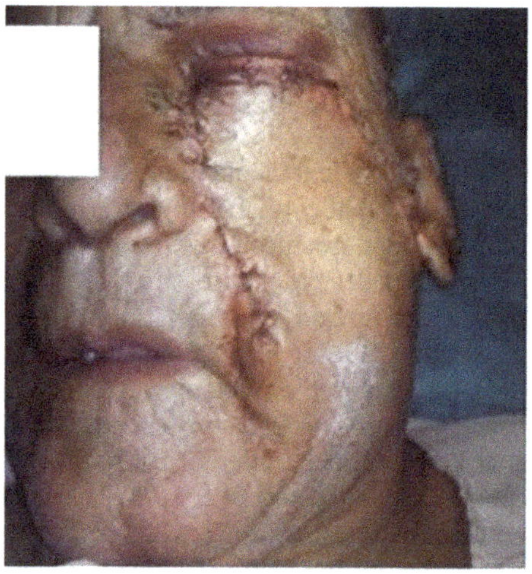

FIGURE 4: Immediate post op. Simultaneous primary closure of the donor site.

4. Discussion

Reconstruction of cheek defects is a complex procedure and needs a lot of consideration with respect to esthetic and functionality and respecting the adjacent anatomic subunits. A useful classification of cheek defects was given by Roth et al. Based on the location of the defect, it can be categorized into three zones. Zone 1 refers to suborbital defects, Zone 2 includes defects in preauricular/temporal areas, and Zone 3 is the perioral, lower cheek and lateral mandibular region. A straightforward algorithm for this flap design was recently published by Al Shetawi et al. in a series of cases [7].

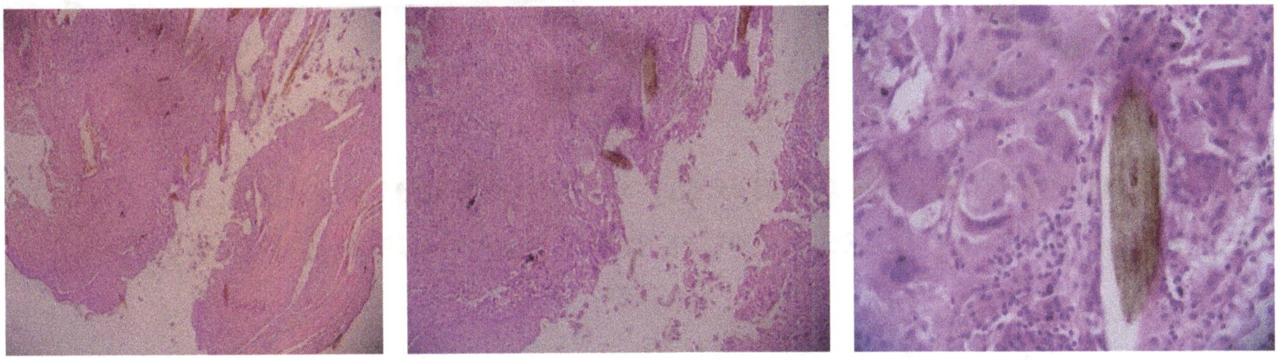

(a) (b) (c)

FIGURE 3: Hematoxylin-eosin stained slides of a specimen of pilonidal sinus obtained from the scalp of a 46-year-old patient. (a) 40, (b) 100, and (c) 400 times magnification images.

After treatment, all patients should be followed up for recurrence [8, 10]. For the purpose of avoiding recurrence, there should not be any PS tissue left after the surgery, and there should also be no dead space remaining or wound infection which affects the recovery process [8, 9]. However, no method of treatment can entirely prevent recurrence and relapse; rates or relapse vary between 2 and 40% [8, 10].

Scalp PS with infection is rare, and the recurrence risk is very low after excision. Recurrence was observed in one case in the literature [5]. In cases of a developing acute pilonidal abscess or fistula formation, drainage with debridement and abscess cultures should be performed [10].

Aerobic and/or anaerobic bacteria can reproduce in abscess cultures. According to culture and antibiogram results, patients should be given an appropriate antibiotic agent to prevent dissemination to surrounding tissue. Antibiotic treatment selection can be changed according to the results of culture [8, 10]. Daily dressings should be performed. When malignancy is determined, extensive resection with flap reconstruction and regional lymph node dissection are performed in accordance with the principles of oncologic surgery. After surgery, radiotherapy and chemotherapy should be applied. However, in these cases, the relapse rate is high and the prognosis is poor [11].

In our case, the totally excised mass was examined by pathology and precisely diagnosed as a pilonidal sinus. Follow-up examinations performed 2 years later showed no complications and no recurrence.

As a result, during the process of diagnosing scalp masses, scalp PS should be considered. Although scalp PS are rare, differential diagnosis is crucial. For treatment, proper surgical techniques should be performed and monitoring should be focused on postsurgical complications and recurrence.

References

[1] J. Kueper, T. Evers, K. Wietelmann, D. Doll, J. Roffeis, and P. Schwabe, "Sinus pilonidalis in patients of German military hospitals: a review," *GMS Interdisciplinary Plastic and Reconstructive Surgery DGPW*, vol. 4, article Doc02, 2015.

[2] F. Çiftci and I. Abdurrahman, "A different disease: extrasacrococcygeal pilonidal sinuses etiopathogenesis," *International Journal of Clinical and Experimental Medicine*, vol. 8, no. 7, pp. 11567–11571, 2015.

[3] D. G. Moyer, "Pilonidal cyst of the scalp," *Archives of Dermatology*, vol. 105, no. 4, pp. 578–579, 1972.

[4] N. Sion-Vardy, L. Osyntsov, E. Cagnano, A. Osyntsov, D. Vardy, and D. Benharroch, "Unexpected location of pilonidal sinuses," *Clinical and Experimental Dermatology*, vol. 34, no. 8, pp. e599–e601, 2009.

[5] O. A. Nalbant and E. Nalbant, "Pilonidal sinus of the scalp: a case report and review of the literature," *Balkan Medical Journal*, vol. 28, no. 4, pp. 445–447, 2011.

[6] M. Kosaka, M. Kida, H. Mori, and H. Kamiishi, "Pilonidal cyst of the scalp due to single minor trauma," *Dermatologic Surgery*, vol. 33, no. 4, pp. 505–507, 2007.

[7] F. Pehlivanli, G. Karaca, M. R. Pekcici, K. Yildirim, and B. Karaca, "Pilonidal sinus disease of the scalp," *American Surgeon*, vol. 78, no. 4, pp. E242–E243, 2012.

[8] A. Onder, S. Girgin, M. Kapan et al., "Pilonidal sinus disease: risk factors for postoperative complications and recurrence," *International Surgery*, vol. 97, no. 3, pp. 224–229, 2012.

[9] V. O. Gul, S. Destek, S. Ozer et al., "Minimally invasive surgical approach to complicated recurrent pilonidal sinus," *Case Reports in Surgery*, vol. 2015, Article ID 759316, 3 pages, 2015.

[10] G. T. Fahrni, R. N. Vuille-Dit-Bille, S. Leu et al., "Five-year follow-up and recurrence rates following surgery for acute and chronic pilonidal disease: a survey of 421 cases," *Wounds*, vol. 28, no. 1, pp. 20–26, 2016.

[11] D. Sharma, A. Pratap, A. Ghosh, and V. K. Shukla, "Malignant transformation of a pilonidal sinus," *Surgery*, vol. 145, no. 2, pp. 243–244, 2009.

13

Maxillomandibular Transverse Osteodistraction: A Multidisciplinary Case Report with 30-Month Follow-Up

G. Turatti,[1] A. Bruni,[2,3] M. Savoini,[4] M. Giordano,[1] and G. Gerbino[4]

[1]*Odontostomatology OU, Martini Hospital, Via Tofane 71, Turin 10141, Italy*
[2]*CIR Dental School, Department of Surgical Sciences, Università degli Studi di Torino, Via Nizza 230, Turin 10126, Italy*
[3]*Department of Mechanical and Aerospatial Engineering (DIMEAS), Politecnico di Torino, C.so Duca degli Abruzzi 24, Turin 10129, Italy*
[4]*Division of Maxillofacial Surgery, Department of Surgical Sciences, Università degli studi di Torino, Città della Salute e delle Scienza Hospital, Corso A.M. Dogliotti 14, Turin 10126, Italy*

Correspondence should be addressed to A. Bruni; alessandro.bruni@polito.it

G. Turatti and A. Bruni contributed equally to this work.

Academic Editor: Hüsamettin Oktay

Aim. To describe a multidisciplinary treatment to correct a severe II class malocclusion with reduced both maxillary and mandibular transverse dimensions and dental crowding. *Case Report.* A 17-year-old young woman presented with an increased overjet complaining chiefly of forwardly placed upper front teeth and unpleasant smile aesthetics. The patient facially exhibited a gently convex profile, severe mentalis strain on lip closure, and dark buccal corridors. The intraoral assessment indicates Class II molar relationship bilaterally, mandibular and maxillary anterior crowding, and narrow shape of upper and lower arches. The cephalometric evaluation of the lateral radiograph of the skull evidences a skeletal Class II with a reduction of lower face height. Based upon the diagnostic records and consultation with the patient, surgically assisted expansion of both arches using bone-borne distractors, comprehensive orthodontic treatment, and combined jaw surgery was planned. *Results.* This approach permitted achieving most of the desired objectives in approximately 30 months. The follow-up records 30 months after treatment conclusion showed a stable occlusion. No complications were clinically and radiographically noticeable during the follow-up.

1. Introduction

Transverse deficiencies are a common finding among populations [1]: in selected patients, concurrent osteodistraction of both arches represents a viable option [2–4] to treat severe maxillomandibular transverse deficiency and dental crowding.

Historically, the mandibular arch dimension has always been considered immutable.

The synostosis of the mandibular symphysis occurs during the first year after delivery, and the use of orthodontic devices (e.g., lingual arches [5], functional appliances [6], Schwarz plates, and archwires [7]) has proved inadequate to gain more than 6-8 mm in the lower arch [8, 9]. Several methods exist to overcome this limit (e.g., through interproximal enamel reduction, extracting teeth, or even using bone anchorages to lower the lateral sectors [8]). However, the stability of these treatments is often unpredictable and can result in adverse side effects [10].

Distraction osteogenesis is the biological process of new bone formation between bone segments that are gradually separated by incremental traction after an intentional surgical bone fracture [10].

The first *Mandibular Symphyseal Distraction Osteogenesis* (MSDO) was performed by Guerrero in 1997 [11] and subsequently described under various nomenclature, e.g., Mandibular Midline (Osteo-) Distraction (MMD) and Transmandibular Symphyseal (Osteo-) Distraction (TMSD).

This treatment modality, compared to the abovementioned ones, improves aesthetics and function, shortens treatment time, and appears stable over time [11].

The fusion of midpalatal suture has a variable timing: it occurs generally after the age of 15 [12].

Surgically Assisted Rapid Palatal Expansion (SARPE), also mentioned as *Surgically Assisted Rapid Maxillary Expansion* (SARME), is a widely accepted procedure for skeletally mature patients with maxillary transverse deficiency.

The first *SARPE* was performed by Brown in 1938 [13, 14] to prevent unwanted effects of orthopedic or orthodontic expansion in skeletally mature patients (e.g., buccal tipping of posterior teeth, extrusion, periodontal membrane compression, buccal root resorption, alveolar bone bending, fenestration of the buccal cortex, palatal tissue necrosis, pain, and instability of the expansion [15]) by surgically releasing the closed sutures resisting the expansion forces.

The most frequent indications for a simultaneous bimaxillary osteodistraction, mentioned as *Maxillomandibular Transverse Osteodistraction* (MMTOD), are severe (maxillary-) mandibular transverse deficiency, severe (maxillary-) mandibular anterior crowding [11], uni- [16] and bilateral buccal crossbite, impacted anterior teeth with insufficient space and hugely tipped teeth [17], and obstructive sleep apnea syndrome [18].

In this case report, the focus is on the orthodontic and surgical procedure, the distractor devices, the distraction sequence, the skeletal and aesthetic outcome, the stability after a 30-month follow-up, treatment-related difficulties, and complications.

2. Case Report

In September 2013, a 17-year-old female came to the Department of Orthodontics at the Martini Hospital in Torino with the chief complaint of prominent upper teeth and crooked mandibular and maxillary incisors with difficulty in maintenance of oral hygiene.

2.1. History. She reported CCE (common childhood exanthemas) when she was a child. She was in good general health, without any allergies. The patient's oral health was good. Before treatment, complete orthodontic and radiographic documentation was requested. No previous orthodontic treatment was performed; no TMJ problems were reported. The first step was to conduct thorough extraoral and intraoral examinations.

2.2. Assessment

2.2.1. Extraoral Assessment. During the extraoral clinical examination, a mandibular retrusion and severe mentalis strain on lip closure were verified; the profile was reasonably convex; and the nasolabial angle was moderately closed. The face shape was oval with moderate mandibular asymmetry to the right side; smile arch appeared to be flattened with an excessive amount of gingival display during forced smiling; and dark buccal corridors were found (Figure 1).

2.2.2. Intraoral Assessment. Intraorally, a narrow shape of the upper arch and the lower arch, a bilateral Class II molar and canine relationship, increased overjet (OVJ: 12.7 mm) and overbite (OVB: 7.2 mm), a dental crowding in both dental arches (slight in the upper, severe in the lower), and deviation of the superior midline to the right of 4 mm and inferior midline to the right of 6 mm were detected. In the mandibular arch, lack of space was noted (Figure 1).

2.2.3. Dental Cast Assessment. The dental cast analysis also showed an increased OVJ and OVB and enhanced Spee's curve (Figure 2).

2.2.4. Radiographic Assessment. Radiographically, a complete permanent dentition with unerupted third molars was observed (Figure 1).

The cephalometric evaluation of the lateral radiograph of the skull (Figure 3(a); Table 1, T0) showed that the patient had a skeletal Class II pattern (Wits: 5.7 mm) with a slightly retruded position of the maxilla (SNA: 77.1°) and mandible (SNB: 75.8°). The occlusal plane was significantly anteriorly upward pitched (Mand plane-Occ plane: 23.6°).

The maxillary incisors were protruded (A1 to APo plane: 2.3 mm) and proclinate (U1-Occ plane: 50.0°; U1-palatal plane: 131.0°), and the mandibular incisors were slightly retruded (L1 to Apo plane: 12.4 mm) and reclined (IMPA: 83.5°).

The cephalometric evaluation of the skull radiograph in the posteroanterior (PA) view showed good symmetry overall (Figure 3(b)).

2.2.5. Diagnosis. No symptoms of TMJ dysfunction were referred (there were neither noises from the joint nor pain identified during mandibular movement; there was a good range of mandibular movement).

The patient was diagnosed as having a skeletal Class II pattern with dental deep bite and severe dental Class II combined with dental crowding, in particular in the anterior part of the lower arch. The accentuated Spee's curve, resulting from an overeruption of lower incisors in association with the anterior labial flaring of the upper incisors, led to the tilting of the occlusal plane anteriorly upward.

2.3. Treatment

2.3.1. Treatment aim. The following treatment objectives were established:

(1) To obtain space in the arches to accommodate the teeth

(2) To expand the maxillary arch to obtain harmony with the mandibular arch

(3) To expand the mandibular arch

(4) To reduce OVJ and OVB

(5) To correct molar and canine Class II dental malocclusion

(6) To restore lip competence at rest and to reduce the mentalis habit

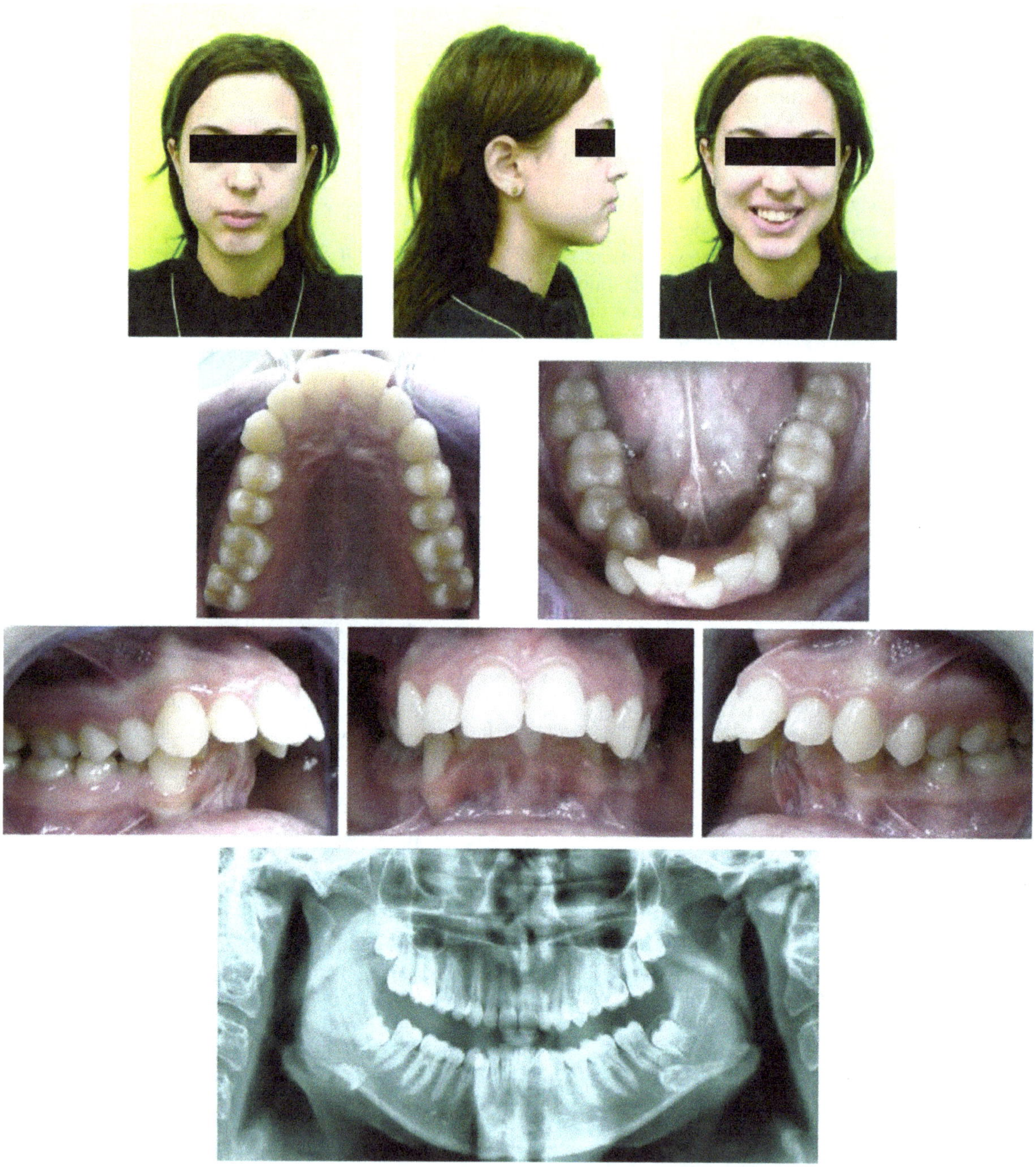

Figure 1: Extraoral photographs (T0), intraoral photographs (T0), and orthopantomogram (T0); T0=pretreatment.

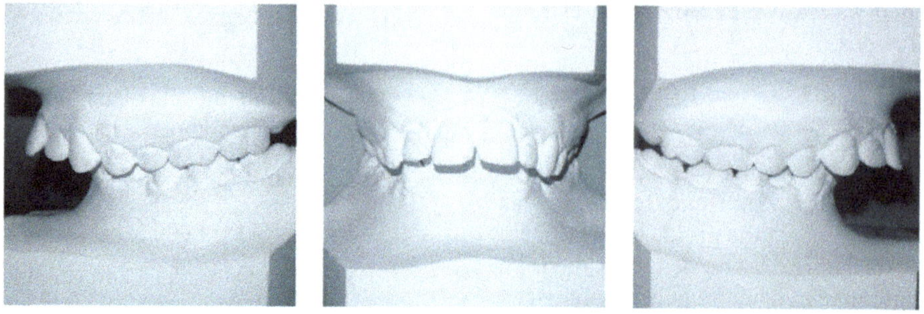

Figure 2: Dental cast models (T0); T0=pretreatment.

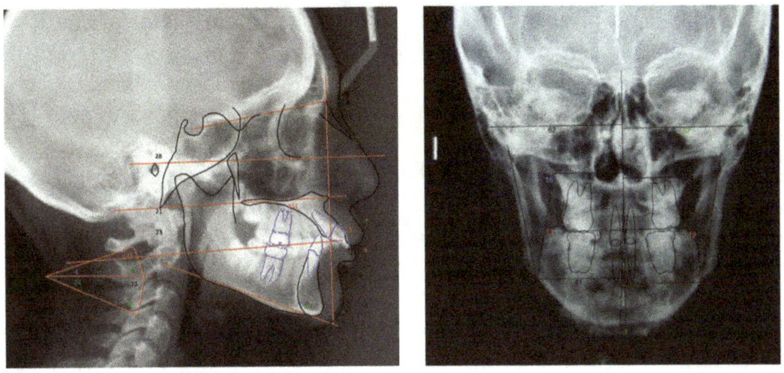

(a) (b)

Figure 3: Cephalometric tracing (T0): (a) cephalometric evaluation of the lateral radiograph of the skull and (b) cephalometric evaluation of the posteroanterior radiograph of the skull; T0=pretreatment.

Table 1: Cephalometric analysis (T0-T2): T0=pretreatment, T2=treatment progress (18 months), and T4=follow-up (30 months after the end of the treatment).

	Measured value T0	Measured value T2	Measured value T4	Norm
SNA	**77.1°**	**83.6°**	***83.1°***	82° ± 3.5°
SNB	**75.8°**	**86.1°**	***80.9°***	80° ± 3°
ANB	**1.4°**	**-2.6°**	***2.2°***	2° ± 2.4°
Maxillary skeletal (A-Na Perp)	**-3.0°**	**5.1°**	***1.6°***	0° ± 3.1°
Mand. skeletal (Pg-Na Perp)	**-5.0°**	**16.5°**	***1.1°***	0° ± 5.3°
Wits appraisal	**5.7** mm	**-4.2** mm	***-0.1°***	0 *mm* ± 1 *mm*
FMA (MP-FH)	**21.1°**	**10.9°**	***20.7°***	26° ± 5°
MP-SN	**30.6°**	**23.3°**	***29.2°***	33° ± 6°
Palatal-Mand angle	**22.7°**	**22.8°**	***23.0°***	28° ± 6°
Palatal-Occ plane	**-1.0°**	**6.3°**	***7.0°***	10° ± 4°
Mand plane-Occ plane	**23.6°**	**16.5°**	***16.0°***	17.4° ± 5°
U1 protrusion (U1-APo)	**2.3** mm	**8.9** mm	***8.6*** mm	0.4 ± 2.0 *mm*
L1 protrusion (L1-Apo)	**12.4** mm	**7.4** mm	***4.5*** mm	3.5 ± 2.3 *mm*
U1-palatal plane	**131.0°**	**120.2°**	***118.4°***	110° ± 5°
U1-Occ plane	**50.0°**	**53.4°**	***54.6°***	57.5° ± 7°
L1-Occ plane	**72.9°**	**58.6°**	***60.6°***	72° ± 5°
IMPA	**83.5°**	**105.0°**	***103.4°***	95° ± 7°

(7) To improve facial and smile aesthetics reducing buccal corridors

The expected compliance was good.

2.3.2. Treatment Plan. Based on the diagnostic records and consultation with the patient, the following plan was developed:

(1) Extraction of 1.8, 2.8, 3.8, and 4.8

(2) Surgically Assisted Rapid Palatal Expansion (SARPE) using bone-borne transpalatal distractor (TPD) and MMD using bone-borne transmandibular distractor (TMD).

(3) Comprehensive orthodontic treatment with particular attention paid to anterior teeth position and relationship

(4) Surgical planning reevaluation of the orthodontic results

(5) Corrective combined jaw surgery: usual bimaxillary advancement procedure with deliberate counterclockwise rotation of the occlusal plane including LeFort I osteotomy of the maxilla for anterior maxillary impaction and advancing; Bilateral Sagittal Split Osteotomy (BSSO) for increasing lower jaw length to provide better balance to the facial features

(6) Postsurgical orthodontics and periodontal follow-up

2.3.3. Treatment Progress. After the removal of the wisdom teeth, a Surgically Assisted Rapid Palatal Expansion using bone-anchored TPD and a Surgically Assisted Mandibular Midline Distraction procedure using bone-anchored TMD were performed.

Both surgical procedures were carried out under general anesthesia with nasotracheal intubation.

The surgical technique and distraction protocol used for SARPE was performed according to Ramieri et al. [19].

A flattened horseshoe-shaped incision was executed high in the vestibule from approximately the second premolar to the second premolar ensuring excellent exposure of the osteotomy site. The surgical cutting of the bone was performed from the piriform aperture to the pterygomaxillary suture, approximately 8 mm above the apices of the teeth. A vertical corticotomy from the anterior nasal spine to the alveolar crest was made using a surgical bur. The maxilla was downfractured sagittaly using a thin, straight osteotome. Pterygomaxillary suture disjunction was obtained using curved osteotomes.

A bone-borne distraction device (TPD™, Surgi-Tec NV, Brugge, Belgium) was subsequently placed to the palatal vault, through small mucosal incisions nearby second premolars, and fixed with 7 mm screws.

The surgical technique used for Surgically Assisted Rapid Mandibular Expansion was performed according to Mommaerts et al. [4]. A labial vestibular incision was carried out in order to gain access for the step osteotomy, consisting of two vertical osteotomies (interdental between canine and later incisor; in the basal bony midline) connected by a horizontal subapical osteotomy. A bone-borne distraction device (TMD™, Surgi-Tec NV, Bruges, Belgium) was subsequently placed on the mandibular symphysis.

The whole surgical procedure had taken approximately 80 minutes.

The patient was hospitalized for one night and was discharged the next morning with antibiotic, analgesic, and corticosteroid therapy. No complication after surgical procedures was reported.

After seven days, the maxillary distractor was activated (0.33 mm/day for the first ten days; 0.66/day thenceforth for an additional seven days); concomitant activation of the mandibular distraction device was performed (2×0.5 mm/day for ten days).

After starting the expansion procedure, the amount of the widening was clinically evaluated weekly: the spacing between the maxillary central incisors, the mandibular lateral incisor, and canines was the first sign of disjunction of the bone halves.

Total expansion of 8 mm, assessed by measuring the maxillary intermolar width as the distance between the mesial fossae of the maxillary first molars, was achieved in the upper arch. Total expansion of 5 mm, assessed by measuring the mandibular intercanine width as the distance from cusp tip to cusp tip of the mandibular canines, was achieved in the lower arch.

After the postoperative activation phase, both expansion devices were locked with a securing screw to prevent their deactivation (Figure 4) and to ensure the consolidation phase.

The patient's clinical status was assessed 15 days after expansion in progress: no teeth mobility, no gingival recession, no periodontal pockets, unaltered teeth vitality, and good hygiene with a suitable plaque without bleeding on probing control were detected.

After the surgically assisted widening of both the maxilla and the mandible, a fixed appliance (SW Roth prescription, $0.022'' \times 0.028''$ slots) was used to align the dentition during the consolidation phase. Before starting the active orthodontic treatment, a segmented arch-wire was used to control undesired movements of the lower incisors.

Both the distractors were removed under local anesthesia: the mandibular one was removed after about 120 days, and the maxillary one was removed after about 180 days. The orthodontic treatment continued following these stages:

(1) *Aligning stage*: a lingual arch was mounted mandibulary after removing the upper and lower distractors to control the intermolar width and rotations. In both arches, .012 NiTi archwires were used. During this stage, an active coil was positioned between 35 and 33 and between 45 and 43 to create space for 34 and 44

(2) *Levelling stage*: a TPB was mounted maxillary. NiTi archwires of successive cross-sections were used for about ten months in order to complete the alignment

(3) *Working stage*: the maxillary and mandibular arches were coordinated, the maxillary and mandibular midlines were aligned, spaces were closed, and the maxillary and mandibular occlusal planes were paralleled. The OVJ and OVB were improved

A panoramic radiograph to evaluate the position of the roots and a lateral radiograph of the skull that showed a clockwise rotation of the maxillomandibular complex were taken. Also, the clinical examination showed excessive incisal exposure during the smile (Figure 5).

Presurgical orthodontic results were reevaluated together with the orthognathic surgery team of the University of Turin to decide the proper treatment plan.

In order to improve aesthetics (correction of excessive tooth exposure at rest and increase of soft tissue support with skeletal facial expansion) and improve dental and occlusal relationship, maxillomandibular osteotomies were planned with the agreement of the patient. A total of 4 mm of maxillary impaction and 7 mm of mandibular advancement were programmed. The following corrective combined jaw surgery was performed: LeFort I osteotomy of the maxilla with differential maxillary impaction and advancing simultaneously with a *Bilateral Sagittal Split Osteotomy* (BSSO), achieving a slight counterclockwise rotation of the occlusal plane.

A lateral radiograph of the skull was requested to do tracing for cephalometric evaluation: comparison of the cephalometric analysis before and after surgery demonstrated an improvement in the sagittal skeletal and dental values (Figure 6; Table 1, T2).

(4) *Detailing and finishing stage*: after surgery, the patient was monitored closely for one month and

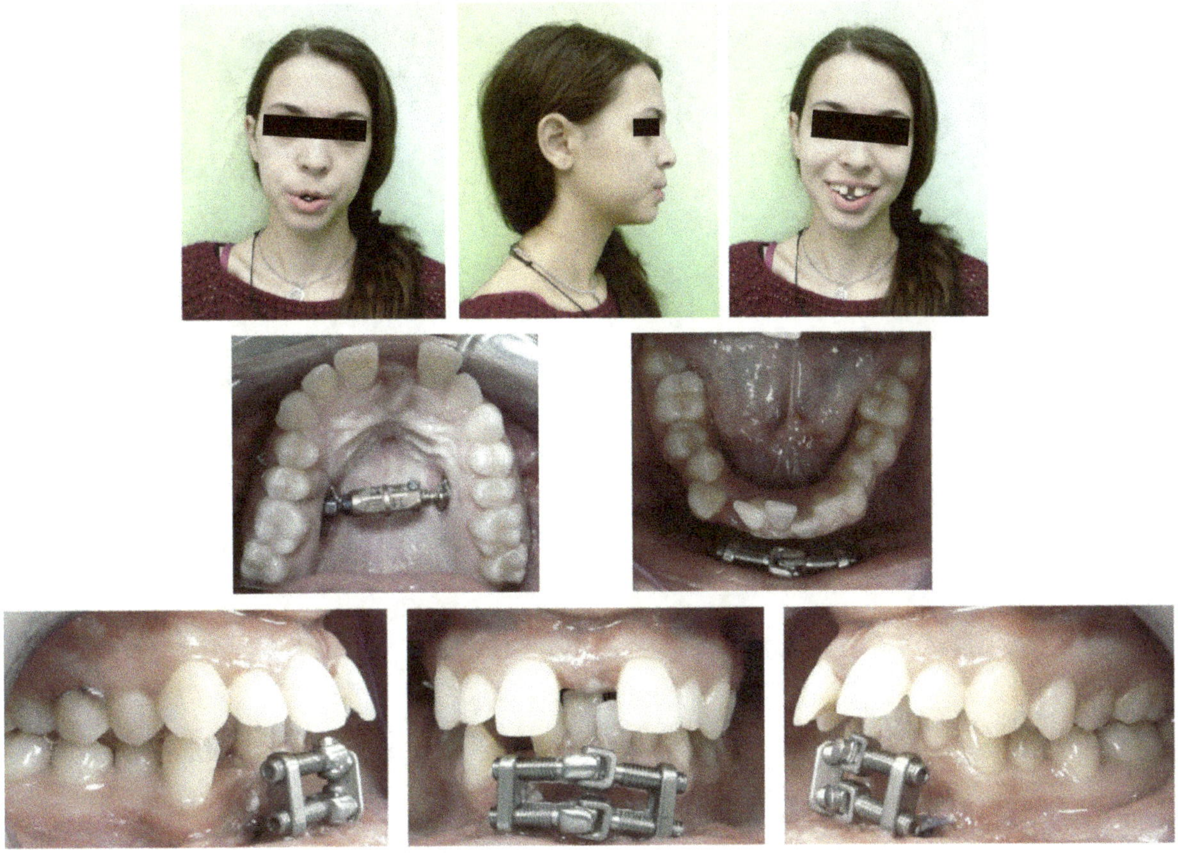

FIGURE 4: Extraoral photographs (T1) and intraoral photographs (T1); T1=treatment progress (1 month).

was then referred for postsurgical orthodontics. At that point, with the same archwires placed, she wore light posterior vertical elastics and bilateral II class elastics full time for three months. The postoperative stage was aimed at additional finalization; therefore, coordination of the maxillary and mandibular arches were followed by finishing and detailing of the occlusion

It was decided that the treatment goals were achieved, and active treatment could be completed. Approximately 30 months spread out over 62 appointments was the comprehensive active treatment time.

2.4. Summary

2.4.1. Treatment Results. On the day of debonding, extra- and intraoral photographs were taken along with impressions and occlusion wax to build the final plaster models. For the retention, it was decided to use a Hawley appliance for the upper teeth and a bonded retainer for the lower teeth.

Review of the treatment outcome with clinical examination, extra- and intraoral photographs (Figure 7), and the final plaster models showed the following outcomes:

(i) Mandibular symmetrization, improvement of smile arch aesthetic, reduction of buccal corridors, and an improved lower third projection

(ii) Correction of the dental Class II was achieved

(iii) Correction of arch shapes was observed

(iv) Significant reduction of the lip incompetence was obtained

(v) Mentalis habit was reduced

2.4.2. Follow-Up. Approximately 30 months after debonding, the shapes of the arches and occlusion appeared to be stable, even though a moderate amount of relapse occurred (Figure 8). Both cephalometric evaluations of the lateral radiograph of the skull (Figure 9(a); Table 1, T4) and the posteroanterior radiograph of the skull (Figure 9(b)) showed a nonsignificant difference compared to postsurgery assessment except for sagittal jaw relationship that exhibited a considerable relapse (Table 1, T2 and T4).

3. Discussion

In selected adult patients, the simultaneous osteodistraction of both the maxilla and mandible represent a viable option to obtain satisfactory and stable outcomes.

The basic requirements for an optimal result of osteodistraction are minimally traumatic osteotomies, stable mechanical fixation across osteotomies, an adequate latency period before lengthening (to establish repair processes), suitable rhythm and amplitude of lengthening, a realistic goal

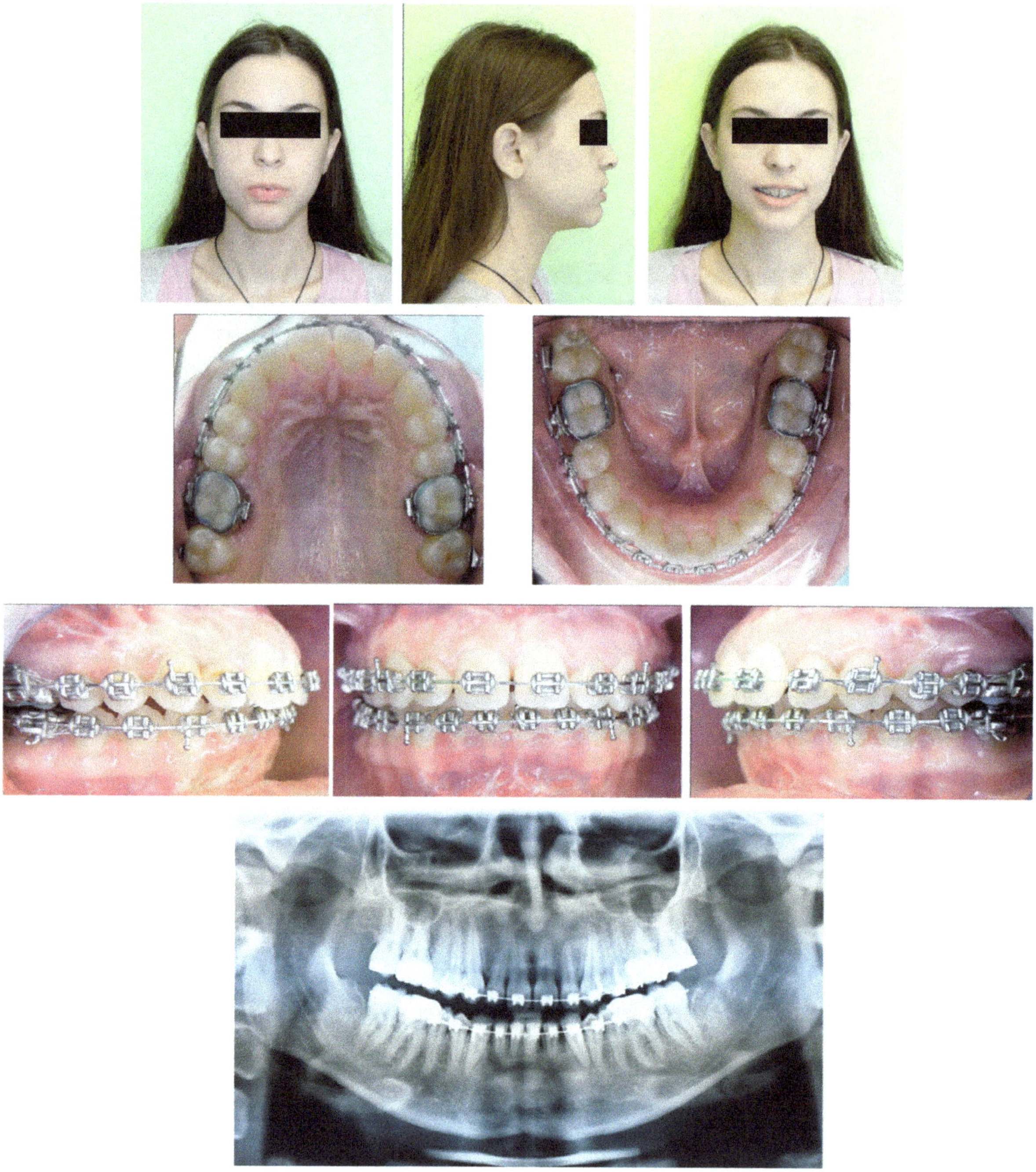

FIGURE 5: Extraoral photographs (T2), intraoral photographs (T2), and orthopantomogram (T2); T2=treatment progress (18 months).

regarding the extent of lengthening, and sufficient time for the callus to mature before frame or nail removal [20].

The use of proper appliances, careful surgery and follow-up, and cooperation between the surgical and orthodontic teams are the key to success in this demanding approach.

Discomfort, apical trauma, and local infections are the main disadvantages of TMD, as reported in the literature [4, 21].

Lip and cheek irritation, as well as speech and eating difficulties are commonly related to osteodistraction devices. Gingival recession, gingivitis, and irritation of the mucosa often represent soft tissue complications [22, 23].

Concerning the present case, several treatment alternatives were explored. Nevertheless, dental compensation could not be achieved because severe crowding in the lower arch cannot be properly fixed with Interproximal Enamel Reduction (IPR) and inclination of the mandibular incisors. As an alternative, the extraction of one mandibular central incisor could be considered.

Therefore, TMD was the best option for mandibular expansion and arch form improvement.

Concerning the upper arch, the severe inclination of the maxillary incisors reduces the chances to solve the crowding only with IPR.

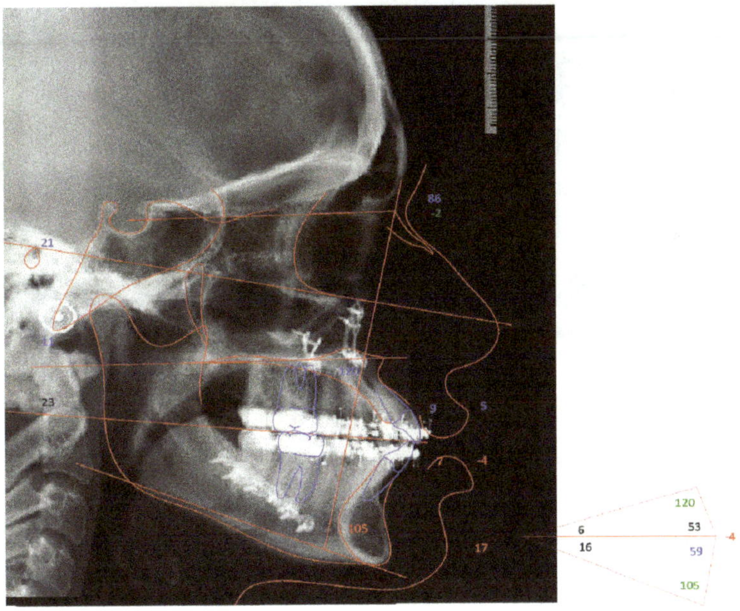

Figure 6: Cephalometric tracing (T2); T2=treatment progress (18 months).

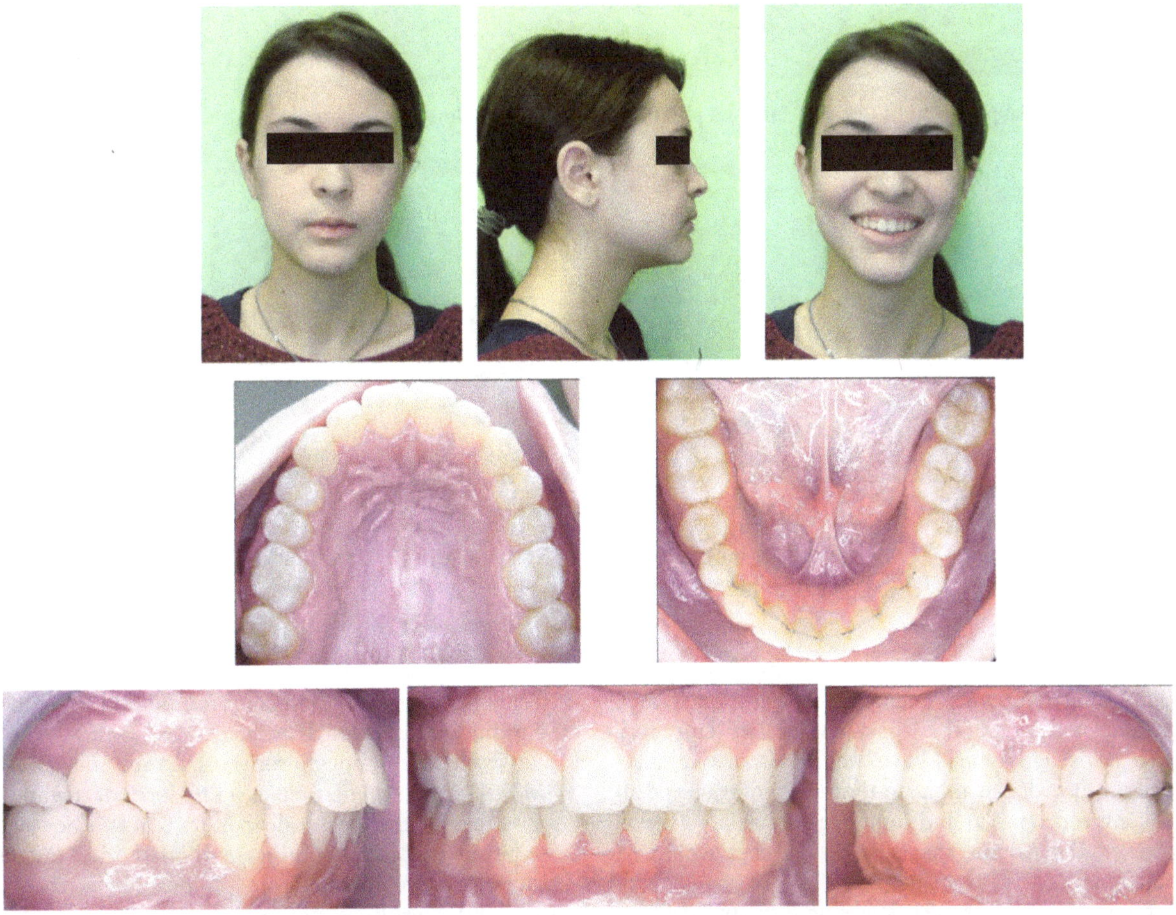

Figure 7: Extraoral photographs (T3) and intraoral photographs (T3); T3=posttreatment (36 months).

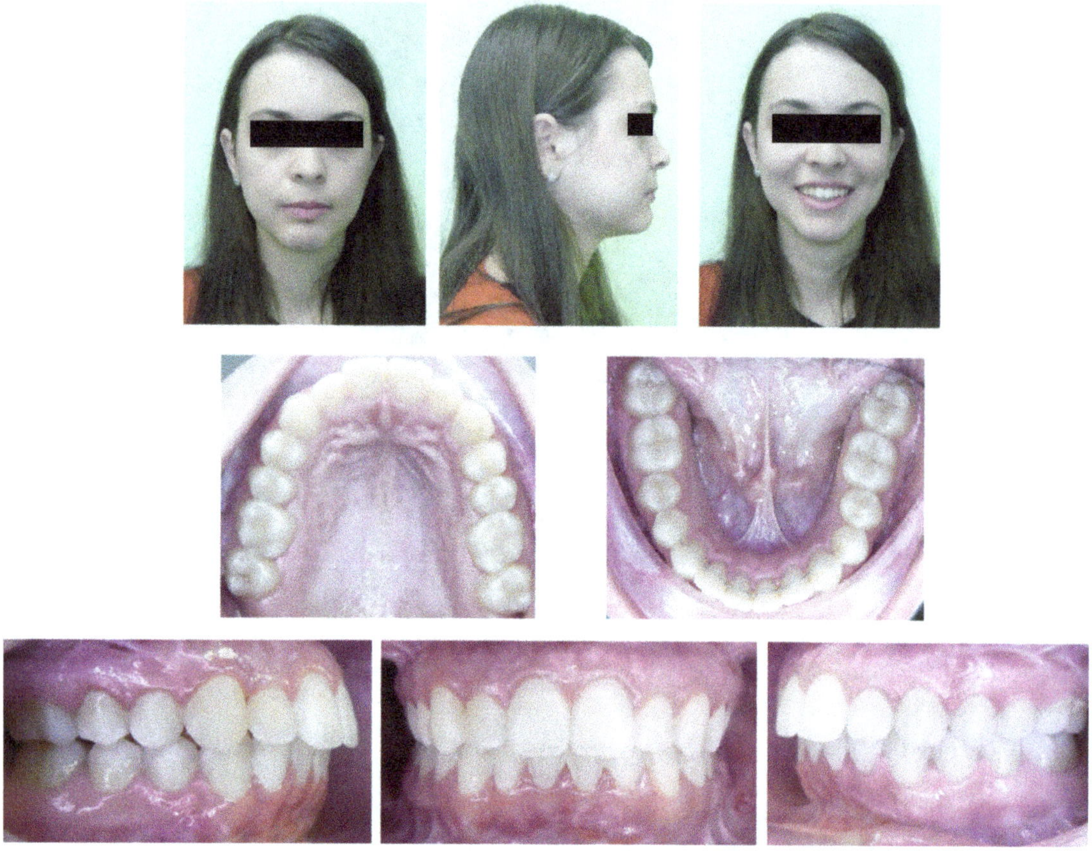

FIGURE 8: Extraoral photographs (T4) and intraoral photographs (T4); T4=follow-up (30 months after the end of the treatment).

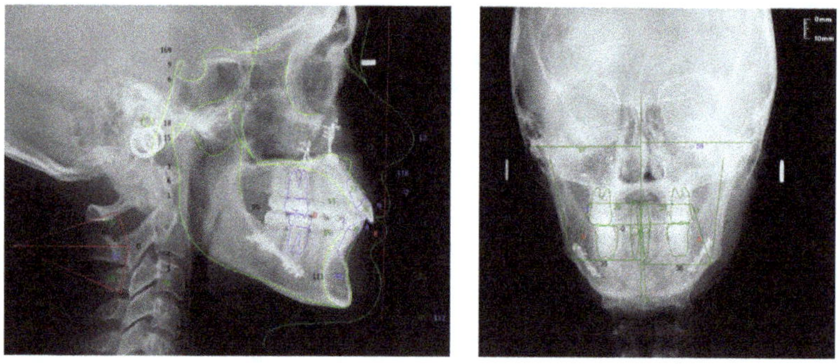

(a) (b)

FIGURE 9: Cephalometric tracing (T4): (a) cephalometric evaluation of the lateral radiograph of the skull and (b) cephalometric evaluation of the posteroanterior radiograph of the skull; T4=follow-up (30 months after the end of the treatment).

Anterior tooth retraction after molar distalization and retraction using temporary anchorage devices (such as a zygoma anchor device [24] or palatally located temporary anchorage device [25]) might have been an alternative treatment option in order to mitigate the severe overjet and to secure an enhanced molar and canine relationship.

However, the narrow shape of both arches would be left unaltered.

Therefore, SARPE was the best option for maxillary arch expansion and arch form improvement.

Extraction of two bicuspids in both arches was aimed at obtaining sufficient space to correct the severe crowding and to increase OVJ properly; this treatment option was rejected because this would compromise both the occlusion, the profile, and the dental aesthetics.

Overall, even though some care must be considered, MMTOD can be recognized as a safe form of treatment.

As regards the type of distractors that can be used, they can be divided into tooth-borne, bone-borne, and hybrid devices, mainly differing from the position of the fixation points and the stiffness of the appliance.

Tooth-borne devices induce less parallel expansion than bone-borne distractors because they apply their vector above the center of resistance: this difference implies an increase of anterior mandible widening when using the tooth-borne devices as compared when using the bone-borne and hybrid distractors.

The parallel expansion of the hemimandibles [26] leads to bone regeneration both at the basal and alveolar level, and it is crucial to reduce relapse.

Ideally, a basal bone widening would decrease the long-term relapse [27, 28].

The rigidity of a distractor defines the parallel movement of segments and the quantity of micromotion between segments.

The choice of bone-borne appliances is preferable because of a biomechanical advantage (vector applied close to the center of resistance) and a clinical advantage (smaller loss of anchorage and less skeletal relapse both during and after expansion and lower incidences of cortical fenestration and buccal root compared to tooth-borne distractors [29]; reduced risk of craniomandibular disorders minimizing lateral displacement of the condyle [30]).

In this case, the enlargement of the transversal diameter was obtained from the canines to the first and second premolars leading to a "fan-shaped" maxilla.

The symphyseal osteodistraction demonstrated parallel movements along the lower jaw, leading to a "square-shaped" mandible.

The slight bimaxillary advancement was deemed necessary to achieve completely the aesthetic goals of the treatment completely, with operational control of facial height and projection.

We decided to increase the facial projections with a slight undercorrection of the facial height in order to leave the patient's face slightly long from a qualitative standpoint, with the elimination of the lip strain and an attractive smile with the elimination of buccal corridors because of the previous maxillomandibular transversal expansion.

The Hawley retainer for the upper arch was selected to promote postorthodontic settling of the posterior occlusion of the patient [31]; this is a bonded retainer for the lower arch because of the slightly better stability over removable retainers and more acceptability to wear. A multistranded stainless steel wire was preferred over a fiber-reinforced composite retainer because of the absence of aesthetic concerns or allergy to metals [32].

The follow-up showed satisfactory long-term stability even though significant skeletal relapse was reported in the literature [33].

4. Conclusions

The Maxillomandibular Transverse Osteodistraction technique associated with orthognathic surgery described here could obtain both functional and aesthetic results in patients with reduced maxillary and mandibular transverse dimensions and severe dental crowding.

Abbreviations

MSDO: Mandibular symphyseal distraction osteogenesis
MMD: Mandibular midline (osteo-) distraction
TMSD: Transmandibular symphyseal (osteo-) distraction
SARPE: Surgically assisted rapid palatal expansion
SARME: Surgically assisted rapid maxillary expansion
MMTOD: Maxillomandibular transverse osteodistraction
CCE: Common childhood exanthemas
TMJ: Temporomandibular joint
OVJ: Overjet
OVB: Overbite
TPD: Transpalatal distractor
TMD: Transmandibular distractor
BSSO: Bilateral sagittal split osteotomy
IPR: Interproximal enamel reduction.

Authors' Contributions

Turatti G. and Bruni A. equally contributed to this work.

References

[1] P. Gandini, A. Schiavi, D. Camassa, and M. Manuelli, "Statistical survey of malocclusion in school age children," *Mondo Ortodontico*, vol. 14, no. 1, pp. 73–78, 1989.

[2] M. Bayram, M. Ozer, S. Arici, and A. Alkan, "Nonextraction treatment with rapid maxillary expansion and mandibular symphyseal distraction osteogenesis and vertical skeletal dimensions," *The Angle Orthodontist*, vol. 77, no. 2, pp. 266–272, 2007.

[3] S. Malkoç, S. Üşümez, and H. J. A. J. Işeri, "Long-term effects of symphyseal distraction and rapid maxillary expansion on pharyngeal airway dimensions, tongue, and hyoid position," *American Journal of Orthodontics and Dentofacial Orthopedics*, vol. 132, no. 6, pp. 769–775, 2007.

[4] M. Y. Mommaerts, Y. J. E. Spaey, P. E. G. S. Correia, and G. R. J. Swennen, "Morbidity related to transmandibular distraction osteogenesis for patients with developmental deformities," *Journal of Cranio-Maxillofacial Surgery*, vol. 36, no. 4, pp. 192–197, 2008.

[5] C. Burstone, "Precision lingual arches. Active applications," *Journal of Clinical Orthodontics*, vol. 23, no. 2, pp. 101–109, 1989.

[6] P. D. McDougall, J. A. McNamara, and J. M. Dierkes, "Arch width development in Class II patients treated with the Frankel appliance," *American Journal of Orthodontics*, vol. 82, no. 1, pp. 10–22, 1982.

[7] M. Weinberg and C. Sadowsky, "Resolution of mandibular arch crowding in growing patients with Class I malocclusions treated nonextraction," *American Journal of Orthodontics and Dentofacial Orthopedics*, vol. 110, no. 4, pp. 359–364, 1996.

[8] L. Pascon, C. Bazert, and E. Bardinet, "Contribution of mandibular symphyseal distraction osteogenesis to our therapeutic strategies," *Journal of Dentofacial Anomalies and Orthodontics*, vol. 19, no. 3, p. 305, 2016.

[9] G. J. C. D. H. Sperber, *Facial Skeleton*, BC Decker Inc., Ontario, Canada, 2001.

[10] J. W. King, J. C. Wallace, D. L. Winter, and J. A. Niculescu, "Long-term skeletal and dental stability of mandibular symphyseal distraction osteogenesis with a hybrid distractor,"

American Journal of Orthodontics and Dentofacial Orthopedics, vol. 141, no. 1, pp. 60–70, 2012.

[11] C. Guerrero, W. Bell, G. Contasti, and A. Rodriguez, "Mandibular widening by intraoral distraction osteogenesis," *British Journal of Oral and Maxillofacial Surgery*, vol. 35, no. 6, pp. 383–392, 1997.

[12] A. Haas, "Long-term posttreatment evaluation of rapid palatal expansion," *The Angle Orthodontist*, vol. 50, no. 3, pp. 189–217, 1980.

[13] G. Brown, *The Surgery of Oral and Facial Diseases and Malformations*, Kimpton, London, 1938.

[14] N. J. Betts, R. L. Vanarsdall, H. D. Barber, K. Higgins-Barber, and R. J. Fonseca, "Diagnosis and treatment of transverse maxillary deficiency," *The International Journal of Adult Orthodontics and Orthognathic Surgery*, vol. 10, pp. 75–96, 1995.

[15] L. Suri and P. Taneja, "Surgically assisted rapid palatal expansion: a literature review," *American Journal of Orthodontics and Dentofacial Orthopedics*, vol. 133, no. 2, pp. 290–302, 2008.

[16] J. W. King and J. C. Wallace, "Unilateral Brodie bite treated with distraction osteogenesis," *American Journal of Orthodontics and Dentofacial Orthopedics*, vol. 125, no. 4, pp. 500–509, 2004.

[17] W. R. Proffit, R. P. White, and D. M. Sarver, *Contemporary Treatment of Dentofacial Deformity*, Mosby, 2003.

[18] F. A. Bianchi, G. Gerbino, M. Corsico et al., "Soft, hard-tissues and pharyngeal airway volume changes following maxillo-mandibular transverse osteodistraction: computed tomography and three-dimensional laser scanner evaluation," *Journal of Cranio-Maxillofacial Surgery*, vol. 45, no. 1, pp. 47–55, 2017.

[19] G. A. Ramieri, M. C. Spada, M. Austa, S. D. Bianchi, and S. Berrone, "Transverse maxillary distraction with a bone-anchored appliance: dento- periodontal effects and clinical and radiological results," *International Journal of Oral and Maxillofacial Surgery*, vol. 34, no. 4, pp. 357–363, 2005.

[20] Z. S. AI-Aql, A. S. Alagl, D. T. Graves, L. C. Gerstenfeld, and T. A. Einhorn, "Molecular mechanisms controlling bone formation during fracture healing and distraction osteogenesis," *Journal of Dental Research*, vol. 87, pp. 107–118, 2008.

[21] J. von Bremen, D. Schäfer, W. Kater, and S. Ruf, "Complications during mandibular midline Distraction," *The Angle Orthodontist*, vol. 78, no. 1, pp. 20–24, 2008.

[22] A. Alkan, M. Özer, B. Baş et al., "Mandibular symphyseal distraction osteogenesis: review of three techniques," *International Journal of Oral and Maxillofacial Surgery*, vol. 36, no. 2, pp. 111–117, 2007.

[23] T. Gunbay, M. C. Akay, A. Aras, and M. Gomel, "Effects of transmandibular symphyseal distraction on teeth, bone, and temporomandibular joint," *Journal of Oral and Maxillofacial Surgery*, vol. 67, no. 10, pp. 2254–2265, 2009.

[24] M. A. Cornelis and H. J. de Clerck, "Maxillary molar distalization with miniplates assessed on digital models: a prospective clinical trial," *American Journal of Orthodontics and Dentofacial Orthopedics*, vol. 132, no. 3, pp. 373–377, 2007.

[25] M. Nienkemper, B. Wilmes, A. Pauls, S. Yamaguchi, B. Ludwig, and D. Drescher, "Treatment efficiency of mini-implant-borne distalization depending on age and second-molar eruption," *Journal of Orofacial Orthopedics / Fortschritte der Kieferorthopädie*, vol. 75, pp. 118–132, 2014.

[26] G. Raoul, T. Wojcik, and J. Ferri, "Outcome of mandibular symphyseal distraction osteogenesis with bone-borne devices," *Journal of Craniofacial Surgery*, vol. 20, no. 2, pp. 488–493, 2009.

[27] R. Conley and H. Legan, "Mandibular symphyseal distraction osteogenesis: diagnosis and treatment planning considerations," *The Angle Orthodontist*, vol. 73, pp. 3–11, 2003.

[28] M. Del Santo, C. A. Guerrero, P. H. Buschang, J. D. English, M. L. Samchukov, and W. H. Bell, "Long-term skeletal and dental effects of mandibular symphyseal distraction osteogenesis," *American Journal of Orthodontics and Dentofacial Orthopedics*, vol. 118, no. 5, pp. 485–493, 2000.

[29] M. Mommaerts, "Transpalatal distraction as a method of maxillary expansion," *British Journal of Oral and Maxillofacial Surgery*, vol. 37, no. 4, pp. 268–272, 1999.

[30] M. Y. Mommaerts, R. Polsbroek, G. Santler, P. E. G. S. Correia, J. V. S. Abeloos, and N. Ali, "Anterior transmandibular osteodistraction: clinical and model observations," *Journal of Cranio-Maxillofacial Surgery*, vol. 33, no. 5, pp. 318–325, 2005.

[31] E. M. Bauer, R. Behrents, D. R. Oliver, and P. H. Buschang, "Posterior occlusion changes with a Hawley vs Perfector and Hawley retainer: a follow-up study," *The Angle Orthodontist*, vol. 80, no. 5, pp. 853–860, 2010.

[32] A. Lucchese, M. Manuelli, L. Bassani et al., "Fiber reinforced composites orthodontic retainers," *Minerva Stomatologica*, vol. 64, no. 6, pp. 323–333, 2015.

[33] G. Rossini, B. Vinci, R. Rizzo, T. M. D. Pinho, and A. Deregibus, "Mandibular distraction osteogenesis: a systematic review of stability and the effects on hard and soft tissues," *International Journal of Oral and Maxillofacial Surgery*, vol. 45, no. 11, pp. 1438–1444, 2016.

14

Intranasal Ectopic Tooth in Adult and Pediatric Patients: A Report of Two Cases

Isabela Polesi Bergamaschi,[1] Bernardo Olsson,[1] Aline Monise Sebastiani,[1,2,3] Guilherme dos Santos Trento,[2] Nelson Luis Barbosa Rebellato,[1] Leandro Eduardo Klüppel,[1,2] Delson Joao da Costa,[1] and Rafaela Scariot[1,2,3]

[1]*Department of Stomatology, Department of Oral and Maxillofacial Surgery, Federal University of Paraná, Curitiba, Brazil*
[2]*Cleft Lip and Palate Integral Care Center, Trabalhador Hospital, Curitiba, Brazil*
[3]*School of Health Sciences, Department of Oral and Maxillofacial Surgery, Positivo University, Curitiba, Brazil*

Correspondence should be addressed to Rafaela Scariot; rafaela_scariot@yahoo.com.br

Academic Editor: Eleftherios Xenos

The aim of this study was to report two rare cases of ectopic tooth into the nasal cavity. The first case reports a 32-year-old female patient with the main complaint of having a tooth inside her nose. According to her, this condition causes pain and sporadic nosebleed. The patient had a facial trauma when she was 6 years old. The second case refers to an 8-year-old girl with left incomplete unilateral cleft lip and palate. The main complaint was left-sided nasal obstruction by a white hard mass. The treatment for both cases was surgical removal of the ectopic erupted tooth under general anesthesia. In conclusion, we can state that the surgical removal of intranasal tooth is a safe procedure and improves patient's quality of life.

1. Introduction

An aberrant tooth can be found in sites outside of the oral cavity and can be a supernumerary, deciduous, or permanent tooth [1]. The maxillary sinus and palate are the most frequently affected sites, while the mandibular condyle, coronoid process, orbits, and facial skin are affected much more rarely [1, 2]. The presence of supernumerary or ectopic teeth is not an uncommon fact, which occurs in 1% of the general population. However, the presence of teeth in the nasal cavity is a rare phenomenon, regardless of etiology [3]. The presence of teeth in the nasal cavity in cleft individuals is a rare phenomenon and obscure etiology and occurs in 0.1-1% of the general population [4]. Medeiros et al. found a prevalence of 0.48% intranasal teeth in children with complete cleft lip and palate [5].

The exact etiology of eruption of a tooth into the nasal cavity remains obscure. A few theories have been proposed to explain it, including the theory of developmental origin, which states that ectopic eruption may occur either due to reversion to the dentition of extinct primates having three pairs of incisor teeth, defect in migration of neural crest derivatives destined to reach the jaw bones, or due to a flaw in the multistep epithelial-mesenchymal interaction [6]. Other causes include developmental disturbances such as cleft lip and palate, trauma, or cystic lesions leading to tooth displacement, genetic factors, persistent deciduous teeth, and supernumerary teeth [7].

The purpose of this paper is to report two rare cases of ectopic tooth into the nasal cavity, with different etiologies, one caused by childhood trauma, while the other is associated with cleft lip and palate.

2. Case Report 1

A 32-year-old female patient, presenting normal facial growth, was referred to the Oral and Maxillofacial Surgery Service at Federal University of Paraná, Curitiba/PR, with the main complaint of having a tooth inside her nose. She reported this condition causes pain and sporadic nosebleed,

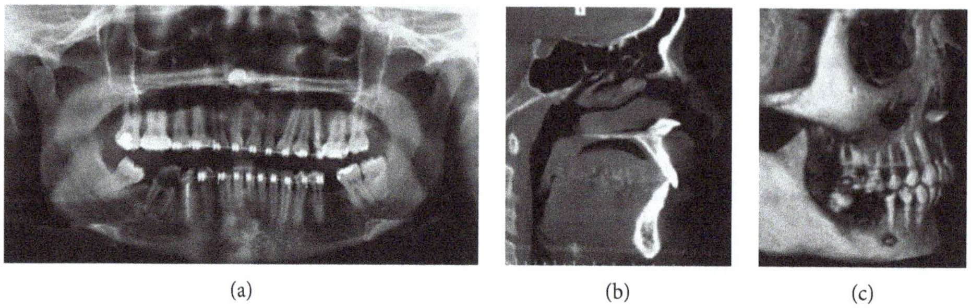

Figure 1: (a) Panoramic radiograph shows an ectopic tooth in the nasal cavity. (b) Sagittal cut of CT scan showing the horizontal orientation of the right superior incisor tooth inside the nasal nostril. (c) 3D reconstruction of CT scan showing the ectopic position of element 11.

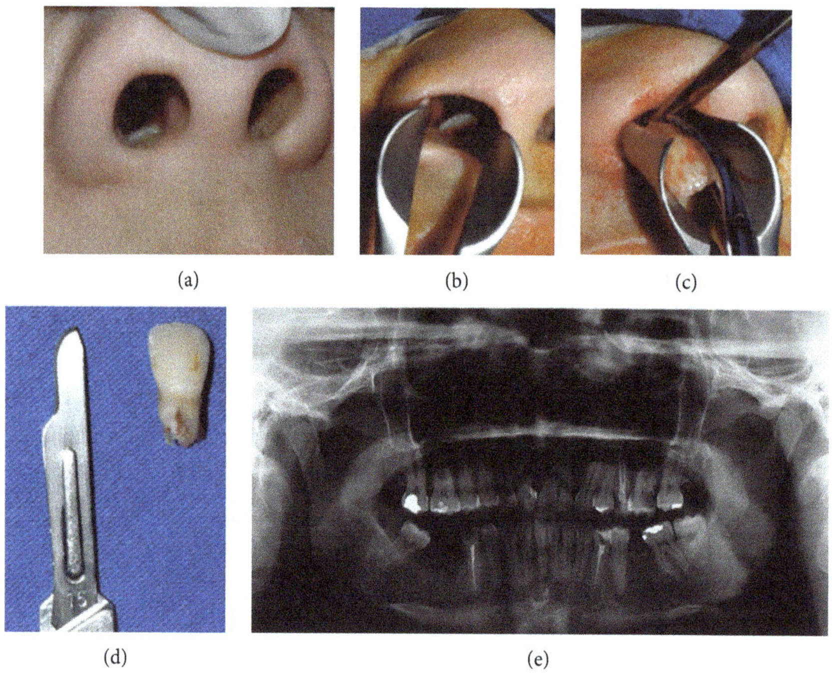

Figure 2: (a) Preoperative picture showing the exposition of the ectopic tooth inside the right nostril. (b, c) With the aid of nasal speculum, the tooth was removed by intranasal approach. (d) Tooth removed. (e) Panoramic radiograph confirms the complete removal of the element 11.

especially on cold days. Patient's clinical history revealed that she had a facial trauma when she was six years old, affecting her superior anterior teeth, which was the etiological factor of the ectopic position of the tooth.

She had no history of systemic diseases or previous surgical procedures, although she was allergic to cephalexin. On clinical examination, raising the nasal tip, it was possible to observe the crown of the maxillary central incisor inside the right nostril.

The patient was submitted to a panoramic radiography, which showed the presence of a radiopaque mass similar to an incisor tooth on the right nasal cavity. For detailed radiographic examination, a computed tomography (CT) was requested and a high-density area was found located in a nasal nostril, horizontally arranged, incomplete rhizogenesis, with the crown facing to the exit of the nasal cavity (Figure 1).

The surgical removal of the ectopic tooth was performed under general anesthesia, mainly because of the potential transoperative bleeding. After infiltration of local anesthesia with a vasoconstrictor, the tooth was removed using an intranasal approach with the aid of nasal speculum. Succeeding the extraction, nasal packing was placed to prevent postoperative epistaxis, which was removed 12 hours later, with no complications (Figure 2).

One-year follow-up shows resolution of the patient's main complaint, who reports a better breathing, no more nosebleed, or bad smells.

3. Case Report 2

An 8-year-old girl with left incomplete unilateral cleft lip and palate was referred to the Cleft Lip and Palate Integral Care Center (CAIF) with left-sided nasal obstruction due to an intranasal hard white mass surrounded by granulation tissue. The patient had no pain or any other complaints regarding the white mass, but because it was hypothesized to be an

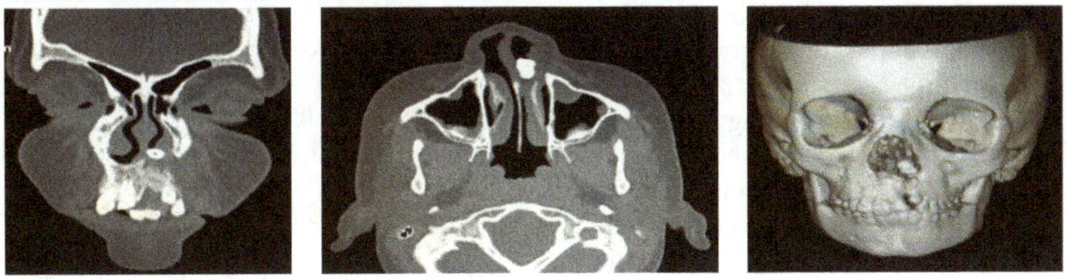

(a) (b) (c)

FIGURE 3: (a, b) CT scan showing intranasal location and soft tissue surrounding the dysmorphic tooth. (c) 3D reconstruction of CT scan showing the ectopic position of element 21.

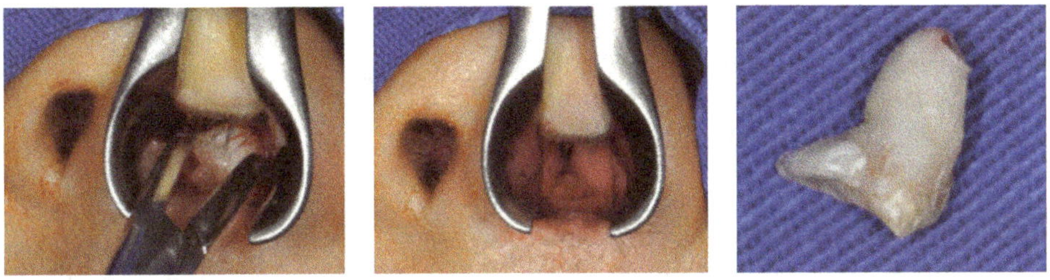

(a) (b) (c)

FIGURE 4: (a) Nasal speculum provided direct access to the toothlike structure removal with a Kelly hemostatic forceps. (b) Hemostasis obtained after the toothlike structure has been removed. No stiches were needed. (c) Ectopic tooth removed.

ectopic eruption of a dysmorphic lateral incisor with no possibility of orthodontic traction, the patient was advised to surgically remove the dysmorphic tooth. Intraoral examination and CT scan assured the hypothesis of ectopic eruption since the left lateral incisor was missing and the radiopacity of the mass matched the radiopacity of other teeth. The patient's surgical history was cheiloplasty at 4 months old, palatoplasty at 1 year old, microotological surgery and tonsillectomy at 5 years old, septoplasty at 6 years old, adenoidectomy at 7 years old, and alveoloplasty and autogenous iliac crest bone craft for oronasal fistula repair at 8 years old. No comorbidities were elicited.

CT scan revealed a radiopaque mass situated in the middle of the palatal cleft towards the left nasal cavity. Despite the superior portion, the dysmorphic lateral incisor was inserted in soft tissue (Figure 3). The tooth removal surgery was under general anesthesia because the patient was not cooperative.

Because the dysmorphic tooth had no bone insertion and could be accessed using a nasal speculum, Kelly hemostatic forceps were chosen to remove the tooth (Figure 4). Hemostasis was obtained only by gauze pressure for a few seconds; no stiches were needed. Findings by nude eye examination confirmed a 10 millimeter wide toothlike structure (Figure 4). On two weeks of follow-up and postsurgery CT scan examination, the patient still had no complaints and the left airway was normal compared to the opposite side, respectively. One year follow-up and the patient still has no complaint.

4. Discussion

Intranasal tooth represents a small portion of all reported cases of ectopic eruption in the literature. Although the occurrence of supernumerary teeth is rare, up to 1% [4], it overcomes the prevalence of deciduous and permanent teeth found in the nasal cavity [2, 8]. In this report, we show two rare cases of permanent teeth found intranasally, one in a 32-year-old woman and the other in an 8-year-old girl. The age range reported for detecting the nasal tooth is broad, from 3 to 62 years [7, 9]. This range is broad due to different conditions that lead the patient to seek treatment [1]. The two cases in this report are examples of conditions: early detection happened because the patient was under treatment for cleft lip and palate, whereas late detection, at 32 years, happened due to professional misinformation provided to the patient, leading her to treat only the symptoms, not the cause of pain and nasal bleeding.

Both cases agree with previous reports regarding no predisposition for left or right nostril [7], no occurrence in both nostrils [2], and symptoms such as nasal obstruction and epistaxis [2, 8]. The lack in pattern for left or right nostril could be explained by the possible etiology of the ectopic eruption: obstruction by the time of eruption caused by persistent deciduous teeth; no space in the arc; intrusive luxation; facial deformities, such as cleft palate; cysts; and genetic predisposition [5]. Despite crowded dentition, trauma (i.e., intrusive luxation) [10], and facial deformities (i.e., cleft palate [5, 11]), the other possible etiologies do not have a predilection for left, right, or anterior region.

The 32-year-old woman reported a traumatic injury involving her teeth when she was 6 years old, age when the front incisor are in eruption route [6] and Nolla stage 7 (complete crown and 1/3 of the root's development) [12]. On the other hand, the 8-year-old girl's mother said that the white mass appeared after 3 months her daughter had been through iliac crest bone craft for oronasal fistula repair. Although both conditions are different, both are capable of causing tooth displacement [6, 13]. Since cleft palate has a multifactorial etiology, including environmental and genetic factors [11], genetic predisposition as an etiology for the ectopic eruption of the dysmorphic tooth in the case 2 cannot be neglected. We did not have access to previous CT scans or other radiographic images to determine whether or not trauma and maxilla crafting were the main causes of tooth ectopic eruption. Despite the lack of previous CT scans or other radiographic images, the patients' age suggests that Nolla stage in both of them could be classified as 7 or 8 [12], which could be a facilitating factor for the tooth displacement.

To accomplish a precise diagnosis in both cases, CT scans were requested for both patients in order to make a differential diagnosis between tooth in the nasal cavity, benign tumors, rhinolith [4, 6, 9, 14], and calcified inflammatory lesions due to tuberculosis and syphilis [9]. These hypotheses were negated by matching clinical and tomographic findings [2]. Another hypothesis that could be taken into consideration is an ectopic eruption of a supernumerary tooth [1]. Theories have been developed to explain the formation of a supernumerary tooth [1], including theories involving single nucleotide polymorphisms [15] and dental lamina hyperactivity [1, 16]. Clinically, both patients had missing permanent tooth. Tomographic examination showed matching radiopacity between normal teeth and the investigated teeth [2, 14]. Although histological examination has been performed by other authors to confirm the diagnosis of a tooth in the nasal cavity [6], the authors did not find it relevant as a method for differential diagnosis since both patients had a history of a missing permanent tooth in the oral cavity related to trauma or tissue manipulation in the area.

To solve symptoms and prevent further complications, surgically removing the tooth has been proposed as treatment [2, 6, 9, 14]. When the tooth is not inserted in the bone, the procedure becomes simple, but it still has important possible major complications, such as infection [17] and hemorrhage [18], that indicate general anesthesia as a safer protocol to be followed [17, 18].

Finally, intranasal ectopic tooth is somehow rare but is potentially harmful when left untreated; thus, surgically removing the intranasal ectopic tooth is important to improve patient's quality of life. Furthermore, the diagnosis is simple, fast, and cheap.

Acknowledgments

The authors thank Coordenação de Aperfeiçoamento de Pessoal de Nível Superior–Brazil (CAPES; No. 001) for its partial financial support.

References

[1] L. D. Rajab and M. A. Hamdan, "Supernumerary teeth: review of the literature and a survey of 152 cases," *International Journal of Paediatric Dentistry.*, vol. 12, no. 4, pp. 244–254, 2002.

[2] I. H. Lin, C. F. Hwang, C. Y. Su, Y. F. Kao, and J. P. Peng, "Intranasal tooth: report of three cases," *Chang Gung medical journal.*, vol. 27, no. 5, pp. 385–389, 2004.

[3] O. HFd, M. B. Vieira, W. M. S. Buhaten, C. A. Neves, G. P. Seronni, and M. O. Dossi, "Tooth in nasal cavity of non-traumatic etiology: uncommon affection," *International Archives of Otorhinolaryngology*, vol. 13, no. 2, pp. 201–203, 2009.

[4] R. A. Smith, N. C. Gordon, and S. F. De Luchi, "Intranasal Teeth: Report of two cases and review of the literature," *Oral Surgery, Oral Medicine, and Oral Pathology*, vol. 47, no. 2, pp. 120–122, 1979.

[5] A. S. Medeiros, M. R. Gomide, B. Costa, C. F. Carrara, and L. T. das Neves, "Prevalence of intranasal ectopic teeth in children with complete unilateral and bilateral cleft lip and palate," *The Cleft Palate-Craniofacial Journal*, vol. 37, no. 3, pp. 271–273, 2000.

[6] M. Agrawal, T. S. Khan, T. Gupta, and S. Khanna, "Intranasal tooth: ectopic eruption 1 year after maxillofacial trauma," *BMJ Case Reports.*, vol. 2014, no. aug06 1, article bcr2014204432, 2014.

[7] Y. K. Gupta and N. Shah, "Intranasal tooth as a complication of cleft lip and alveolus in a four year old child: case report and literature review," *International Journal of Paediatric Dentistry.*, vol. 11, no. 3, pp. 221–224, 2001.

[8] C. Yu, D. Gu, J. An, and Y. Tang, "Case presentation of an intranasal ectopic tooth in a pediatric patient," *American Journal of Otolaryngology*, vol. 36, no. 3, pp. 472–474, 2015.

[9] A. Chen, J. K. Huang, S. J. Cheng, and C. Y. Sheu, "Nasal teeth: report of three cases," *AJNR American Journal of Neuroradiology.*, vol. 23, no. 4, pp. 671–673, 2002.

[10] B. R. Chrcanovic, S. C. Bueno, D. T. da Silveira, and A. L. N. Custodio, "Traumatic displacement of maxillary permanent incisor into the nasal cavity," *Oral and Maxillofacial Surgery.*, vol. 14, no. 3, pp. 175–182, 2010.

[11] C. L. Antunes, A. M. Aranha, M. C. Bandeca, C. R. de Musis, A. H. Borges, and E. M. Vieira, "Eruption of impacted teeth after alveolar bone graft in cleft lip and palate region," *The Journal of Contemporary Dental Practice.*, vol. 19, no. 8, pp. 933–936, 2018.

[12] H. M. Park, D. H. Han, and S. H. Baek, "Comparison of tooth development stage of the maxillary anterior teeth before and after secondary alveolar bone graft: unilateral cleft lip and alveolus vs unilateral cleft lip and palate," *The Angle orthodontist.*, vol. 84, no. 6, pp. 989–994, 2014.

[13] E. H. Moreano, D. K. Zich, H. C. Goree, and S. M. Graham, "Nasal tooth," *American Journal of Otolaryngology*, vol. 19, no. 2, pp. 124–126, 1998.

[14] F. P. Lee, "Endoscopic extraction of an intranasal tooth: a review of 13 cases," *The Laryngoscope.*, vol. 111, no. 6, pp. 1027–1031, 2001.

[15] S. Kan, G. Zhu, Y. du et al., "Non-syndromic cleft lip with or without palate-susceptible SNPs is associated with hyperdontia," *Oral diseases*, 2019.

[16] J. Liu, "Characteristics of premaxillary supernumerary teeth: a survey of 112 cases," *ASDC Journal of Dentistry for Children.*, vol. 62, no. 4, pp. 262–265, 1995.

[17] S. Ogane, A. Watanabe, N. Takano, and T. Shibahara, "Case of inverted supernumerary tooth in nasal cavity," *The Bulletin of Tokyo Dental College.*, vol. 58, no. 4, pp. 255–258, 2017.

[18] B. Ray, L. K. Singh, C. J. Das, and T. S. Roy, "Ectopic supernumerary tooth on the inferior nasal concha," *Clinical Anatomy*, vol. 19, no. 1, pp. 68–74, 2005.

15

Total Mandibular Subapical Alveolar Osteotomy to Correct Class II Division I Dentofacial Deformity

Rafael Correia Cavalcante,[1] Isabela Polesi Bergamaschi,[1] Aline Monise Sebastiani,[2] Fabiano Galina,[1] Marina Fanderuff,[1] Delson João da Costa,[1] Nelson Luis Barbosa Rebellato,[1] Rafaela Scariot,[1,2] and Leandro Eduardo Klüppel[1]

[1]*Oral and Maxillofacial Surgery Department, Federal University of Parana, Curitiba, Brazil*
[2]*School of Health Science, Positivo University, Curitiba, Brazil*

Correspondence should be addressed to Rafaela Scariot; rafaela_scariot@yahoo.com.br

Academic Editor: Mario Ganau

Introduction. Class II division I malocclusions are the most common dentofacial deformities seen in clinical practice. Severe cases or cases in which growth has ceased may require full correction combining orthodontic and surgical treatment. We report a case of a total mandibular subapical alveolar osteotomy, performed to correct a class II division I dentofacial deformity. *Case Report.* A 19-year-old female patient was referred to the oral and maxillofacial surgery department at the Federal University of Paraná with chin aesthetic complaints as well as class II malocclusion. The proposed treatment was total mandibular subapical alveolar osteotomy, retaining the chin position and eliminating the need for genioplasty, since, although the patient presented with a class II dentofacial deformity, the chin was well positioned. Under general anesthesia, a "V-shaped" incision was conducted from the right retromolar region to the left retromolar region. A ring of cortical bone was removed around the mental foramen, with the aim to create a space around the mental nerve. Fixation was conducted with plates and screws of the 2.0 system. The patient on six-year follow-up showed osteotomy stability, a better overall occlusion, and outcome satisfaction.

1. Introduction

Class II division I malocclusions are the most common dentofacial deformities seen in clinical practice and are reported to occur in 13% of the population. Combined orthodontic and surgical treatment in cases of severe class II dentofacial deformities is a routine procedure in these orthodontic patients. Mild to moderate class II dentofacial deformities in young patients (whose growth has not ceased) can only be managed with orthodontic treatment [1]. Moderate or severe mandibular retrusion cases, however, are commonly treated with bilateral mandibular ramus sagittal split osteotomy (BSSO). Depending on the nature of the problem and its severity, surgical correction of class II division I malocclusion can involve one or both jaws [2, 3].

The specific mandibular osteotomy technique to correct this type of deformity was first described by Hofer in 1942 [4]; however, surgery was limited to the anterior mandibular region alone. Hofer's original technique was modified and popularized by Kole only in 1959 [3]. The total mandibular subapical alveolar osteotomy (TMAO) was developed by MacIntosh in 1974 [4], mainly for the correction of anterior open bite. Dietz et al. [5] and Murray [6] reported further modifications to the total mandibular osteotomy technique, which included a horizontal and medial ramus cut above the lingula. The main indications of TMAO are as follows: class II division I incisor relationship, particularly in cases where the chin is well positioned at the beginning of the treatment [1, 7], pogonion kept in the same position to increase the lower facial height [8]; class II division II low-angle malocclusion uncorrected by orthodontic treatment alone, especially in patients that need advancement but have an excessive mental projection [9]; mandibular vertical alveolar deficiency; anterior open bite; mandibular ramus sagittal split osteotomy relapse; cases of condylar agenesis and hypoplasia; lateral open bite [4, 10]; and in cases that need a profound change in the mentolabial sulcus [1, 11].

Pangrazio-Kulbersh et al. [11] compared the stability between the total mandibular subapical osteotomy and bilateral sagittal split ramus osteotomy (BSSO) for correction of class II subjects. Stability yielded long-term results with both techniques. Mandibular advancement with the use of BSSO associated with rigid fixation has been shown to improve stability by resisting slippage at the osteotomy site because of the stretch of the paramandibular connective tissues, suggesting high stability. A reduction in relapse is also observed with TMAO because the suprahyoid muscles are not disturbed during the alveolar segment advancement. The authors suggest, however, that total TMAO is the procedure of choice in those cases where a profound change in labiomental sulcus is needed. Changes in the profile that resulted from TMAO appear to be more satisfactory than those which resulted from BSSO associated with genioplasty. A reduction of chin could yield a squarer mandible in patients who are already brachycephalic with increased bigonial width. The other advantage is the possibility of anterior, vertical, and posterior repositioning of the mobilized mandibular alveolar segment [12]. TMAO is a meticulous procedure that requires time and care with mental nerves. In addition to the risk of paresthesia, it has a risk of loss of pulp vitality and one or more teeth or even the entire dentoalveolar segment [4]. According to Scheideman et al. [13], Zisser and Gattinger [14], and Allen et al. [15], TMAO has no long-term deleterious effects on pulp vitality nor the alveolar segment.

The mandibular technique more commonly used to correct mandibular deficiencies is BSSO because it is a versatile and easy technique. However, other surgical techniques must be considered under certain conditions and in specific clinical cases. Although TMAO is an alternative for correction of mandibular deficiency, only a few cases have been reported in literature. The aim of the present study is to report a case of class II division I dentofacial deformity with good projection of chin, corrected through total subapical mandibular osteotomy.

2. Case Report

A 19-year-old, white female patient was referred to the oral and maxillofacial surgery department at the Federal University of Paraná as she complained regarding her aesthetics and malocclusion. Facial analysis showed a well-positioned maxilla despite a hypodivergent face pattern, with a reduction of tooth exposure upon smiling, and favorable chin projection associated with accentuated and deep labiomental fold due to retrusion of the inferior alveolar segment (Figures 1 and 2). There was also a shortening of the lower third of the face. There was no transversal deformity. Preoperative imaging exams showed a favorable position of the maxilla associated with good inclination of maxillary and mandibular incisors. A class II malocclusion with a deep bite in association with accentuated curve of Spee (COS) was found. The chin (pogonion) was well positioned (Figure 3). The lower third molar was extracted six months before the time of orthognathic surgery. Different treatment options to correct the mandibular retrusion were offered to the patient: bilateral sagittal split ramus osteotomy (BSSO) associated with backward genioplasty or total subapical mandibular osteotomy (TMAO) which would keep the chin in position and eliminate the need for genioplasty. Another option was combined orthognathic surgery on the mandible with BSSO or TMAO, associated with forward and downward repositioning of the maxilla. The patient chose the total subapical mandibular osteotomy procedure only.

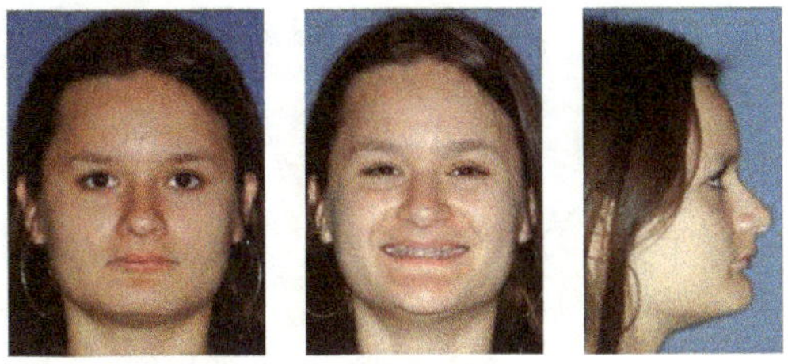

(a) (b) (c)

Figure 1: (a–c) Preoperative facial images showed a well-positioned maxilla and favorable chin projection associated with a deep labiomental sulcus.

After 39 months of orthodontic treatment, surgery was performed under general anesthesia. After a local bupivacaine 0.5% infiltration, a "V" incision was conducted from the right to the left retromolar region, and a mucoperiosteal flap was carefully detached to maintain the mental nerve integrity (Figure 4(a)). A ring of cortical bone was removed around the mental foramen, aiming to create a space around it. A gradual and careful removal of the buccal cortical bone with a drill, exposing the inferior alveolar neurovascular bundle and letting it free in all of its extension from the foramen to retromolar region, was done (Figure 4(b)), different from the original technique [5]. Once the inferior alveolar neurovascular bundle was viewed in its entirety, it was carefully removed from the inferior dental canal and repositioned either inferiorly or superiorly. After the repositioning, a reciprocate saw was carefully used to conduct an osteotomy from the mental foramen to the retromolar region to divide the lingual cortical bone from the basal bone, taking care to avoid damage to the posterior teeth's apices (Figure 4(c)). The posterior vertical cut on the posterior body area behind the second molar was also done with 5 mm to safety margin of the tooth. The osteotomy was conducted until the parasymphyseal region, through the buccal and lingual plates, approximately 5 mm below the apices of the anterior teeth, taking care not to damage them. It is crucial to avoid as much

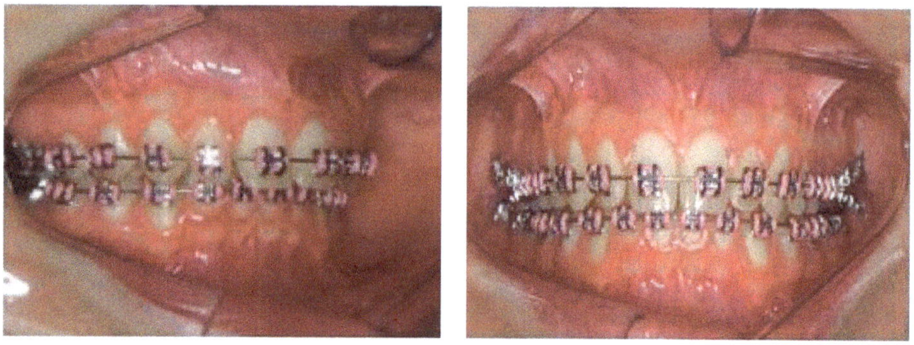

(a) (b)

FIGURE 2: (a, b) Preoperative intraoral images showing a deep bite and retrusion of the inferior alveolar segment.

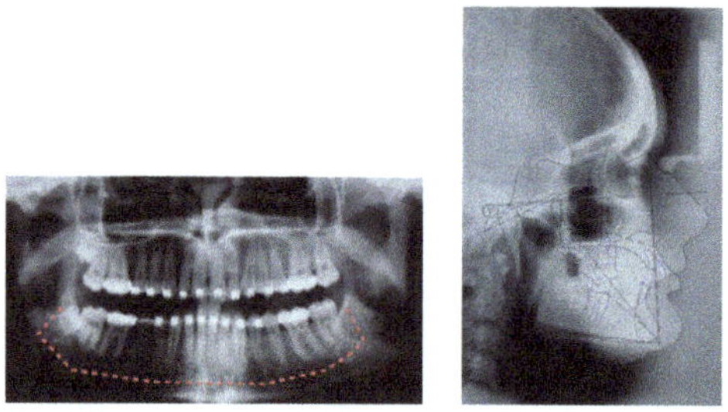

(a) (b)

FIGURE 3: (a) Preoperative panoramic radiography with subapical osteotomy simulation. (b). Digital cephalometric tracing of preoperative lateral radiograph using Dolphin Imaging Software.

possible damage to the lingual mucosa when cutting the lingual cortical bone due to the fact that it is the main pedicle supplying nutrition to the dentoalveolar segment after the osteotomy is completed (Figure 4(d)). After the dentoalveolar segment containing the entire lower dentition was mobilized, it was repositioned to the desired site and stabilized with miniplates and screws of the system 2.0. The conducted incision was closed with absorbable sutures (Figure 4(e)). Panoramic radiograph and cephalometric radiograph showed occlusal stability as well as the condyle in the right position after surgery (Figure 5). Postoperative orthodontics consisted of intercuspidation and adjustment of the COS, since an intentional open bite in the bicuspid area was left during surgery to allow increase of the anterior facial height. The patient finished orthodontic treatment after 12 months. In Table 1, it is possible to observe the measurements obtained from the lateral radiograph, pre- and postoperatively. Improvement in the measurements related to overjet, facial axis, jaw angle, inferior sulcus to H-line, and occlusal plane is noteworthy.

The six-year follow-up showed stability of the osteotomized segments with maintenance of plates and screws. Occlusal stability was also observed, associated with a 49 mm mouth opening. The labiomental sulcus was observed to be less deep in comparison to the preoperative stage. Patient reported of paresthesia in the mental region, which was expected, due to incisal nerve sectioning. The resolution of the main aesthetic complaint of the patient, which was a deep labiomental sulcus, was achieved through the TMAO (Figures 6, 7, and 8).

3. Discussion

Cases where total subapical mandibular osteotomy (TMAO) technique was used to correct class II patients are relatively few. The bilateral sagittal split ramus osteotomy (BSSO), on the other hand, is a widely used technique and has been an extensively described technique for mandibular retrusion correction [1]. Some of the reasons for this may be surgical complexity in bilateral dissection of inferior alveolar nerves, more probability for nerve lesions posttotal subapical mandibular osteotomy, and longer operative time when compared to the BSSO (1.5–2 times long) [1, 2, 16–18]. Boye et al. [1] stated that TMAO is a technique that allows mandibular advancement with excellent aesthetic and functional results in class II patients with good chin position. According to the author, patients subjected to BSSO had more postoperative pain and swelling than those subjected to TMAO, due to the fact that in the TMAO there is no fracture of the basal bone which favors postoperative repair. However, due to possible complications, this technique should only be performed by experienced surgeons and in cases with complete indications. In the present case report, the BSSO technique was not chosen due to the fact that the patient's soft tissue projection of chin was in good position; however, the dentoalveolar segment was retracted. As mentioned earlier, the use of this technique would result in an accentuated projection of the pogonion, so another retrusion/impaction genioplasty surgery would be necessary. Other option for the patient was the use of Kole modification osteotomy technique to obtain a better chin, but this technique is more used to correct anterior open bite, and there would be a need for bone graft if significant movement is planned [19]. In the present case report, the patient was able to open and close her mouth with little discomfort from the immediate postoperative period, and as mentioned earlier, swelling was less when compared to the traditional approach [1, 2, 6, 7].

There are a few recent studies with the use of TMAO. Pangrazio-Kulbersh et al. [11] compared the BSSO with TMAO in patients with skeletal and dental class II. Twenty

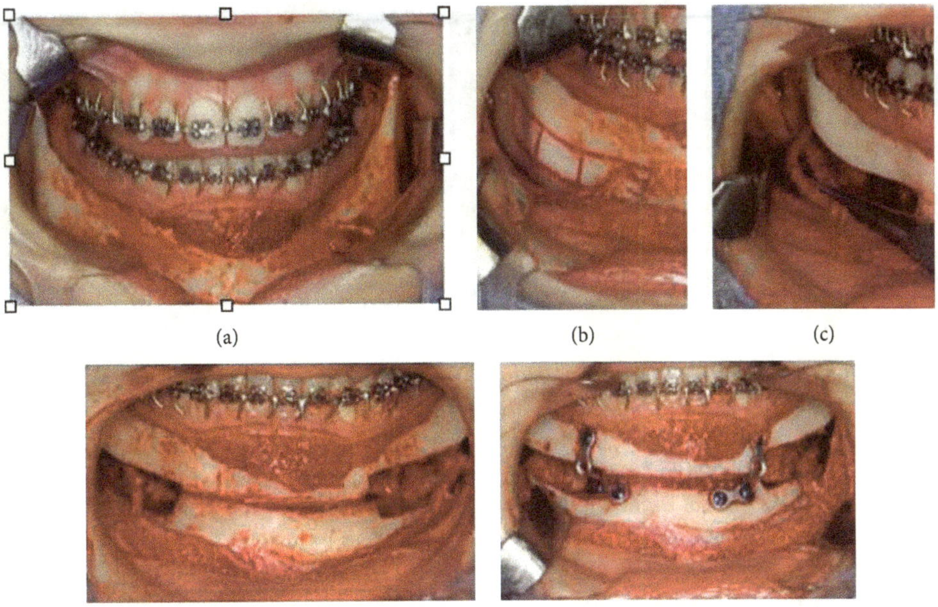

(a) (b) (c) (d) (e)

Figure 4: Surgical technique. (a) A "V" incision was conducted from the right to left retromolar region, and a mucoperiosteal flap was carefully detached to maintain the mental nerve integrity. (b) A ring of cortical bone was removed around the mental foramen, aiming to create a space around it. A gradual and careful removal of the buccal cortical bone with a drill exposed the inferior alveolar neurovascular bundle and let it free in all of its extension from the foramen to the retromolar region. (c) Once the inferior alveolar neurovascular bundle was viewed in its entirety, it was carefully removed from the inferior dental canal and repositioned either inferiorly or superiorly to it. (d) After nerve repositioning, a reciprocate saw was carefully used to conduct an osteotomy from the mental foramen to the retromolar region, to divide the lingual cortical bone from the basal bone, careful to avoid damage to the posterior teeth's apices. (e) After the dentoalveolar segment containing the entire lower dentition was mobilized, it was repositioned to the desired site and stabilized with miniplates and screws of the system 2.0.

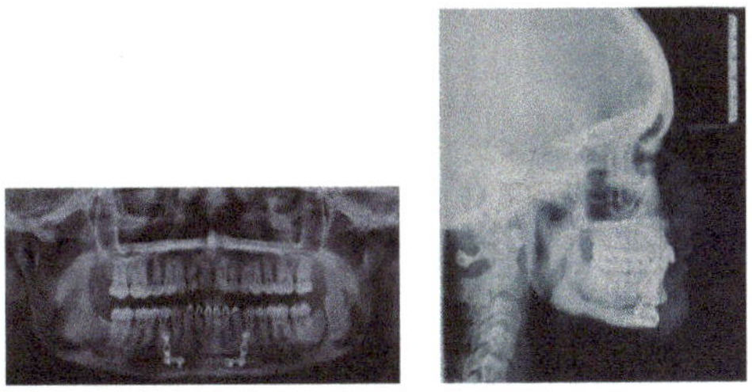

(a) (b)

Figure 5: (a) Postoperative panoramic radiograph. (b) Digital cephalometric tracing of postoperative lateral radiograph using Dolphin Imaging Software.

patients with mandibular retrognathia were treated with BSSO, and the other twenty with dentoalveolar retrusion were treated with TMAO. Both techniques yielded long-term stability even though TMAO had better results in reducing the depth of the mentolabial sulcus. This finding has proven a clinical significance in using TMAO for those patients in whom an alteration in the mentolabial sulcus is desired. In deep bite cases, total subapical mandibular osteotomy also increased the lower facial height [7, 8, 20], just like the BSSO since the mandible rotates downwards and forwards. None of the hard tissue changes were significantly different between the 2 procedures, except for a large increase in anterior facial height observed in the BSSO group [1].

Table 1: Values from the digital cephalometric tracing done in the lateral radiograph, comparing pre- and postoperative measurements, using Dolphin Imaging Software.

Cephalometric measurements	Preoperative values	Postoperative values	Norms
SNA (°)	85.5	86.2	82.0 ± 1.0
SNB (°)	80.1	84.7	80.9 ± 1.1
ANB (°)	5.4	1.5	1.6 ± 2.5
Overjet (mm)	7.0	2.2	2.5 ± 1.8
Overbite (mm)	3.5	3.4	2.5 ± 0.5
Lower face height (ANS-Xi-Pm) (°)	34.9	35.9	45 ± 2.5
FMA (MP-FH) (°)	9.8	13.8	23.9 ± 3.1
SN-GoGn (°)	13.0	17.6	32.9 ± 3.8
Facial axis-Ricketts (NaBa-PtGn) (°)	104.7	98.5	90.0 ± 4.2
Gonial/jaw angle (Ar-Go-Me) (°)	113.1	119.4	122.9 ± 1.5
Chin thickness (Pg-Pg′) (mm)	12.6	16.4	13.9 ± 0.4
Inferior Sulcus to H-Line (mm)	8.4	4.8	4.0 ± 2.2
Occlusal plane to SN (°)	5.0	10.0	14.4 ± 3.7

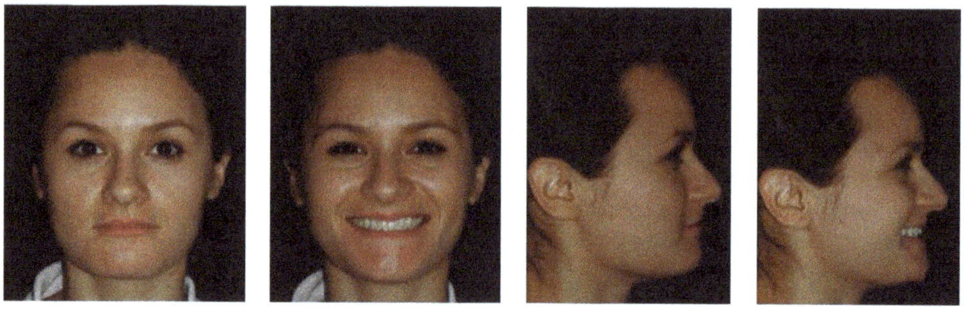

(a) (b) (c) (d)

FIGURE 6: Correction of deep bite and dental retrusion associated with occlusal stability (6-year follow-up).

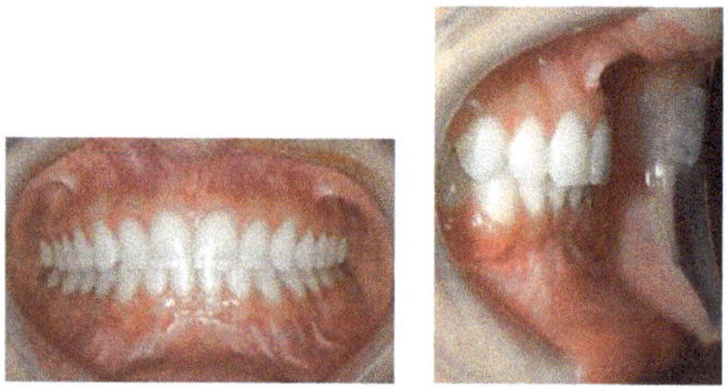

(a) (b)

FIGURE 7: Occlusal stability associated with aesthetic face (6-year follow-up).

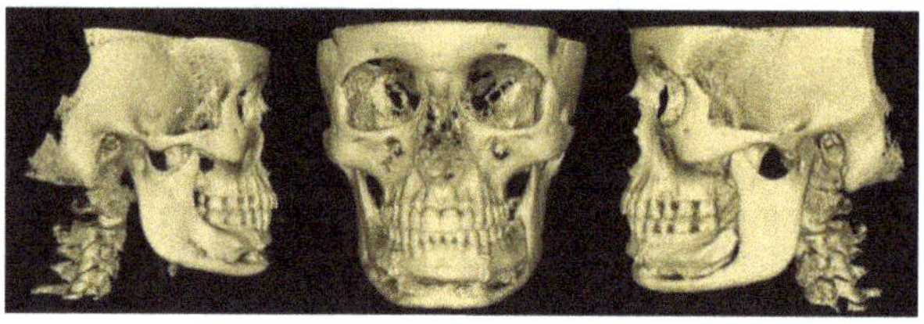

FIGURE 8: Reconstructed computerized tomography images showing bone deposition and stability of the osteotomized segments (6-year follow-up).

More anterior displacements of the mandibular incisors, second molars, and pogonion were also observed in the BSSO group. Eliades and Hegdvedt [21] treated a class II division II skeletal discrepancy by using a combination of BSSO and TMAO over the standard BSSO accompanied by the genioplasty technique. The authors suggested that the main advantage of BSSO-TMAO technique over BSSO-genioplasty combination is the relatively decreased advancement required, because the surgical movement is limited to the extent dictated by the maxilla-mandibular skeletal relationship, as opposed to the dental relationship (dental overjet). Mohammed-Ali et al. [10] proposed a modification in TMAO osteotomy involving a different technique of decortication of the inferior alveolar nerve. The authors suggested that this modification is efficient in reducing what otherwise would be a time-consuming process.

Drawbacks associated with the total mandibular subapical osteotomy include the following: the risk of inferior alveolar nerve and dental root damage and the fact that this procedure is technically laborious and time consuming. To minimize these risks, piezosurgery has proven to be a valid alternative to the use of drills or traditional instrumentation. It is helpful and safe for conducting different surgical procedures involving removal of a bone in close proximity to noble structures, such as nerves and blood vessels. Peripheral nerves exposed in direct contact with piezosurgery were not transected. Functional and structural damage related to the force applied on the nerve, rather than to the ultrasonic microvibrations, was observed [22]. Even though piezosurgery was not used in the case reported in this paper, the team highly recommends it. In our case report, post-TMAO, the patient reported of mild paresthesia in the mental region, which was expected, but not affecting her quality of life. She did not report of difficulty in masticatory function and phonation nor in personal relationships.

4. Conclusion

TMAO allowed the anteroposterior and vertical correction of the malocclusion and elimination of deep labiomental sulcus, and no complications in the dentoalveolar portion were observed. The authors believe that when fully indicated and well conducted, TMAO will result in excellent functional and aesthetic results, with stability of the osteotomized segments maintained with plates and screws. Occlusal stability was also observed, associated with a 49 mm mouth opening. Patient reported of paresthesia in the mental region, which was expected.

References

[1] T. Boye, P. Doyle, F. McKeown, and J. Sandler, "Total subapical mandibular osteotomy to correct class 2 division 1 dento-facial deformity," *Journal of Cranio-Maxillo-Facial Surgery*, vol. 40, no. 3, pp. 238–242, 2012.

[2] R. Trauner and H. Obwegeser, "The surgical correction of mandibular prognathism and retrognathia with consideration of genioplasty: part I. Surgical procedures to correct mandibular prognathism and reshaping of the chin," *Oral Surgery, Oral Medicine, Oral Pathology*, vol. 10, no. 7, pp. 677–689, 1957.

[3] H. Kole, "Surgical operations on the alveolar ridge to correct occlusal abnormalities," *Oral Surgery, Oral Medicine, and Oral Pathology*, vol. 12, no. 3, pp. 277–288, 1959.

[4] R. B. MacIntosh, "Total mandibular alveolar osteotomy: encouraging experiences with an infrequently indicated procedure," *Journal of Maxillofacial Surgery*, vol. 2, no. 4, pp. 210–218, 1974.

[5] V. S. Dietz, A. A. Gianelly, and D. F. Booth, "Surgical orthodontics in the treatment of a class II, division 2 malocclusion: a case report," *American Journal of Orthodontics*, vol. 71, no. 3, pp. 309–316, 1977.

[6] R. B. Murray, "Mandibular sagittal subapical osteotomy: a case study," *American Journal of Orthodontics*, vol. 77, no. 5, pp. 469–485, 1980.

[7] W. H. Bell, J. D. Jacobs, and H. L. Legan, "Treatment of class II deep bite by orthodontic and surgical means," *American Journal of Orthodontics*, vol. 85, no. 1, pp. 1–20, 1984.

[8] D. F. Booth, V. Dietz, and A. A. Gianelly, "Correction of class II malocclusion by combined sagittal ramus and subapical body osteotomy," *Journal of Oral Surgery*, vol. 34, no. 7, pp. 630–634, 1976.

[9] A. S. Herford, D. E. Stringer, and R. Tandon, "Orthognathic surgery," *An Issue of Oral and Maxillofacial Clinics of North America*, pp. 480–492, Elsevier, 2004.

[10] R. I. Mohammed-Ali, A. Schache, S. Walsh, and K. Sneddon, "Total mandibular subapical osteotomy: modification of the technique," *The British Journal of Oral & Maxillofacial Surgery*, vol. 47, no. 8, pp. 629-630, 2009.

[11] V. Pangrazio-Kulbersh, J. L. Berger, R. Kaczynski, and M. Shunock, "Stability of skeletal class II correction with 2 surgical techniques: the sagittal split ramus osteotomy and the total mandibular subapical alveolar osteotomy," *American Journal of Orthodontics and Dentofacial Orthopedics*, vol. 120, no. 2, pp. 134–143, 2001.

[12] V. Pangrazio-Kulbersh and R. B. MacIntosh, "Total mandibular alveolar osteotomy: an alternate choice to other surgical procedures," *American Journal of Orthodontics*, vol. 87, no. 4, pp. 319–337, 1985.

[13] G. B. Scheideman, H. Kawamura, R. A. Finn, and W. H. Bell, "Wound healing after anterior and posterior subapical osteotomy," *Journal of Oral and Maxillofacial Surgery*, vol. 43, no. 6, pp. 408–416, 1985.

[14] G. Zisser and B. Gattinger, "Histologic investigation of pulpal changes following maxillary and mandibular alveolar osteotomies in the dog," *Journal of Oral and Maxillofacial Surgery*, vol. 40, no. 6, pp. 332–339, 1982.

[15] R. Allen, P. L. Sadowsky, and C. F. Cox, "Resorption patterns following intentional vital root transection in Macaca mulatta," *The International Journal of Adult Orthodontics and Orthognathic Surgery*, vol. 9, no. 2, pp. 119–127, 1994.

[16] J. E. Van Sickels and C. M. Flanary, "Stability associated with mandibular advancement treated by rigid osseous fixation," *Journal of Oral and Maxillofacial Surgery*, vol. 43, no. 5, pp. 338–341, 1985.

[17] G. W. Arnett, "A redefinition of bilateral sagittal osteotomy (BSO) advancement relapse," *American Journal of Orthodontics and Dentofacial Orthopedics*, vol. 104, no. 5, pp. 506–515, 1993.

[18] I. M. Watzke, T. A. Turvey, C. Phillips, and W. R. Proffit, "Stability of mandibular advancement after sagittal osteotomy with screw or wire fixation: a comparative study," *Journal of Oral and Maxillofacial Surgery*, vol. 48, no. 2, pp. 108–121, 1990.

[19] J. Kloosterman, "Köle's osteotomy, a follow-up study," *Journal of Maxillofacial Surgery*, vol. 13, no. 2, pp. 59–63, 1985.

[20] W. H. Bell, "Correction of the short-face syndrome-vertical maxillary deficiency: a preliminary report," *Journal of Oral Surgery*, vol. 35, no. 2, pp. 110–120, 1977.

[21] T. Eliades and A. K. Hegdvedt, "Orthodontic-surgical correction of a class II, division 2 malocclusion," *American Journal of Orthodontics and Dentofacial Orthopedics*, vol. 110, no. 4, pp. 351–357, 1996.

[22] P. Scolozzi and G. Herzog, "Total mandibular subapical osteotomy and Le Fort I osteotomy using piezosurgery and computer-aided designed and manufactured surgical splints: a favorable combination of three techniques in the management of severe mouth asymmetry in Parry-Romberg syndrome," *Journal of Oral and Maxillofacial Surgery*, vol. 72, no. 5, pp. 991–999, 2014.

16

Reconstruction of the Adult Hemifacial Microsomia Patient with Temporomandibular Joint Total Joint Prosthesis and Orthognathic Surgery

Piero Cascone,[1] Valentino Vellone,[1] Valerio Ramieri,[1] Emanuela Basile,[1] Achille Tarsitano,[2] and Claudio Marchetti[2]

[1]*Sapienza Università di Roma, Via del Policlinico, Roma, Italy*
[2]*Department of Biomedical and Neuromotor Sciences, Maxillofacial Surgery Unit, S. Orsola-Malpighi Hospital, Alma Mater Studiorum University of Bologna, Bologna, Italy*

Correspondence should be addressed to Valentino Vellone; valentino.vellone@gmail.com

Academic Editor: Fabio Roccia

Background. HFM patients' reconstruction has always been a challenge for maxillofacial surgeons, and numerous reconstructive techniques have been described. Surgical treatment depends on the patient's age and contemplates Temporomandibular Joint (TMJ) reconstruction in conjunction with orthognathic surgery, usually necessary following completion of growth to maximize the functional and esthetic results. Distraction osteogenesis had gained popularity as valid alternative in growing patients, but the two primary methods to reconstruct the TMJs involve the use of autogenous, using free or microvascular bone grafts, or alloplastic graft, but there is no widely accepted method. *Methods.* The increasing use of temporomandibular prosthesis for temporomandibular problems has led us to use them even in HFM. A case of female nongrowing patients with HFM type IIb treated with temporomandibular prosthesis in an all-in-one protocol is presented. *Results.* Incisal opening, measured with BioPAK system (Bioresearch Inc., Milwaukee, USA), was 21.4 mm in the presurgical period and 32.2 mm after all-in-one procedure, for an increase of 50.5%. Excursive movement to the right side was 2.2 mm in the presurgical period and was 1.5 mm after surgery, for a decrease of 31.8%. Left excursion movement changed from 5 mm to 6.1 mm, for an increase of 22.0%. *Conclusions.* The TMJ Concepts patient-fitted TJP in conjunction with orthognathic surgery for TMJ and jaw reconstruction is a valid option for patients with HFM.

1. Introduction

Hemifacial microsomia (HFM) is the second most common facial birth defect after cleft lip and palate. The estimated incidence is of 1 of every 4000 to 5600 live births.

The aetiology and pathogenesis of hemifacial microsomia are still unknown.

The two proposed etiopathogenic theories include hematoma of the stapedial artery during fetal development and abnormal neural crest migration. Both models explain the variable and asymmetric nature of this condition.

The clinical presentation is variable, and many classification systems have been developed.

Figueroa and Pruzansky [1], subsequently modified by Vento et al. [2], described three mandibular types. In type I, the temporomandibular joint and ramus are well formed but smaller than normal. In type II, the temporomandibular joint, ramus, and glenoid fossa are hypoplastic and malformed. In type III, the entire ramus is missing.

Kaban et al. [3] added a subdivision of type II, identifying type IIa as a ramus with abnormal size and shape and type IIb as a ramus and TMJ with abnormal size, shape, and function. This classification system may be the most useful to the surgeon in the preoperative evaluation because of its simplicity and inclusion of the TMJ anatomy and function.

HFM patients' reconstruction has always been a challenge for maxillofacial surgeons, and numerous reconstructive techniques have been described.

Surgical treatment depends on the patient's age and contemplates TMJ reconstruction in conjunction with orthognathic surgery, usually necessary following completion of growth to maximize the functional and esthetic results [4].

TMJ and jaw reconstruction in patients with HFM has been described using autogenous tissue such as rib graft or sternoclavicular graft alone or in conjunction with orthognathic surgery in patients with various degrees of deformity, but without high-quality outcomes documentation.

It must be remembered that most of the patients reconstructed with an autogenous graft require at least one additional maxillomandibular surgical procedure due to the high percentage of ankylosis, fracture, variable growth behavior, resorption, infection, and donor side morbity [5].

Another option for early intervention is the use of distraction osteogenesis but requires multiple operations to place and remove the distractors, and this can lead to difficulty in controlling the vector of growth.

Improving the predictability of results and limiting correction of the jaw and TMJ deformities to 1, major operation can best be achieved by waiting until growth is complete, provided that the patient is functionally and psychologically stable [4].

The development of custom-fitted total joint prosthesis (TJP) provides an additional option to aid in reconstruction of the HFM patient in conjunction with orthognathic surgical procedures [6].

A case of female nongrowing patient with HFM type IIb treated with temporomandibular prosthesis in an all-in-one protocol is presented.

2. Case Description

A 22-year-old female with left side hemifacial microsomia (type IIb) was referred to the Maxillo-Facial Surgery Department at the Sapienza Università di Roma for evaluation and treatment.

Clinical examination and 3-dimensional CT scans showed unilateral hypoplasia of the mandibular condyle, ramus, and body; retrognathic mandible deviated toward the ipsilateral side; large occlusal plane angle with a hyperdivergent facial morphology; hypoplasia of the ipsilateral maxilla and temporal bone; Class II skeletal and Class II occlusal relation; canting of the occlusal plane; ear anomalies and ipsilateral soft tissue deficiency affecting skin, subcutaneous, muscular, and glandular tissues; decreased ipsilateral facial height.

Following completion of clinical, cephalometric, dental model, and radiographic imaging analyses, the treatment plan included the following:

(1) Presurgical orthodontics to align and level the maxillary and mandibular arches.

(2) Surgery

  (a) Right mandibular ramus sagittal split osteotomy to advance the mandible in a counterclockwise rotation.

  (b) Left TMJ reconstruction to advancement the mandible in a counterclockwise direction with custom-fitted total joint prostheses (TMJ Concepts, Ventura, California, USA).

  (c) Maxillary osteotomies to advance the maxilla in a counterclockwise direction and level the occlusal plane transversely with rigid fixation and bone grafting.

(3) Postsurgical orthodontics to refine and retain the occlusion.

A CT scan was acquired, and a 3-D stereolithic model was produced for a better evaluation and to simulate subsequent mandibular surgery.

The bone thickness, confirmed by CT scan (Figure 1), in temporal root of the zygomatic arch and glenoid fossa were adequate for the fixation of the fossa component of the prosthesis.

The custom-made prosthesis was developed basing on 3-dimensional virtual program (Dolphin 11.5, Dolphin Imaging and Management Solutions, Chatsworth, CA, USA) and stereolithographic model.

The sagittal split osteotomy was performed to reposition the mandible in the predetermined new position based on the clinical evaluation, dental model analysis, and the prediction tracing.

The mandible was moved downward in the back, advanced in a counterclockwise direction, transversely levelled and fixed with quick-cure acrylic (Figure 1).

A LeFort I osteotomy was performed to correct the canting.

A wax disc was recreated to reconstruct as much as possible the vertical dimension after the sagittal split osteotomy.

Before surgery, dental models mounted on an anatomic articulator were used to replicate the mandibular repositioning performed on the 3-dimensional plastic model for the construction of the intermediate surgical occlusal splint necessary for precise positioning of the mandible at surgery.

Intermediate splint construction was required to improve the accuracy of a patient's surgery and outcome according to "mandible first" surgical sequence.

2.1. Surgical Technique. In the operating room, the same time of model surgery was followed.

Sagittal split osteotomy on the right side was performed.

The left side was approached through an external preauricular and submandibular incision with reflection of the musculature, and mobilization of the mandible.

The dissection was carried down to the temporal bone anterior to the internal meatus and extended medially. A subperiosteal tunnel was created over the hypoplastic ramus to connect to the base of the temporal bone.

The TMJ fossa component of the TJP was placed and secured to the temporal bone with screws.

The mandibular component was inserted through the submandibular incision, and the condyle was seated into the fossa component and secured to the ramus with bicortical screws. The incisions were closed.

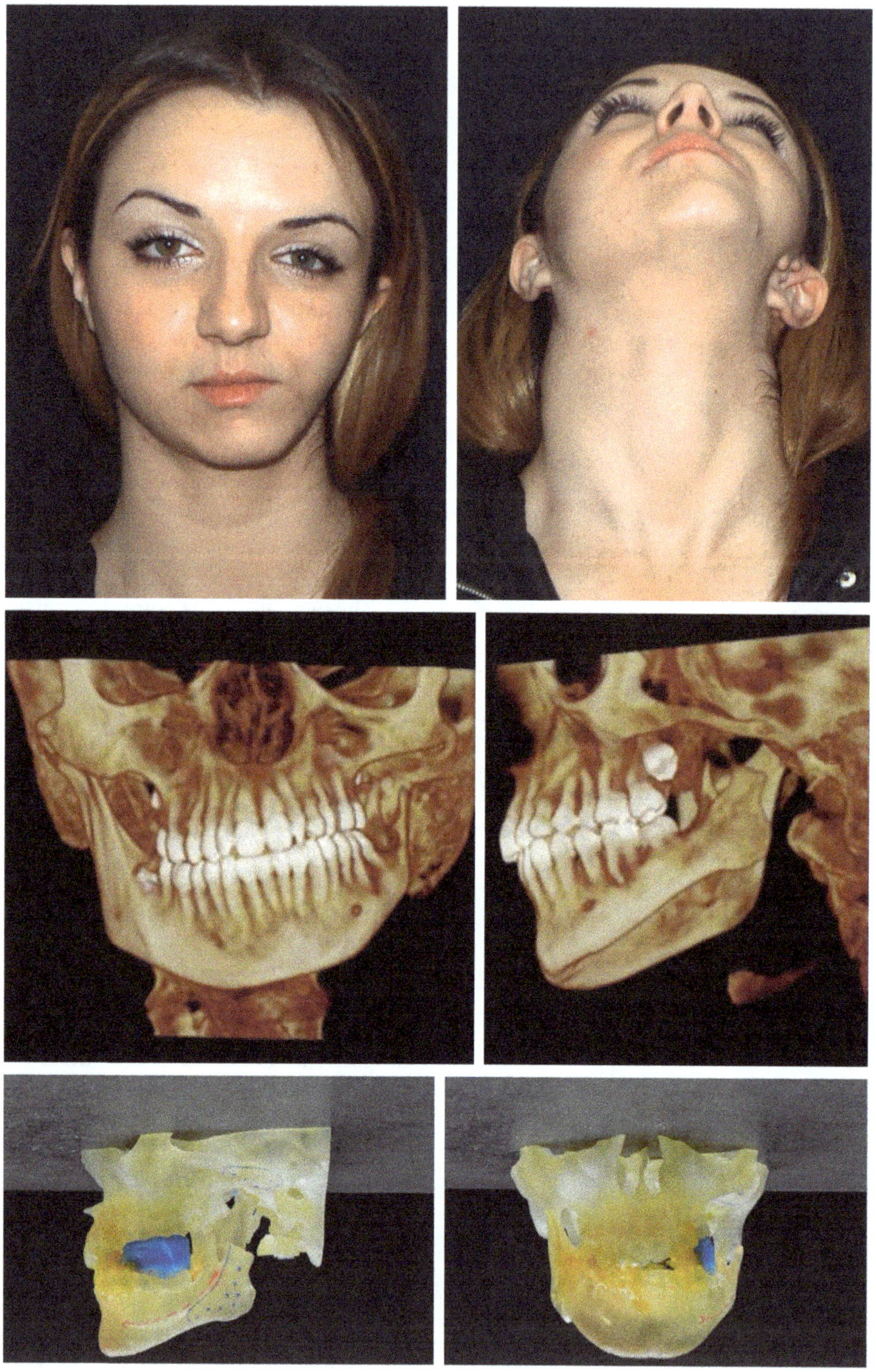

Figure 1: Patient presurgery in frontal view and axial view. 3D CT scan pre surgery in frontal and left lateral views. 3-dimensional plastic model of the patient's jaws, TMJs, and cranial base structures repositioned and fixed with quick-cure acrylic.

A separate set of instruments was used to maintain sterility of the TMJ area.

Moreover, surgical gloves were changed every time that surgeons passed from mouth to TMJ area.

A prefabricated intermediate occlusal splint was placed in order to position the mandible into its final predetermined position.

Intermaxillary fixation was performed, and mandibular sagittal split osteotomy stabilized with bicortical screws, and the oral incision closed.

The IMF and occlusal splint were removed. Through a maxillary vestibular incision, the maxillary osteotomies were completed. The maxilla was downfractured, mobilized 6 millimetres down in the left side and fixed with four bone plates, with 2 screws above and 2 screws below the osteotomy site for each plate. A laminar, cortical, heterologous bone graft (Tecnoss Medical Devices, Giaveno, Italy) was used to fill the osteotomy's gap.

The final occlusion was established and secured with IMF.

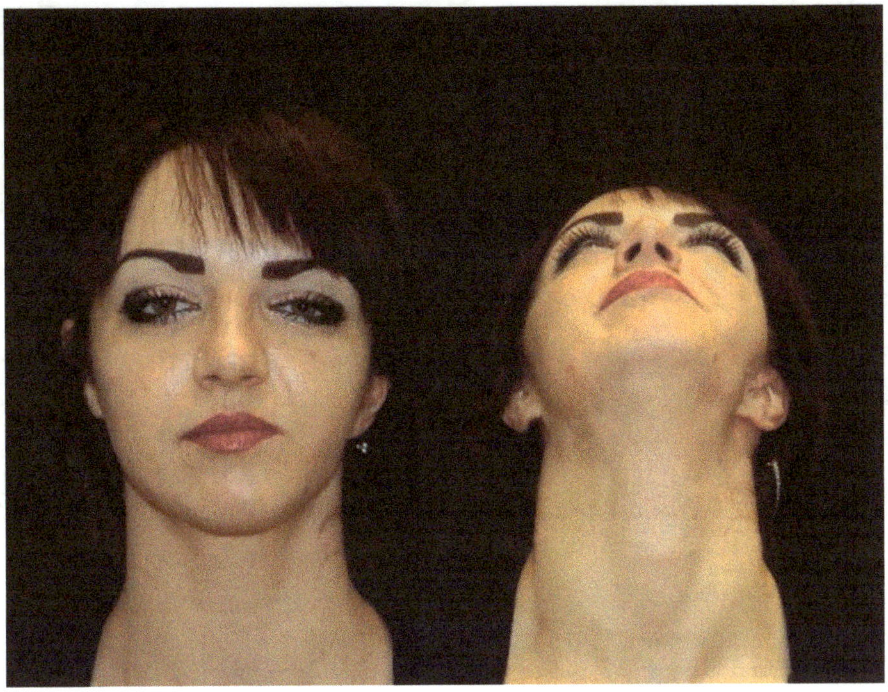

FIGURE 2: Patient 1 year after surgery in frontal and axial views.

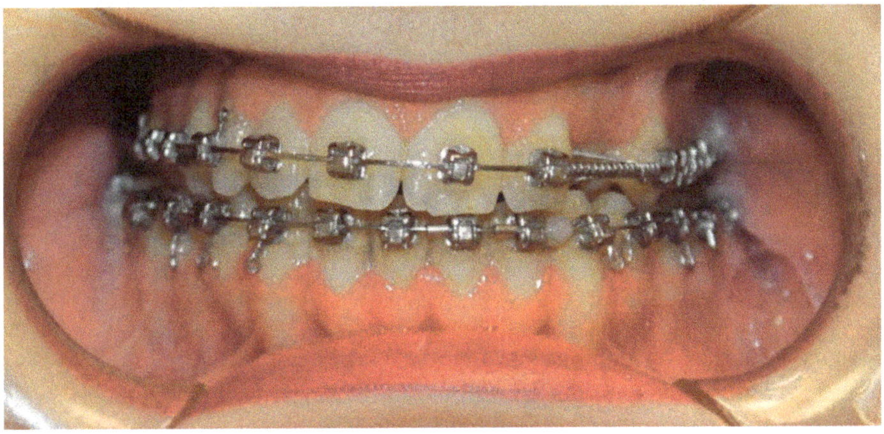

FIGURE 3: Patient occlusion 1 year after surgery.

As refinements, genioplasty and lipofilling procedure was performed.

The IMF was removed, and light elastics were applied to guide the occlusion and decrease the stress on the muscles of mastication (Figures 2–4).

3. Results

Incisal opening, measured with BioPAK system (Bioresearch Inc., Milwaukee, USA), was 21.4 mm in the presurgical period and 32.2 mm after 1-year follow-up, for an increase of 50.5%. Excursive movement to the right side was 2.2 mm in the presurgical period and was 1.5 mm after surgery, for a decrease of 31.8%. Left excursion movement changed from 5 mm to 6.1 mm, for an increase of 22.0%.

4. Discussion

Management of hemifacial microsomia is controversial. Numerous reconstructive techniques have been described.

Early surgical intervention to lengthen the ramus on the affected side has often been advocated as a method to prevent maxillary compensatory deformity.

Unfortunately, mandibular distraction osteogenesis requires multiple operations to place and remove the distractors, and this can lead to difficulty in controlling the vector of growth; furthermore, very few long-term reports are available.

Anyway, the two primary methods to reconstruct the TMJs involve the use of autogenous tissues (i.e., rib or sternoclavicular grafts (SCGs)) versus alloplastic total joint prosthetic devices.

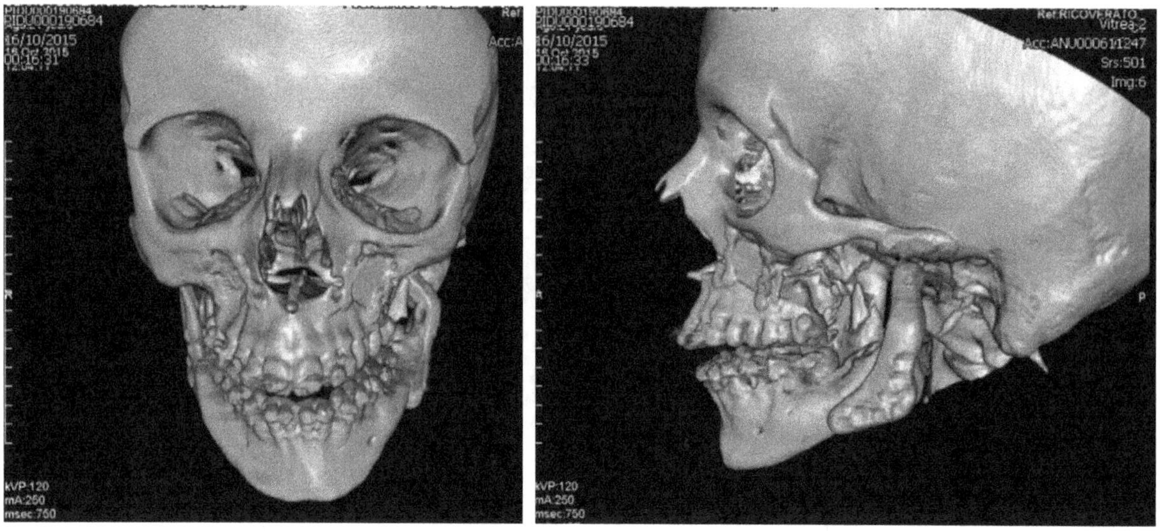

Figure 4: 3D CT scan after surgery in frontal and lateral views.

Autologous bone grafting techniques are well established and accepted. A costochondral bone graft is the most commonly used autogenous replacement for mandibular ramus/condyle defects, especially in growing children.

Theoretically, the costochondral grafts keep a "growth potential" but has been shown to be unpredictable or resulting in ankyloses, due to allograft and/or fixation failure or for an uncooperative patient nature with postreconstruction physical therapy.

Recent studies have even questioned the necessity for using a cartilaginous graft to restore and maintain mandibular growth.

Peltomäki et al. [7] in investigations of mandibular growth after costochondral grafting supported previous experiments with regard to the inability of the graft to adapt to the growth velocity of the new environment. If autogenous grafts fail to incorporate into the host bone, fail to grow, grow horizontally rather than vertically, or more commonly become ankylosed; under these circumstances, the patient basically becomes disabled—unable to eat foods because they cannot open their mouths wide enough. These and other issues can lead to social ostracization, depression, and very poor life quality.

Improving the predictability of results and limiting correction of the jaw and TMJ deformities to 1, major operation can best be achieved by waiting until growth is complete, provided that the patient is functionally and psychologically stable [4].

The introduction of alloplastic TJR has improved the quality of life for many adult orthopedic and TMJ patients with unsalvageable functional and anatomical joint pathology [8, 9]. However, these devices, because they are a biomechanical rather than biological nature, have a finite life-span making them an unattractive alternative in the growing patient.

Taking into consideration the information available for autogenous tissue grafting, the use of alloplastic TMJ TJR may be an option in type II HFM onwards [10].

A further advantage for TJR is the possibility, when zygomatic arch and glenoid fossa are absent, to plan the fossa component custom-fitted to the base of the skull and lateral temporal bone morphology.

Correction of the transversal anomaly of HFM has always been difficult because of deficiencies of facial skeleton and the overlying soft tissue.

The concept and technique of using TMJ TJP for TMJ reconstruction and simultaneous mandibular advancement with counterclockwise rotation of the maxillomandibular complex was developed by Wolford et al. in 1990 and was first used for HFM in 1997 [6].

This operation permits to solve many HFM-related problems at one time while multiple TMJ operations create scar tissue and interrupt normal blood flow and normal physiologic nutritional distribution to the anatomic structures.

Concern has been raised about the longevity of TMJ TJR devices.

The longevity of prosthesis for any joint is dependent on materials, design, stability, and functional loading.

It is difficult to determine the functional load for the TMJ prosthesis. For the average adult, the biting forces generated at the molars is approximately 60 pounds (27 kg) and that for the incisors is 35 pounds (15 kg) [11].

Although the life expectancy of TMJ Concepts TMJ TJR devices is still unknown [12], it should be longer than their orthopedic joint counterparts.

Potential risks and concerns using TJPs include (1) an unknown functional service life of the TMJ Concepts TJP; (2) surgical risks associated with TMJ reconstruction; (3) infection; and (4) development of hypersensitivity to the materials in the prostheses.

5. Conclusions

The TMJ Concepts patient-fitted TJP in conjunction with orthognathic surgery for TMJ and jaw reconstruction is a valid option for patients with HFM because (1) no bone graft donor site is required; (2) it does not require reconstruction of the glenoid fossa; (3) it is a patient-fitted device to meet a patient's specific anatomic requirements for mandibular advancement, vertical lengthening, and TMJ reconstruction; and (4) treatment results are highly predictable and stable in relation to skeletal and occlusal stability, TMJ function, improved facial balance, and comfort.

Consent

The patient agreed to publish clinical pictures.

References

[1] A. A. Figueroa and S. Pruzansky, "The external ear, mandible and other components of hemifacial microsomia," *Journal of Maxillofacial Surgery*, vol. 10, pp. 200–211, 1982.

[2] A. R. Vento, R. A. LaBrie, and J. B. Mulliken, "The O.M.E.N.S. classification of hemifacial microsomia," *Cleft Palate-Craniofacial Journal*, vol. 28, no. 1, pp. 68–77, 1991.

[3] L. B. Kaban, B. L. Padwa, and J. B. Mulliken, "Surgical correction of mandibular hypoplasia in hemifacial microsomia: the case for treatment in early childhood," *Journal of Oral and Maxillofacial Surgery*, vol. 56, pp. 628–638, 1998.

[4] L. M. Wolford and D. E. Perez, "Surgical management of congenital deformities with temporomandibular joint malformation," *Oral and Maxillofacial Surgery Clinics of North America*, vol. 27, no. 1, pp. 137–154, 2015.

[5] N. S. Zanakis, K. Gavakos, M. Faippea, A. Karamanos, and N. Zotalis, "Application of custom-made TMJ prosthesis in hemifacial microsomia," *International Journal of Oral and Maxillofacial Surgery*, vol. 38, no. 9, pp. 988–992, 2009.

[6] L. M. Wolford, T. C. Bourland, D. Odrigues, D. E. Perez, and E. Limoeiro, "Successful reconstruction of nongrowing hemifacial microsomia patients with unilateral temporomandibular joint total joint prosthesis and orthognathic surgery," *Journal of Oral and Maxillofacial Surgery*, vol. 70, no. 12, pp. 2835–2853, 2012.

[7] T. Peltomäki, L. A. Quevedo, G. Jeldes, and O. Rönning, "Histology of surgically removed overgrown osteochondral rib grafts," *Journal of Cranio-Maxillofacial Surgery*, vol. 30, no. 6, pp. 355–360, 2002.

[8] L. G. Mercuri and A. Giobbie-Hurder, "Long-term outcomes after total alloplastic temporomandibular joint reconstruction following exposure to failed materials," *Journal of Oral and Maxillofacial Surgery*, vol. 62, no. 9, pp. 1088–1096, 2004.

[9] L. G. Mercuri, "Alloplastic temporomandibular joint replacement: rationale for the use of custom devices," *International Journal of Oral and Maxillofacial Surgery*, vol. 41, no. 9, pp. 1033–1040, 2012.

[10] A. Westermark, P. Hedén, E. Aagaard, and C. P. Cornelius, "The use of TMJ Concepts prostheses to reconstruct patients with major temporomandibular joint and mandibular defects," *International Journal of Oral and Maxillofacial Surgery*, vol. 40, no. 5, pp. 487–496, 2011.

[11] L. M. Wolford, L. G. Mercuri, E. D. Schneiderman, R. Movahed, and W. Allen, "Twenty-year follow-up study on a patient-fitted temporomandibular joint prosthesis: the Techmedica/TMJ Concepts device," *Journal of Oral and Maxillofacial Surgery*, vol. 73, no. 5, pp. 952–960, 2015.

[12] L. Ciocca, A. Tarsitano, C. Marchetti, and R. Scotti, "A CAD–CAM-prototyped temporomandibular condyle connected to a bony plate to support a free fibula flap in patients undergoing mandiblectomy: a pilot study with 5 years of follow up," *Journal of Cranio-Maxillofacial Surgery*, vol. 44, no. 7, pp. 811–819, 2016.

17

Giant Parotid Pleomorphic Adenoma with Atypical Histological Presentation and Long-Term Recurrence-Free Follow-Up after Surgery: A Case Report and Review of the Literature

Mohammed AlKindi,[1] **Sundar Ramalingam**,[1] **Lujain Abdulmajeed Hakeem**,[1] **and Manal A. AlSheddi**[2]

[1]*Department of Oral and Maxillofacial Surgery, College of Dentistry, King Saud University, Riyadh, Saudi Arabia*
[2]*Department of Basic Sciences, College of Dentistry, Princess Nourah Bint Abdulrahman University, Riyadh, Saudi Arabia*

Correspondence should be addressed to Sundar Ramalingam; sundar.ksu@gmail.com

Academic Editor: Pravinkumar G. Patil

Salivary gland tumors (SGT) comprise 3% of all head and neck tumors, are mostly benign, and arise frequently in the parotid gland. Pleomorphic adenoma (PA) is the commonest SGT, representing 60-70% of all benign parotid tumors. Clinically, parotid PA presents as irregular, lobulated, asymptomatic, slow-growing preauricular mass, involving both superficial and deep lobes, and could grow to gigantic proportions. Histologically, PA has epithelial and mesenchymal elements in chondromyxoid matrix and is managed surgically. Based on a review of 43 cases reported in English literature since 1995, giant parotid PA is reported as large as 35 cm (diameter) and 7.3 kg (resected weight). Although rare, 10 cases of malignant transformation were reported in the review. Surgical management included extracapsular dissection (ECD), superficial parotidectomy, and total parotidectomy for benign tumors, and adjuvant radiation or chemotherapy for malignant tumors. We further present the case of a 36-year-old healthy male with slow-growing and asymptomatic giant parotid PA, of 4-year duration. The patient presented with firm, lobulated preauricular swelling, provisionally diagnosed as PA based on radiographic and cytological findings. The tumor was resected through ECD, and the patient had uneventful postoperative recovery and a 7-year recurrence-free follow-up period. Histological examination revealed epimyoepithelial proliferation punctuated by chondromyxoid areas, with extensive squamous metaplasia and keratin cysts. To the best of knowledge from indexed literature, giant parotid PA is rarely reported in Saudi Arabia. In addition to its rarity, this case is reported for its benign nature despite atypical histological presentation, successful surgical management without complications, and long-term recurrence-free follow-up. Based on this report, clinicians must be aware of atypical histological presentations associated with PA and plan suitable surgical management and follow-up to avoid morbidity. Nevertheless, attempts must be made to diagnose and manage these lesions at an early stage and before they reach gigantic proportions.

1. Introduction

Neoplastic lesions of the salivary glands are uncommon and comprise less than 3% of all reported head and neck tumors [1, 2]. Nearly 80% of the reported salivary gland tumors (SGT) are benign and occur predominantly in major salivary glands, with the parotid gland being the commonest site (70–80%) [2, 3]. Often presenting as slow-growing, painless masses, tumors involving major salivary glands are rarely aggressive or malignant (<10%). On the contrary, tumors of minor salivary glands while occurring rarely have a preponderance to be malignant (80–90%) [2, 3]. Pleomorphic adenoma (PA) is the commonest SGT, accounting for almost 60–80% of all benign SGT and 60–70% of all parotid gland tumors [1, 3]. Clinically, PA presents as an irregular, rubbery, lobulated, slow-growing mass without any associated pain or discomfort. The presenting complaint is typically related to unpleasant or unesthetic facial appearance, which when disregarded can lead to patients reporting with huge lesions [4]. Reports in the literature suggest resected dimensions of PA to be frequently in the range of 2 cm to 6 cm and rarely reaching even up to 25–35 cm [4, 5].

As the name suggests, PA is histologically categorized as a benign mixed (pleomorphic) tumor of ductal and myoepithelial cell origin. Owing to the pluripotential nature of myoepithelial cells, the tumor is composed of epithelial and fibrous, myxoid, and cartilaginous mesenchymal elements surrounded by a pseudocapsule, with occasional squamous metaplasia [3, 4, 6]. While the diagnosis of PA is based primarily on clinical and histological findings, the mainstay of management is by surgical excision [1, 4]. Depending upon their size and depth of involvement, parotid PA is surgically managed either by superficial parotidectomy (SP), extracapsular dissection (ECD), or total parotidectomy (TP). All of the above procedures carry the risk of postoperative facial nerve paralysis and Frey's syndrome [1, 7]. Recurrence is usually associated with inadequate clearance and incomplete removal of pseudocapsule, and malignant transformation has been reported with large, long-standing PA [4, 7].

Although uncommon, giant pleomorphic adenomas of the parotid gland have been reported. An electronic search of the English-language articles through the Medline, Scopus, and Google Scholar databases revealed 43 reports of giant parotid PA since 1995 [4, 8–32], with sizes ranging up to 28-33 cm [15, 18, 27] and tumor mass ranging up to 6.85–7.3 kg [10, 27]. Major reasons for patients reporting with large PA are lack of resources, inaccessibility to medical facilities, fear of surgical procedure, and poor awareness, compounded by an asymptomatic and slow-growing lesion [4]. The aim of this paper is to add to the existing scientific literature, a case of giant parotid PA treated surgically by ECD, followed by uneventful postoperative recovery and a 7-year recurrence-free follow-up. This paper also attempts to highlight the benign nature of parotid PA, despite the atypical histological presentation, which could be associated with it.

2. Case Report

A 36-year-old healthy male patient reported to the oral and maxillofacial surgery outpatient clinic at the College of Dentistry and Dental University Hospital, King Saud University, in October 2012. The patient sought medical attention for a slow-growing, painless swelling in the right preauricular region. History revealed that the patient noticed the swelling almost 4 years ago, and since then, it had gradually increased in size with no obvious symptoms or changes to the overlying skin. Upon interviewing, the patient reported no relevant medical or surgical history and mentioned fear of surgery and absence of discomfort as reasons for delaying medical consultation, in spite of an unesthetic facial appearance.

Clinical examination revealed a firm, nontender, nodular, and mobile swelling with apparently normal overlying skin. The swelling extended superoinferiorly from the level of the external ear to the lower border of the mandible and anteroposteriorly from the angle of the mouth to the posterior border of the mandible. There was no lymph node involvement or facial nerve deficit (Figure 1). Preoperative computed tomography (CT), magnetic resonance imaging (MRI), and fine-needle aspiration cytology (FNAC) were ordered. CT with contrast revealed a well-defined mass lesion in the superficial lobe of the right parotid gland, without any underlying bony erosion and normal-appearing pharynx, larynx, and parapharyngeal spaces. While confirming the CT findings, head and neck MRI further demonstrated a well-demarcated, heterogeneous, mass lesion measuring 10 × 7 × 8 cm in maximum dimension (Figure 2). FNAC showed numerous scattered groups and clusters of plasmacytoid myoepithelial cells, associated with a chondromyxoid matrix. A provisional diagnosis of PA with no malignant tendency was arrived at based on CT, MRI, and FNAC findings.

Surgical removal of the right parotid SGT under general anesthesia was planned and explained to the patient. Following informed consent, the lesion was excised completely through ECD, with preservation of all branches of the facial nerve. The right parotid gland was approached using a cervically extended preauricular skin incision. A clearly discernible plane of dissection around the tumor was used for dissecting the tumor mass, without any iatrogenic damage to the facial nerve branches. Owing to the long-standing nature, multiple small feeder vessels had to be ligated circumferentially around the tumor to achieve hemostasis. The intraoperative period was unremarkable, and the patient did not require any blood transfusions (Figure 3). The resected mass was bilobed and ovoid in shape with a final dimension of 7 × 13 × 7 cm and weighing 1.2 kg.

Histopathological examination of the excised specimen gave a gross appearance of a partially encapsulated mass containing myoepithelial and ductal proliferation. There was marked stromal hyalinization, squamous metaplasia, and keratinization. Some epithelial islands exhibited papillary configuration, along with large cysts and inflammation. Chondromyxoid changes and fibrosis were evident throughout the tumor. Certain foci of tumor islands were seen approaching and breaking through it. Hematoxylin and eosin (H&E) stained sections revealed a partially encapsulated tumor with variable histopathological features and focal effacement of the fibrous capsule. The tumor typically showed epithelial/myoepithelial proliferation punctuated by chondromyxoid areas. Aggregates of plasmacytoid myoepithelial cells as well as ducal differentiation surrounded by clear myoepithelial cells were evident. Based on the above findings, a final diagnosis of benign PA was reached. While the tumor sections showed no evidence of malignant change, there was extensive squamous metaplasia and keratin cyst formation, which were atypical for PA (Figure 4). The patient was therefore advised close follow-up, once every month for the first year postoperatively and subsequently once in six months.

At 6 weeks postsurgery, the patient had unremarkable wound healing without any neurological deficit of the facial nerve (Figure 5). As of December 2019, the patient had a recurrence-free follow-up period of 7 years and presented with normal activity of muscles of facial expression, indicating the absence of any long-term facial nerve weakness (Figure 6).

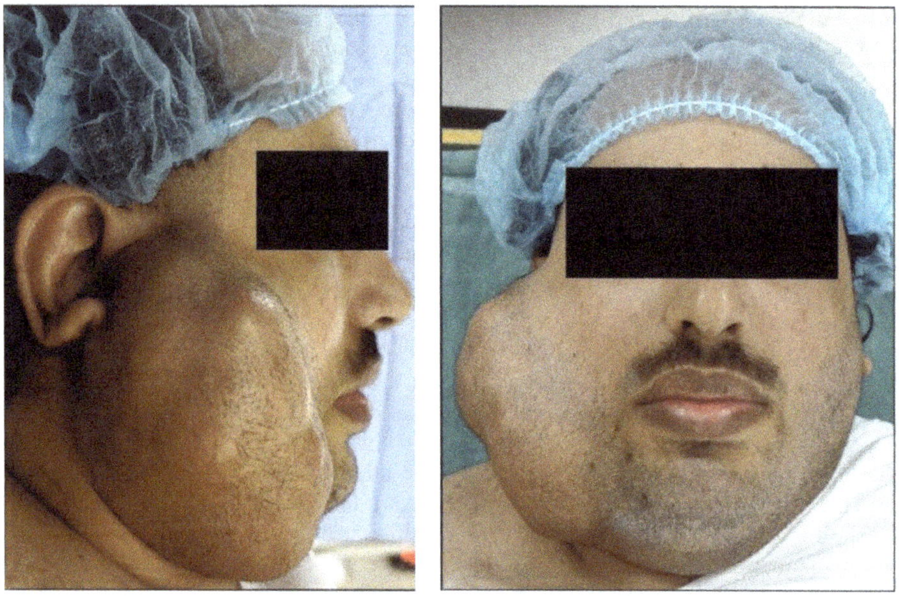

(a) (b)

FIGURE 1: Preoperative clinical photograph of the right preauricular swelling. (a) Right lateral facial view shows the swelling extending superoinferiorly from a point anterior to the helix of the external ear until the lower border of the mandible; anteroposteriorly, the swelling is seen extending from the angle of the mouth to the posterior border of the mandible; the ear lobe is deflected outward and elevated, and the skin overlying the swelling appears free of any ulceration, puckering, or discharge. (b) Frontal facial view shows the swelling causing facial asymmetry and obliterating the view of most of the right external ear; there is no clinical evidence of facial nerve weakness or deficit.

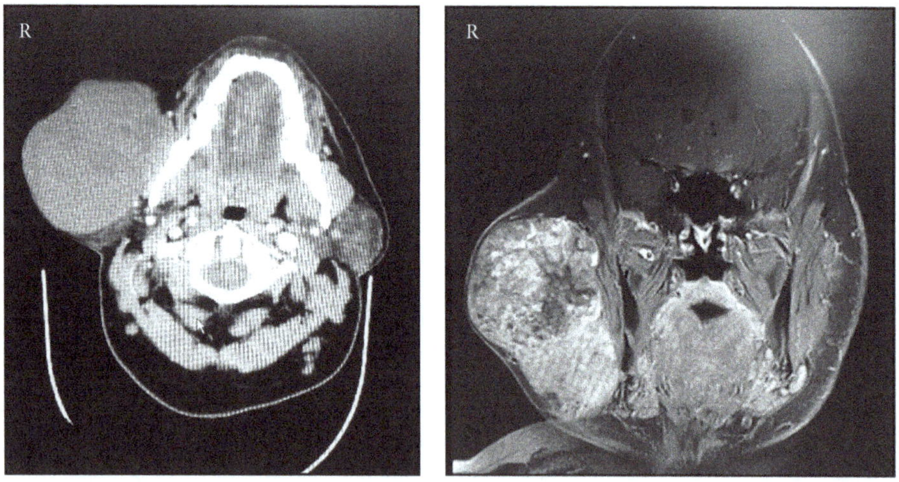

(a) (b)

FIGURE 2: Preoperative radiographic examination of the right preauricular swelling. (a) Contrast-enhanced computed tomography axial section at the level of mandibular teeth shows a well-defined mass lesion in the superficial lobe of the right parotid gland, without any underlying bony erosion and normal-appearing pharynx, larynx, and parapharyngeal spaces. (b) Magnetic resonance imaging coronal section along the posterior border of the mandible shows a large, heterogeneous, well-demarcated solid mass lesion within the right parotid superficial lobe and measuring $10 \times 7 \times 8$ cm at maximum dimensions.

3. Discussion

The parotid gland is the largest salivary gland with an average weight ranging from 0.015 to 0.021 kg and measuring approximately 5.8×3.4 cm in the craniocaudal and ventrodorsal dimensions, respectively. Being the first salivary gland to develop in utero, during the 6th gestational week, it is anatomically located bilaterally between the mastoid process of temporal bone and ramus of the mandible. The terminal branches of the facial nerve are an important anatomic landmark which divide the parotid gland into its superficial and deep lobes [33]. Although SGT are uncommon, they are

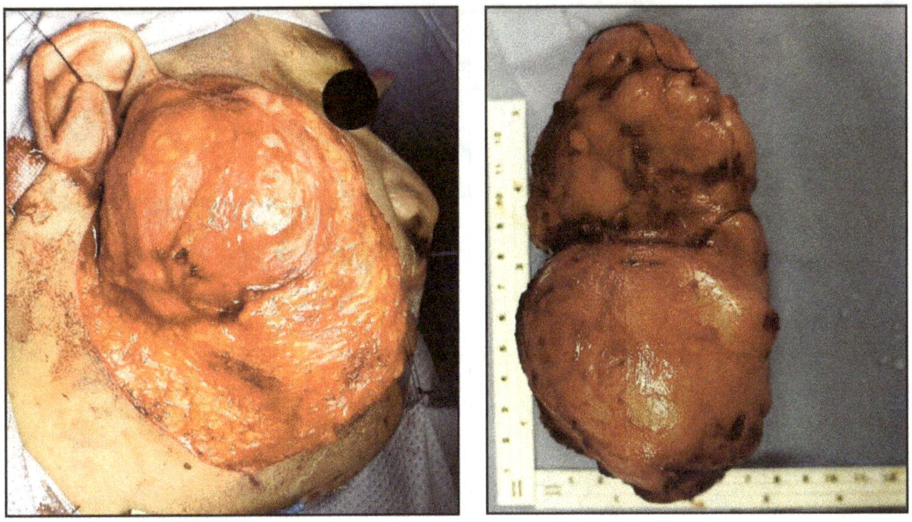

(a) (b)

FIGURE 3: Intraoperative photograph showing (a) the surgical plane for extracapsular dissection of the right parotid tumor and (b) the excised tumor specimen.

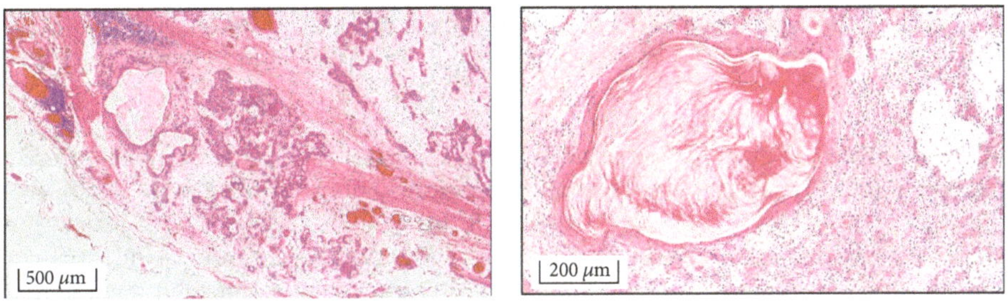

(a) (b)

FIGURE 4: Histological examination of the excised tumor specimen showing (a) a partially encapsulated mass lesion containing myoepithelial and ductal proliferation, with stromal hyalinization, squamous metaplasia, and keratinization; epithelial islands exhibiting papillary configuration, large cysts surrounded by inflammation, focal areas of chondromyxoid changes and fibrosis, and tumor islands approaching and penetrating the capsule are evident (HE original magnification ×4); (b) extensive squamous metaplasia and keratin cyst formation are conspicuous at higher magnification (HE original magnification ×10).

predominantly benign and are reported frequently in the parotid gland [2]. The present report details a case of giant PA in the right parotid gland, along with its surgical management, histological presentation, and long-term recurrence-free follow-up.

Pleomorphic adenoma is the commonest mixed SGT arising in the parotid gland, and several cases have been reported in the literature. Although there are no specific physical criteria outlined in the literature to classify giant parotid PA, the earliest recorded case report dates back to 1863 [27]. In this report, Spence reported a mixed tumor involving lateral face and neck and a resected mass weighing greater than 1 kg [27]. Similarly, Short and Pullar (1956) reviewed and reported a case of giant parotid PA weighing about 2.3 kg [27]. In a report reviewing 31 cases of giant parotid PA over a period of 140 years by Schultz-Coulon, the resected tumor weights ranged from 1.0 to 26.50 kg, with a greater female predilection (64.5%) and only 3 cases of malignant transformation [15]. Based on a review of the 10 largest parotid PA published between 1863 and 1994, Buenting et al. reported resected tumors ranging in weight from 2.83 to 26.50 kg, in patients with age ranging from 25 to 85 years and 90% female predilection [10].

A literature search was conducted to review giant parotid PA cases reported in Medline, Scopus, and Google Scholar databases. The search strategy involved a combination of search keywords including "GIANT", "PAROTID GLAND", and "PLEOMORPHIC ADENOMA", based on which 288 articles were identified from the three databases (Medline—66; Scopus—63; Google Scholar—159). Reviewing their abstracts, articles published in English only were selected based on them reporting a case or series of cases of giant parotid PA, including clinical, radiographic, histological, and surgical outcomes. Twenty-six articles published in English language were identified [4, 8–32] since 1995, and they reported 43 cases of PA in total. While most of the articles selected for review were single case reports, three articles were case series reporting about two cases [16], three cases

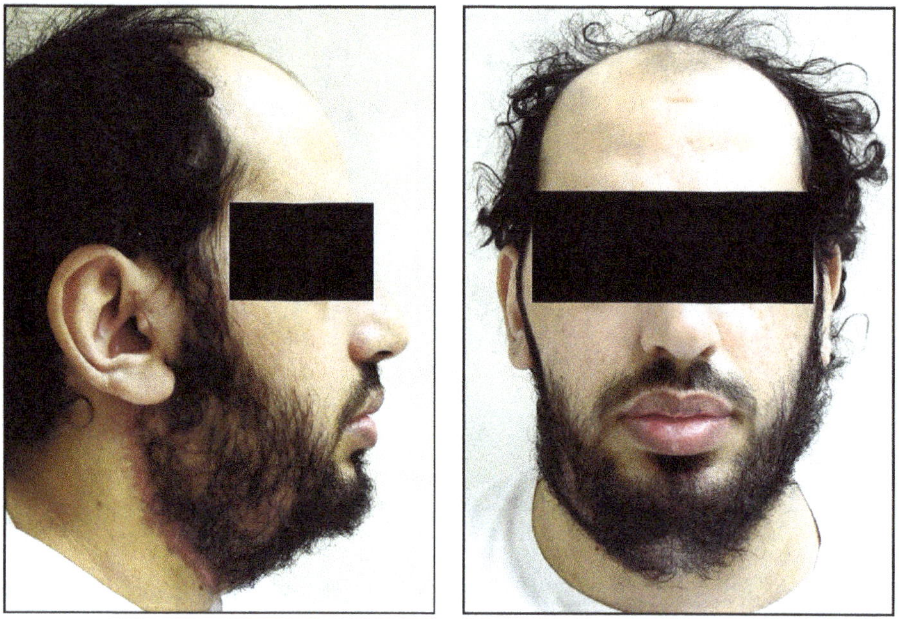

(a) (b)

FIGURE 5: Postoperative clinical photograph taken 6 weeks postsurgery. (a) Lateral facial view shows healing surgical incision without any obvious postoperative sequelae. (b) Symmetric facial appearance observed in the frontal facial view, with no clinical weakness of muscles of facial expression.

[17], and 15 cases [32], respectively. The largest case series in the present review, comprising 15 PA patients, was reported by Pareek et al. [32].

Although majority of the reported cases were in patients aged 45 years or older ($n = 30$, 69.8%), the age at clinical presentation and surgery ranged from 21 to 92 years. The asymptomatic, slow-growing nature of pleomorphic adenoma was evidenced by the fact that the duration from the first observation of lesion to reporting for treatment varied from 5 to 35 years. Demographically, there were more females ($n = 25$, 58.1%) than males, and all reported cases were unilateral, with the right side ($n = 23$, 53.5%) affected more than the left. In terms of clinical dimension, the tumors ranged from 3 to 5 cm in diameter [16, 17], until 35 × 28 cm [27], in two perpendicular planes. The clinical dimensions corroborated with the resected tumor weight, wherein the smallest tumor weighed 0.12 kg [16] and the largest weighed 7.3 kg [27]. Predominant clinical presentation of the tumors was that of a large, lobulated, and pedunculated mass with apparently normal overlying skin. Ulceration of the skin was reported in eight patients, out of which five were reportedly associated with malignant change [15, 23, 24, 30, 32], and the remaining three were due to injury [18, 29, 32]. Anatomically, the tumor more commonly involved the superficial lobe of the parotid gland ($n = 29$, 70.7%) giving rise to the clinical presentation of a large preauricular mass. Nevertheless, when the deep lobe of parotid and parapharyngeal spaces were involved by the tumor, patients presented with an intraoral swelling leading to soft palate displacement, difficulty in swallowing and breathing, and obstructive sleep apnea [11, 13, 16, 17, 22, 25]. While diagnosis was primarily based on clinical and radiographic (USG, CT, and MRI) findings, preoperative diagnosis was established through FNAC in most cases. The clinical, radiographic, surgical, and histological findings in the reviewed case reports are detailed in Table 1.

Preoperative diagnosis of PA is routinely based on clinical findings, supplemented by radiological investigations such as CT, MRI, and USG [2]. The role of FNAC in arriving at a provisional diagnosis has been debated and considered nonrepresentative due to varying histological patterns at different sites within the same tumor [34]. In terms of histopathological diagnosis, the characteristic feature of PA is its histological diversity and differing arrangements of epithelial and mesenchymal tissue elements. Das and Anim [34], based on a study comparing FNAC and histological sections in PA, reported consistent findings of epithelial cells in a myxoid stroma through cytological and histological examination. Nevertheless, they reported better characterization of oncocytic changes such as acini, giant cell and mucus globule formation, and squamous and chondroid metaplasia in histological sections [34]. Preoperative diagnosis of PA in the present case was based on a combination of clinical examination, radiographic investigations, and FNAC. Our radiographic finding (CT and MRI) of well-demarcated, lobulated, and heterogeneous mass lesion involving the parotid gland and FNAC finding of plasmacytoid epithelial cells in a chondromyxoid matrix were in coherence with the majority of cases reported in the review (Table 1). Additionally, necrotic changes [10, 24, 30] and calcifications [4, 30], within the tumor, have also been reported in the literature, based on CT and in association with malignant change [24, 30]. The combination of CT and MRI enables optimum preoperative diagnosis of pleomorphic adenomas and precise planning of the surgical approach for tumor resection [11]. In addition to volumetric information, CT with contrast provides

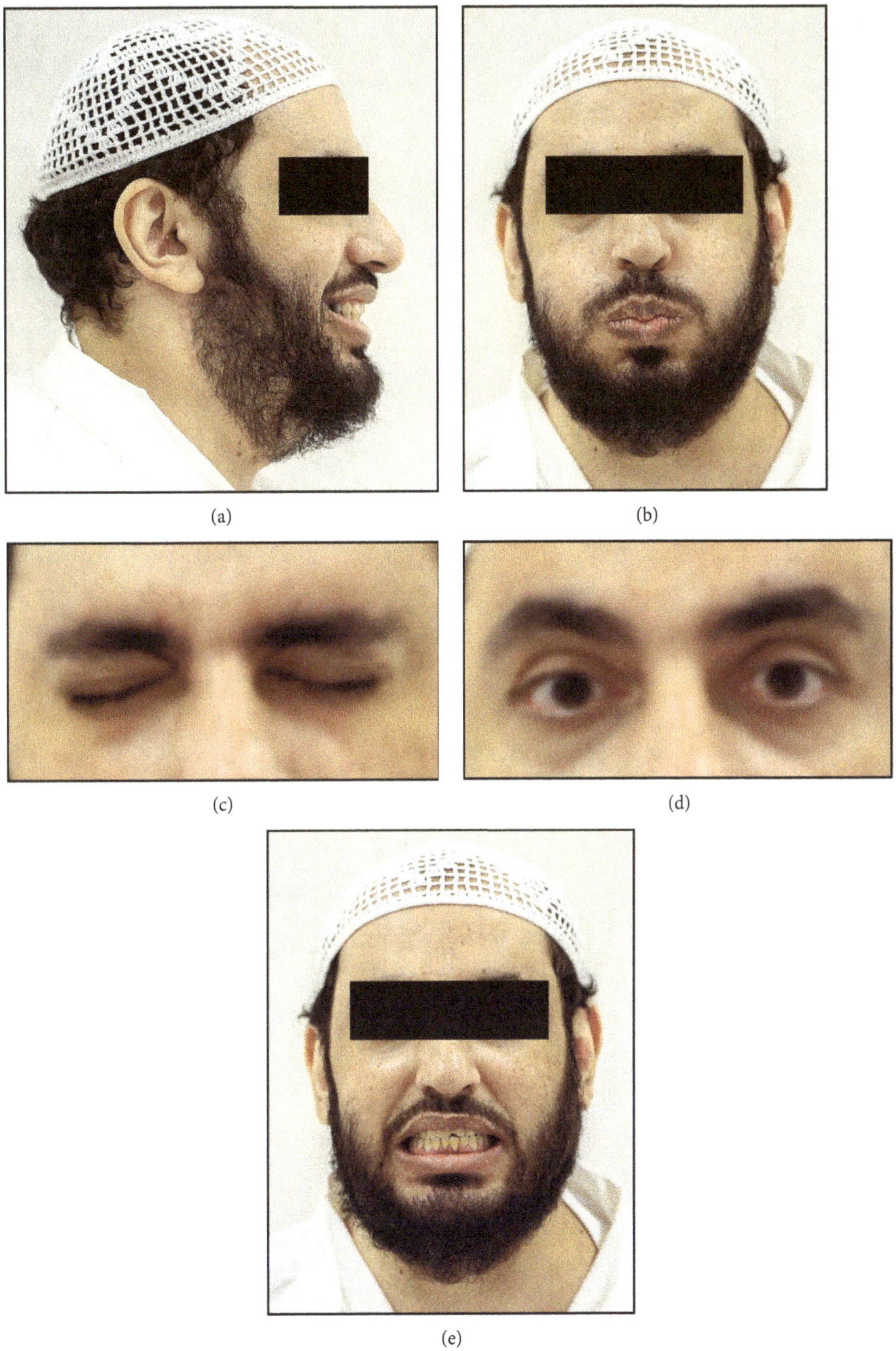

FIGURE 6: Postoperative clinical photograph taken 7 years postsurgery with facial gestures eliciting unrestrained action of different muscles of facial expression. (a) Unremarkable healing of the surgical wound without any scarring and the patient is seen smiling. (b) Frontal facial view showing symmetric appearance and the patient is seen puffing the cheeks. (c, d) Bilateral symmetric eyelid closure and opening. (e) The patient is seen grinning broadly.

knowledge about vascularity of the tumor and MRI shows the relationship of the tumor to surrounding vital structures in the head and neck regions [11].

The treatment of PA irrespective of their size, severity, or malignant potential is only by surgery. Based on our literature review, giant PA involving the superficial lobe of parotid was managed either by SP or ECD [4, 10, 24, 26–29, 31, 32]. On the contrary, TP was reportedly done for tumors exhibiting malignant characteristics [8, 12, 15, 17, 19, 20, 23, 30] and those involving both the deep and superficial lobes [9, 13, 14,

TABLE 1: Review of giant parotid pleomorphic adenoma case reports and their demographic, clinical, radiographic, surgical, and histological findings.

	Patient demographics				Preoperative evaluation		Surgical intervention			Postoperative period		
Author (year)	Age (in years)/gender	Duration of lesion	Affected side	Clinical dimension	Clinical presentation	Investigations	Procedure	Resected dimension	Reason for surgery	Histological findings	Postoperative course	Follow-up
Alvarez-Cañas and Rodilla (1996) [8]	86/F	15 years	Left		Large painless preauricular mass which enlarged suddenly over the past 1 year and associated with facial nerve deficit	Only clinical examination	Total parotidectomy	9.5 × 8 × 7 cm	Sudden increase in size with facial nerve deficit	Mixed malignant transformation of PA with salivary ductal carcinoma and high-grade fibrosarcoma elements		Patient developed local recurrence of tumor and died 6 months after surgery
Lomeo (1996) [9]	74/F	35 years	Left		Large preauricular mass	Only clinical examination	Total parotidectomy		Patient was convinced for surgery by grandchildren	Pleomorphic adenoma		
Buenting et al. (1998) [10]	85/F	20 years	Right		Large, multinodular preauricular mass with evidence of infection. The mass was tensely cystic and had prominent veins near the base	CT showed a parotid mass 14 cm across with extensive necrotic foci and numerous feeding vessels, which were not amenable to embolization	Extracapsular dissection of the tumor mass	26 cm diameter (6.85 kg)	Inadvertent injury to the base of the mass resulting in bleeding and infection	Pleomorphic adenoma with extensive necrosis and cartilaginous metaplasia		1-year recurrence-free follow-up
Rodriguez-Ciurana et al. (2000) [11]	48/F	30 years	Right		Large mass in the submandibular and laterocervical regions, extending intraorally from soft-palate to floor of mouth	MRI showed a mass involving the deep lobe of the parotid gland, extending into parapharyngeal, prestyloid, and submandibular spaces, displacing external and internal carotid arteries and thinning the ramus of mandible. Measuring 6 × 5 × 4 cm. FNAC was indicative of PA	Deep lobe parotidectomy through cervical transparotid approach			Pleomorphic adenoma	Transient facial nerve weakness for 4 weeks	
Manuel (2002) [12]	68/F		Left		Recurrent parotid mass which was incompletely excised earlier and diagnosed as mixed malignant tumor		Total parotidectomy, with removal of facial nerve branches due to tumor infiltration and modified neck dissection		Recurrent lesion in the previously excised tumor site	Carcinosarcoma arising from PA, with residual PA, epimyoepithelial carcinoma, and pleomorphic sarcoma. Multiple metastatic cervical lymph nodes		Patient was operated for metastatic anterior chest wall mass, 7 months postsurgery and had an 18-month disease-free follow-up

Table 1: Continued.

Author (year)	Patient demographics Age (in years)/gender	Duration of lesion	Affected side	Clinical dimension	Preoperative evaluation Clinical presentation	Investigations	Surgical intervention Procedure	Resected dimension	Reason for surgery	Postoperative period Histological findings	Postoperative course	Follow-up
Panoussopoulos et al. (2002) [13]	63/M	30 years	Left	13 × 12 cm	Large, lobulated mass in the submandibular, preauricular, and laterocervical regions, extending intraorally to the lateral pharyngeal wall at the level of tongue	MRI showed a well-defined mass involving both superficial and deep lobes of the parotid gland, and extending into the parapharyngeal space, displacing tissues deep to the tonsil	Total parotidectomy through cervical transparotid approach			Pleomorphic adenoma		
de Silva et al. (2004) [14]	76/M	>30 years	Left	20 × 30 cm	Large, oval preauricular swelling, firm in consistency, with venous engorgement on overlying skin and movable	FNAC was indicative of PA	Total parotidectomy with preservation of facial nerve	20 × 14 × 12 cm (3.5 kg)		Pleomorphic adenoma	Facial nerve deficit observed 1 week postoperatively and recovered 90% by 1 month	1-year recurrence-free follow-up and complete recovery of facial nerve function
Honda et al. (2005) [15]	72/F	20 years	Left		Large, pedunculated preauricular mass extending up to the submandibular region, with a history of rapid growth in preceding 3 months and 2 areas of ulceration with yellowish, foul-smelling discharge in the lower part of the mass. An associated anterior chest wall mass measuring 10 × 8 cm was clinically identified	CT showed a mass with multiple encapsulated nodules involving the entire parotid gland, having several feeder vessels and supplied predominantly by the transverse facial artery. Coincidental finding of abnormal skull base lesion measuring 4 cm in diameter. Chest radiograph revealed multiple metastatic nodules, measuring around 1 cm, in both lungs	Total parotidectomy + simultaneous resection of anterior chest wall mass	33 × 18 × 17.5 cm exophytic tumor (6.051 kg)	Sudden increase in size with ulceration and discharge	Pleomorphic adenoma with focal areas of malignant adenocarcinoma cells with hyperchromatic nuclei and increased mitotic figures. Similar histological findings observed in the resected anterior chest wall mass		Patient died 6 months postsurgery, due to metastatic lung disease

Table 1: Continued.

Author (year)	Patient demographics: Age (in years)/gender	Duration of lesion	Affected side	Clinical dimension	Preoperative evaluation: Clinical presentation	Investigations	Surgical intervention: Procedure	Resected dimension	Reason for surgery	Postoperative period: Histological findings	Postoperative course	Follow-up
Ruiz-Laza et al. (2006) [16]	54/M	5 years	Left	3 cm	Solid mass in preauricular and mandibular angle regions	MRI showed a multilobulated mass measuring 8 cm in diameter and extending from deep lobe of the parotid gland into parapharyngeal space, displacing the pharyngeal airway medially and the jugular and carotid vessels posteriorly. FNAC was indicative of PA	Total parotidectomy through cervical transparotid approach and facial nerve preservation			Pleomorphic adenoma	Postoperative facial nerve deficit which recovered completely in 6 months	3-year recurrence-free follow-up
Ruiz-Laza et al. (2006) [16]	21/M		Right		Intraoral mass occupying the entire soft palate with no other associated symptoms	MRI showed a well-defined mass lesion measuring 6 × 5 × 4 cm in the parapharyngeal space and with apparent continuity to the deep lobe of the parotid gland. FNAC was indicative of PA	Surgical excision of tumor mass only, through intraoral approach and "Double-Y" incision in soft palate	11 × 10 cm (0.12 kg)		Pleomorphic adenoma		3-year recurrence-free follow-up
Sergi et al. (2008) [17]	36/M	1 year	Left	5 cm	Solid preauricular mass	USG showed two hypoechogenic, lobulated masses measuring 2.5 × 1.9 × 1.6 cm in the deep lobe of the parotid gland and 4.4 × 5.1 × 4.6 cm posterior to mandibular ramus. MRI revealed expansive mass measuring about 5 cm in the deep lobe of the parotid gland, extending from mandibular angle to lateral pharyngeal wall medially	Using cervical transparotid approach, superficial and deep lobe parotidectomy performed separately to preserve facial nerve branches			Pleomorphic adenoma	Transient neurological deficit of marginal mandibular branch of facial nerve	

Table 1: Continued.

Author (year)	Patient demographics: Age (in years)/gender	Duration of lesion	Affected side	Clinical dimension	Preoperative evaluation: Clinical presentation	Investigations	Surgical intervention: Procedure	Resected dimension	Reason for surgery	Postoperative period: Histological findings	Postoperative course	Follow-up
Sergi et al. (2008) [17]	42/M		Right	3 cm	Solid preauricular mass	MRI showed a mass in the deep lobe of the parotid gland, extending into parapharyngeal space and displacing the pharyngeal muscles medially. FNAC was indicative of PA	Using cervical transparotid approach, superficial and deep lobe parotidectomy performed separately to preserve facial nerve branches		Increased in size over 2 months	Pleomorphic adenoma		
Sergi et al. (2008) [17]	38/F		Left		No extraoral swelling. Intraoral mass lateral to the soft palate and displacing it across the midline	MRI showed inhomogeneous, expansive mass arising from the deep lobe of the parotid gland and measuring 5.5 × 5.5 cm in the lateral pharyngeal space. The mass was seen displacing the pterygoid and pharyngeal muscles medially. FNAC was indicative of PA	Separate superficial and deep lobe parotidectomy through transcervical, mandibular split approach to preserve facial nerve branches		Pain while swallowing and sensation of foreign body in the throat since 5 months	Pleomorphic adenoma with a nucleus of carcinoma ex-PA	Postoperative radiotherapy	
Takahama et al. (2008) [18]	78/M	>30 years	Right	30 cm	Large, multinodular preauricular mass extending to the submandibular region and crossing the midline. Focal areas of ulceration in the lower part of the mass	Only clinical examination	Total parotidectomy	28 × 20 × 16 cm (4.0 kg)		Pleomorphic adenoma		
Bhutta (2009) [19]	63/F		Left		Slow-growing mass in the left superficial parotid	Only clinical examination	Excision done in 1993, followed by multiple recurrences managed surgically through excision from 1995-2006			Early lesion was suggestive of PA. Recurrent lesions resembled PA with high mitotic rate and no malignancy	45 Gy external beam radiation therapy (in 25 fractions) given in 2000 to prevent recurrence	In 2006, CT showed a right kidney mass, diagnosed as metastasizing PA by histology (typical features of PA with positive Ki67 staining)

Table 1: Continued.

	Patient demographics				Preoperative evaluation		Surgical intervention			Postoperative period		
Author (year)	Age (in years)/gender	Duration of lesion	Affected side	Clinical dimension	Clinical presentation	Investigations	Procedure	Resected dimension	Reason for surgery	Histological findings	Postoperative course	Follow-up
Karpowicz et al. (2010) [20]	45/M		Right		Subcutaneous parotid mass with ipsilateral cervical lymphadenopathy involving multiple nodes. Associated with severe pain and rapid increase in size. Clinically staged as stage Iva malignant disease	Only clinical examination	Total parotidectomy with comprehensive neck dissection	Nonencapsulated tumor measuring about 3.5 cm	Severe pain and rapid increase in size	Malignant epithelial cells in a chondromyxoid stroma indicative of carcinoma ex-PA. Malignant foci included high-grade squamous cell carcinoma and adenocarcinoma. One of the cervical lymph nodes showed evidence of metastatic carcinoma. Immunohistochemistry identified a melanoma component	Two months postsurgery, the patient reported severe pelvic pain, diagnosed as metastatic bone disease through MRI	Patient died 3 months postsurgery due to metastatic disease
Cetin et al. (2012) [21]	55/F	20 years	Left	15 × 15 × 20 cm	Large preauricular mass extending to cervical regions, with overlying skin atrophic and vascular	USG showed a lobulated mass in the parotid gland with both homogeneous and heterogeneous echotextures	Total parotidectomy			Pleomorphic adenoma		
Morariu et al. (2012) [22]	42/M		Right		Large mass arising from the lateral pharyngeal wall, displacing the soft palate and uvula, and narrowing the pharyngeal airway. Associated symptoms of painful swallowing, heavy snoring, and sleep apnea for past 1 year	MRI showed a circumscribed mass lesion 7 × 6 × 4 cm extending from the deep lobe of the parotid gland into the parapharyngeal space with fluid spaces and septation. CT angiogram while showing splayed internal and external carotid arteries, ruled out any abnormal vascularity. Transoral FNAC was indicative of PA	Deep lobe parotidectomy through transparotid approach		Pharyngodynia and nocturnal hypoxia symptoms	Pleomorphic adenoma	Patient reported relief from nocturnal hypoxia, snoring, and sleep apnea symptoms, postoperatively	6-month recurrence-free follow-up

Table 1: Continued.

Author (year)	Patient demographics: Age (in years)/gender	Duration of lesion	Affected side	Preoperative evaluation: Clinical dimension	Clinical presentation	Investigations	Surgical intervention: Procedure	Resected dimension	Reason for surgery	Postoperative period: Histological findings	Postoperative course	Follow-up
Yoshida et al. (2013) [23]	40/F	17 years	Left		Small parotid swelling before 17 years, diagnosed as PA by FNAC. Surgery delayed for 10 years due to patient's fear and then lost to follow-up. Swelling grew rapidly in past 6 months, causing gait disturbance and skin ulceration with foul-smelling, bloody discharge from the lower part of lesion	CT showed a nodular mass arising from the parotid gland and attached in its deeper aspect to the carotid sheath. Evidence of metastasis in chest radiograph owing to bilateral hilar lymphadenopathy and coin-shaped radiolucency in the right lung. Incision biopsy was indicative of PA, with clinical suspicion of malignancy	Total parotidectomy and en bloc resection of the tumor along with the lower portion of the auricle	25 × 28 × 18 cm (4.80 kg)	Rapid growth of tumor in last 6 months with cervical and thoracic scoliosis and gait disturbance	Nearly 80% of the resected tumor sections showed evidence of PA. Sections of the tumor near the ulcerated areas showed undifferentiated malignant cells indicative of carcinoma ex-PA	Postoperative adjuvant chemotherapy for metastasis	6-month follow-up with no local recurrence
Pamuk et al. (2014) [24]	82/F	20 years	Right	13 × 13 × 10 cm	Large, multilobular preauricular mass with areas of ulceration and necrosis on overlying skin	CT showed a giant, exophytic mass in the superficial lobe of the parotid gland with multiple necrotic spaces and enhanced vascularity. Incisional biopsy was indicative of a salivary gland neoplasm without ruling out malignant transformation	Superficial parotidectomy with excision of overlying ulcerated skin	14 × 12 × 9 cm		Pleomorphic adenoma with multiple foci of neoplastic proliferation, along with cellular atypia and necrosis. Final diagnosis carcinoma ex-PA	Postoperative radiotherapy 60 Gy	Patient died 8 months postsurgery due to cerebrovascular accident
Datarkar and Deshpande (2014) [25]	40/F		Right		Large, firm intraoral mass arising from the lateral pharyngeal wall, displacing the soft palate and crossing midline. Associated symptoms of difficulty in swallowing and breathing, and sleep apnea for past 6 months	CT showed parapharyngeal space mass extending medially across the midline and laterally between the posterior border of ramus and styloid process. MRI showed lobulated, homogeneous mass lesion extending	Deep lobe parotidectomy through transcervical, mandibular split osteotomy approach	5.5 × 6.5 × 3.5 cm	Difficulty in swallowing and breathing, and sleep apnea	Pleomorphic adenoma	Patient reported relief from sleep apnea symptoms, postoperatively	

Table 1: Continued.

Author (year)	Patient demographics: Age (in years)/gender	Duration of lesion	Affected side	Clinical dimension	Preoperative evaluation: Clinical presentation	Investigations	Surgical intervention: Procedure	Resected dimension	Reason for surgery	Postoperative period: Histological findings	Postoperative course	Follow-up
						from the deep lobe of the parotid gland with hypointense septae and measuring 5.4 × 6.5 × 3.5 cm, and indenting on lateral pharyngeal wall. No involvement of skull base or intracranial extension was observed. Transoral FNAC was indicative of PA						
Sajid et al. (2015) [26]	47/M	>7 years	Right	26 × 20 cm	Large, nodular preauricular mass extending up to submandibular region inferiorly and anteriorly up to 2 cm posterior to the nasolabial fold	MRI showed a heterogeneous, lobulated mass in the superficial lobe of the parotid gland, extending medially up to sternomastoid and carotid sheath. FNAC was indicative of PA	Superficial parotidectomy with excision of redundant skin	22 × 24 × 12 cm (1.8 kg)		Pleomorphic adenoma		
Tarsitano et al. (2015) [27]	83/M	>30 years	Left	35 × 28 cm	Giant, multinodular, pedunculated mass in the preauricular region, extending up to the cervical region	MRI showed a giant, heterogeneous mass arising from the superficial lobe of the parotid gland, with well-demarcated boundaries and preservation of surrounding tissue planes. CT revealed primary blood supply though facial artery and numerous small feeder vessels. Incisional biopsy confirmed the diagnosis of PA	Extracapsular dissection of the tumor mass	33 × 27 × 16 cm (7.3 kg)	The mass became too big and a hindrance for the patient to ambulate	Pleomorphic adenoma		5-year recurrence-free follow-up

Table 1: Continued.

	Patient demographics			Preoperative evaluation			Surgical intervention			Postoperative period		
Author (year)	Age (in years)/gender	Duration of lesion	Affected side	Clinical dimension	Clinical presentation	Investigations	Procedure	Resected dimension	Reason for surgery	Histological findings	Postoperative course	Follow-up
Akintububo et al. (2016) [4]	60/M	>10 years	Left	25 × 23 × 17 cm	Giant, lobulated, and pedunculated mass in the preauricular region, extending up to cervical region, with firm consistency and measuring almost the size of the patient's head	CT showed a large soft tissue mass arising from the superficial lobe of the parotid gland and presenting with several amorphous calcifications, but without any bony involvement. FNAC was indicative of PA	Superficial parotidectomy	(5.5 kg)	Patient had delayed surgery due to financial constraints	Pleomorphic adenoma with multiple foci of microcalcifications	Reactionary hemorrhage in the immediate postoperative period, managed through exploratory ligation. Transient neurological deficit of the buccal branch of facial nerve	6-month recurrence-free follow-up
Calvo-Henriquez et al. (2016) [28]	72/F	14 years	Right	20 × 15 cm	Giant preauricular mass, fixed to underlying tissues and associated with facial nerve deficit (House-Brackman Grade III)	CT showed a well-defined parotid mass with mixed solid and cystic areas. The mass extended superiorly up to temporal muscle and cervically up to the hyoid bone. FNAC was indicative of mixed tumor of salivary gland origin	Extracapsular dissection of tumor mass along with a superficial skin island	(1.6 kg)			Facial nerve deficit (House-Brackman Grade III) persisted postoperatively	
Swain (2016) [29]	92/M	>25 years	Right	20 × 15 cm	Large, multinodular preauricular mass with skin ulceration due to repeated trauma for past 6 months	CT showed a well-defined mass involving the superficial lobe of the parotid gland. FNAC was indicative of PA	Superficial parotidectomy with preservation of facial nerve branches		Skin ulceration due to repeated trauma for past 6 months	Pleomorphic adenoma		
Chao et al. (2017) [30]	83/F	>20 years	Right		Patient presented with a slow-growing, preauricular mass 1 year ago which was provisionally identified as PA through FNAC. Patient however delayed surgery due to personal reasons. Rapidly proliferating	CT showed a heterogeneous parotid mass measuring 9 × 8.4 cm with foci of necrosis and calcification. The mass was in close proximity to inferior aspect of external auditory canal and was invading	En bloc resection with total parotidectomy. Facial nerve branches except the buccal branch were preserved. The buccal branch was encased in tumor. Selective neck dissection (levels I-III) along with resection of	10.5 cm diameter	Rapid growth with skin ulceration in the last 1 year	True malignant mixed tumor with extensive foci of necrosis and poorly differentiated adenocarcinoma and chondrosarcoma components. No histological evidence of original PA seen	Postoperative radiotherapy 60 Gy	At 3-year follow-up, no loco regional recurrence was observed. Patient however presented with lung and liver nodules on PET scan

TABLE 1: Continued.

	Patient demographics			Preoperative evaluation			Surgical intervention			Postoperative period		
Author (year)	Age (in years)/gender	Duration of lesion	Affected side	Clinical dimension	Clinical presentation	Investigations	Procedure	Resected dimension	Reason for surgery	Histological findings	Postoperative course	Follow-up
					exophytic, firm, multilobulated growth with skin ulceration and bleeding were seen in the same lesion in the last 1 year. Facial nerve function was intact	sternomastoid and masseter muscles. Superficially skin erosion was seen. No evidence of lymph node or bony involvement. FNAC was suggestive of carcinoma ex-PA	infratemporal and parapharyngeal spaces. Soft-tissue reconstruction with anterolateral thigh free flap					
Alnofaie et al. (2020) [31]	25/F	10 years	Right	25 × 25 × 15 cm	Irregular, multilobulated, giant mass with a sessile base in the right parotid region extending to the neck. Overlying skin appeared erythematous with prominent vasculature and no discharge. Swelling was fixed to underlying tissues and facial nerve function was unaffected	CT showed a heterogeneous mass lesion arising from the parotid. MRI showed a lobulated heterogeneous mass with multilocular cystic changes and measuring 12 × 10 × 12 cm. No extension to retromandibular or parapharyngeal spaces. FNAC was suggestive of PA	Superficial parotidectomy with preservation of facial nerve branches	18 × 17 × 11.5 cm (1.5 kg)	Patient was mentally challenged and patient's mother requested surgery as the mass had become too large and hindered daily activities	Pleomorphic adenoma		1-year recurrence-free follow-up
Pareek et al. (2020) [32] (case series comprising 15 giant parotid PA)	30-81 years (mean—50.3)/5 males and 10 females	5-20 years	Right—9; left—6	All lesions were greater than 10 cm in diameter (range 10-25 cm)	Majority of the lesions presented as irregular or ovoid parotid masses with well-defined margins and overlying skin was ulcerated in 2 cases. None of the cases had preoperative facial nerve weakness	A combination of USG, CT, MRI, and FNAC to arrive at a provisional diagnosis of PA. One case was preoperatively diagnosed with malignant change based on FNAC	Total parotidectomy—10; total parotidectomy + neck dissection—1; superficial parotidectomy—3; enucleation—1. Facial nerve preserved in all cases	(2.0-3.5 kg; mean—2.7)	Majority of the patients delayed surgery due to poor awareness and underprivileged socioeconomic status	All cases were histologically confirmed as PA, except one case which showed a malignant change	Transient facial nerve deficit in 2 patients which recovered within 6 months. Postoperative radiotherapy only for the malignant case	Minimum 6-month recurrence-free follow-up

M: male/F: female; CT: computed tomography; MRI: magnetic resonance imaging; FNAC: fine-needle aspiration cytology; PA: pleomorphic adenoma; USG: ultrasonography; PET: positron emission tomography.

16–18, 21, 32] (Table 1). Since the present case was that of a PA involving superficial parotid only (Figures 1 and 2), the patient was surgically managed through ECD (Figure 3), avoiding any iatrogenic damage to the facial nerve (Figure 5). The surgical techniques for resecting PA have evolved over the last century and have essentially focused on preserving anatomic and functional integrity of the facial nerve and its branches [1, 7]. While intracapsular removal was advocated, during the late 19th and early 20th centuries in an attempt to avoid facial nerve injury, the technique was abandoned due to its high risk of recurrence (≥45%) [1, 7]. This leads to the popularity of SP, associated with a very low recurrence rate (≤2%), but still carrying a risk of facial nerve injury, Frey syndrome, and loss of facial contour [1]. In the last 2-3 decades, ECD has gained significance as a surgical technique which involves tumor resection along with the capsule and a thin rim of extracapsular normal tissue, without attempting to identify or dissect the facial nerve and its branches [1]. Based on literature reviews, Kato et al. [1] and Bonavolontà et al. [7] reported that ECD is safe, is economical, and reduces operating time and risk of morbidity. They further considered it as the treatment of choice for mobile, benign tumors involving the superficial lobe of the parotid gland [1, 7]. Moreover, traction due to gravity in giant PA causes the tumor mass to descend away from the facial nerve and its branches, thereby facilitating ease of dissection, as encountered in the present case [10].

Several surgical approaches to remove PA and other benign parotid gland tumors involving the deep lobe and extending to the lateral pharyngeal and parapharyngeal spaces have been reported [11]. These include cervical, cervical-transpharyngeal, infratemporal fossa, parotid-cervical, transoral, and transparotid approaches. In the present review, 9 cases of PA were reportedly involving the deep lobe of parotid and extending into pharyngeal spaces. The cervical-transparotid surgical approach was used for resection in 6 cases [11, 13, 16, 17, 22], a transcervical, split-mandibulotomy approach was used in 2 cases [17, 25], and one case was managed through a transoral approach using "Double-Y" incision in soft palate [16] (Table 1). Postoperative complications following surgical resection of parotid PA are similar to that of other benign SGT [1, 4, 7, 23]. These include hemorrhage, hematoma, seroma, fistula, hypoesthesia, scarring, Frey syndrome, transient facial nerve injury, and facial paralysis [7]. While these complications are reportedly associated with all surgical techniques mentioned before, ECD was associated with a significantly lower risk of hypoesthesia, Frey syndrome, and facial nerve injury and paralysis [7]. Nevertheless, when dealing with large parotid tumors with suspected malignancy, which mandate identification and dissection of facial nerve branches, no significant differences were observed in the outcomes and complications between antegrade and retrograde dissection techniques [30]. Postoperative complications reported in the current review include reactionary hemorrhage immediately after surgery [4] and transient facial nerve deficit which recovered in durations ranging from one month to 6 months [4, 11, 14, 16, 17, 32] (Table 1). Although there were no documented cases of permanent facial nerve injury, Calvo-Henriquez et al. [28] reported a case of preoperative "House-Brackman Grade III" facial nerve deficit, which persisted postoperatively.

In addition to the long-standing nature of the tumor and its large size, the currently reported case also presented with atypical histological findings. While the histological picture was predominantly coherent with that ofPA characterized by epithelial tissue dispersed in a chondroid and myxoid matrix [34], there was marked squamous metaplasia and keratin cyst formation (Figure 4). These findings are unusual in PA of the parotid gland and lead to a high index of suspicion towards a diagnosis of mucoepidermoid carcinoma or squamous cell carcinoma [35]. However, similar findings have been reported in the literature in PA arising in labial and palatal minor salivary glands, wherein malignant transformation is highly suspected and ranges from 2 to 23% [6, 35]. Squamous metaplasia of glandular cells is attributed to hypoxia within the growing tumor and combined with keratin cysts; they mimic cutaneous appendages and are termed as "cystic pleomorphic adenoma with extensive adnexa-like differentiation" [35]. It has further been emphasized that the above findings during the histological examination of suspected pleomorphic adenomas warrant meticulous histopathological evaluation to avoid surgical overtreatment [6, 35]. Analyzing the histological findings in the present review, only one case was associated with cartilaginous metaplasia [10], without any evidence of malignant change, similar to that observed in our case too. Nevertheless, malignant transformation was reported based on final histopathological examination in 10 cases, including 5 cases of carcinoma expleomorphic adenoma (CA-ExPA) [17, 20, 23, 24, 32], one case of adenocarcinoma along with PA [15], 3 cases of mixed malignant tumor arising in PA [8, 12, 30], and one case of metastasizing PA with renal metastasis [19] (Table 1). Interestingly, one of the cases of CA-ExPA also had a malignant melanoma component, arising possibly from melanocytes within parotid tissue [20].

Malignant transformation of PA is reported at around 12% and comprises nearly 4% of all SGT [20]. According to the World Health Organization (WHO) classification of SGT, malignant tumors arising in PA were originally classified either into CA-ExPA or the relatively rare mixed malignant tumor with epithelial and mesenchymal components [8, 12]. While metastasizing PA, with metastatic lesions exhibiting histological characteristics of PA and no malignant change was originally considered a malignant variant, it has been relegated to the benign category as per the WHO classification (2017) of SGT [36]. Although rare, metastasizing PA is frequently associated with multiple recurrences of the primary tumor. Bhutta et al. [19] reported a case of metastatic renal PA, with multiple postsurgical recurrences of the parotid PA in over a decade. Based on a retrospective study of 221 patients with PA and 15 patients with CA-ExPA, Seok et al. [37] reported increasing age, regional lymph node involvement (>5 mm), and MRI apparent diffusion coefficient as the distinguishing clinical and radiographic features of CA-ExPA. In terms of histology, cellular atypia and stromal hyalinization have been regarded as the key delineating features of CA-ExPA from benign PA [36, 38]. Based on immunohistochemistry (IHC), loss of expression of PLAG-

1 (pleomorphic adenoma gene-1) protein and overexpression of Ki-67, p53, and HER-2 (human epidermal growth factor receptor-2) are considered suggestive of malignant transformation in otherwise benign PA [38, 39]. At a molecular genetic level, malignant transformation of PA is further characterized by PLAG-1/HMGA-2 (High Mobility Group AT-Hook 2) fusion and rearrangement, p53 mutation, and HER-2 amplification [36, 38, 39].

In the present review, PA with malignant transformation was treated surgically, followed by radiotherapy for locoregional disease and chemotherapy for distant metastases. Within postoperative follow-up periods ranging from 6 months to 5 years, only one case of recurrent benign PA was reported in the review [19]. Among tumors with malignant change, locoregional recurrence was reported in one case of mixed malignant tumor [8], cervical lymph node metastasis was seen in 2 cases [12, 20], and distant metastasis to the anterior chest wall, lungs, liver, pelvis, and kidney was observed in 5 cases [12, 15, 19, 20, 30]. While there was no mortality associated with benign PA or its surgical treatment, 3 patients with malignant transformation died within 6 months after surgery as a result of metastatic disease [8, 15, 20]. The longest recurrence-free follow-up for a giant parotid PA in the present review was 5 years [27], and this was still lesser than the 7-year recurrence-free follow-up observed in our case.

4. Conclusion

Giant parotid PA is rare, and to the best of our knowledge from indexed literature, this is one of the very few cases reported in this geographical region (Saudi Arabia). Apart from its rarity, the present case is being reported for its long-standing clinical presentation, successful surgical management through ECD without any postoperative complications or facial nerve deficit, atypical histological presentation, and long-term recurrence-free follow-up. In addition to complete tumor removal, ECD helped preserve the integrity of facial nerve branches. Interestingly, the present case of giant parotid PA was benign in spite of associated squamous metaplasia and keratin cyst formation identified histologically in the resected specimen. Nevertheless, this mandated a long-term follow-up of the patient. Therefore, based on this case report, clinicians must be aware of atypical histological presentation associated with parotid PA and plan suitable surgical management and follow-up, to achieve complete tumor removal and avoid morbidity. Lastly, attempts must be made to diagnose and manage PA at an early stage and before they reach gigantic proportions, through better public health care initiatives and creating awareness among all physicians and patients.

Consent

Informed consent was obtained from the patient.

References

[1] M. G. Kato, E. Erkul, S. A. Nguyen et al., "Extracapsular dissection vs superficial parotidectomy of benign parotid lesions," *JAMA Otolaryngology- Head & Neck Surgery*, vol. 143, no. 11, pp. 1092–1097, 2017.

[2] A. Reinheimer, D. S. Vieira, M. M. Cordeiro, and E. R. Rivero, "Retrospective study of 124 cases of salivary gland tumors and literature review," *Journal of Clinical and Experimental Dentistry*, vol. 11, no. 11, pp. e1025–e1032, 2019.

[3] O. E. Ogle, "Salivary gland diseases," *Dental Clinics of North America*, vol. 64, no. 1, pp. 87–104, 2020.

[4] O. B. Akintububo, O. K. Ogundipe, Z. Y. Kaltungo, M. I. Guduf, U. H. Pindiga, and Y. M. Abdullahi, "Giant parotid pleomorphic adenoma in a Nigerian male," *Nigerian Journal of Clinical Practice*, vol. 19, no. 5, pp. 681–684, 2016.

[5] A. Rai, S. Sharma, P. Shrivastava, and M. Singh, "A huge pleomorphic adenoma of the submandibular salivary gland," *BMJ Case Reports*, vol. 2018, 2018.

[6] S. Sharma, M. Mehendiratta, N. Chaudhary, V. Gupta, M. Kohli, and A. Arora, "Squamous metaplasia in pleomorphic adenoma: a diagnostic and prognostic enigma," *Journal of Pathology and Translational Medicine*, vol. 52, no. 6, pp. 411–415, 2018.

[7] P. Bonavolontà, G. Dell'Aversana Orabona, F. Maglitto et al., "Postoperative complications after removal of pleomorphic adenoma from the parotid gland: a long-term follow up of 297 patients from 2002 to 2016 and a review of publications," *The British Journal of Oral & Maxillofacial Surgery*, vol. 57, no. 10, pp. 998–1002, 2019.

[8] C. Alvarez-Cañas and I. G. Rodilla, "True malignant mixed tumor (carcinosarcoma) of the parotid gland," *Oral Surgery, Oral Medicine, Oral Pathology, Oral Radiology, and Endodontology*, vol. 81, no. 4, pp. 454–458, 1996.

[9] P. E. Lomeo, "Giant pleomorphic adenoma of the parotid," *Ear, Nose, & Throat Journal*, vol. 75, p. 402, 1996.

[10] J. E. Buenting, T. L. Smith, and D. K. Holmes, "Giant pleomorphic adenoma of the parotid gland: case report and review of the literature," *Ear, Nose, & Throat Journal*, vol. 77, pp. 634, 637–638, 640, 1998.

[11] J. Rodriguez-Ciurana, C. Rodado, M. Saez, and C. Bassas, "Giant parotid pleomorphic adenoma involving the parapharyngeal space: report of a case," *Journal of Oral and Maxillofacial Surgery : official journal of the American Association of Oral and Maxillofacial Surgeons*, vol. 58, no. 10, pp. 1184–1187, 2000.

[12] S. Manuel, A. Mathews, K. Chandramohan, and M. Pandey, "Carcinosarcoma of the parotid gland with epithelial–myoepithelial carcinoma and pleomorphic sarcoma components," *British Journal of Oral and Maxillofacial Surgery*, vol. 40, no. 6, pp. 480–483, 2002.

[13] D. Panoussopoulos, J. Yotakis, B. Pararas, G. Theodoropoulos, and K. Papadimitriou, "Giant pleomorphic adenoma of the parotid gland involving the parapharyngeal space treated by a totally extraoral transparotid approach," *Journal of Surgical Oncology*, vol. 81, no. 3, pp. 155–157, 2002.

[14] M. N. de Silva, K. M. S. Kosgoda, W. M. Tilakaratne, and P. Murugadas, "A case of giant pleomorphic adenoma of the parotid gland," *Oral Oncology Extra*, vol. 40, no. 3, pp. 43–45, 2004.

[15] T. Honda, Y. Yamamoto, T. Isago, H. Nakazawa, M. Nozaki, and T. Hirayama, "Giant pleomorphic adenoma of the parotid

gland with malignant transformation," *Annals of Plastic Surgery*, vol. 55, no. 5, pp. 524–527, 2005.

[16] L. Ruiz-Laza, P. Infante-Cossio, A. Garcia-Perla, J.-M. Hernandez-Guisado, and J.-L. Gutierrez-Perez, "Giant pleomorphic adenoma in the parapharyngeal space: report of 2 cases," *Journal of Oral and Maxillofacial Surgery*, vol. 64, no. 3, pp. 519–523, 2006.

[17] B. Sergi, A. Limongelli, E. Scarano, A. R. Fetoni, and G. Paludetti, "Giant deep lobe parotid gland pleomorphic adenoma involving the parapharyngeal space. Report of three cases and review of the diagnostic and therapeutic approaches," *Acta Otorhinolaryngologica Italica : Organo Ufficiale della Societa Italiana di Otorinolaringologia e Chirurgia Cervico-Facciale*, vol. 28, no. 5, pp. 261–265, 2008.

[18] A. Takahama Jr., D. E. da Cruz Perez, J. Magrin, O. P. de Almeida, and L. P. Kowalski, "Giant pleomorphic adenoma of the parotid gland," *Medicina Oral, Patologia Oral y Cirugia Bucal*, vol. 13, pp. E58–E60, 2008.

[19] M. F. Bhutta, L. Dunk, A. J. Molyneux, and A. Tewary, "Parotid pleomorphic adenoma with solitary renal metastasis," *British Journal of Oral and Maxillofacial Surgery*, vol. 48, no. 1, pp. 61–63, 2010.

[20] M. K. Karpowicz, B. Shalmon, K. H. Molberg, and A. K. El-Naggar, "Melanoma in a carcinoma ex pleomorphic adenoma of the parotid gland: a case report and putative histogenesis," *Human Pathology*, vol. 42, no. 9, pp. 1355–1358, 2011.

[21] M. A. Cetin, A. Ikinciogullari, G. Saygi, H. G. Hatipoglu, S. Koseoglu, and H. Dere, "Giant pleomorphic adenoma of the parotid gland," *The Turkish Journal of Ear Nose and Throat*, vol. 22, no. 2, pp. 116–118, 2012.

[22] I. Morariu, A. Dias, and A. Curran, "Giant parotid pleomorphic adenoma in parapharyngeal space causing severe obstructive sleep apnoea," *Irish Medical Journal*, vol. 105, no. 6, pp. 184-185, 2012.

[23] N. Yoshida, M. Hara, H. Kanazawa, and Y. Iino, "Large carcinoma ex pleomorphic adenoma of the parotid gland: a case report and review of literature," *Journal of Oral and Maxillofacial Surgery*, vol. 71, no. 12, pp. 2196.e1–2196.e6, 2013.

[24] A. E. Pamuk, C. Cabbarzade, H. Uner, R. Ö. Günaydın, and K. Kosemehmetoglu, "A neglected giant parotid gland mass: excision and reconstruction with facial nerve preservation," *Otolaryngologia Polska*, vol. 68, no. 6, pp. 333–337, 2014.

[25] A. N. Datarkar and A. Deshpande, "Giant parapharyngeal space pleomorphic adenoma of the deep lobe of parotid presenting as obstructive sleep apnoea: a case report & review of the diagnostic and therapeutic approaches," *Journal of Maxillofacial and Oral Surgery*, vol. 14, no. 3, pp. 532–537, 2015.

[26] M. Sajid, S. Rehman, and J. Misbah, "Giant pleomorphic adenoma of the parotid gland," *Journal of the College of Physicians and Surgeons–Pakistan*, vol. 25, Supplement 2, pp. S110–S111, 2015.

[27] A. Tarsitano, A. Pizzigallo, F. Giorgini, and C. Marchetti, "Giant pleomorphic adenoma of the parotid gland: an unusual case presentation and literature review," *Acta Otorhinolaryngologica Italica : Organo Ufficiale della Societa Italiana di Otorinolaringologia e Chirurgia Cervico-Facciale*, vol. 35, no. 4, pp. 293–296, 2015.

[28] C. E. Calvo-Henriquez, A. Telmo-Mella, C. Dios-Loureiro, and C. Martin-Martin, "Giant pleomorphic adenoma of the parotid gland," *Acta Otorrinolaringologica Espanola*, vol. 67, no. 6, pp. e40–e41, 2016.

[29] S. K. Swain, M. C. Sahu, and S. Mishra, "An ulcerated giant pleomorphic adenoma of the parotid gland – a case report," *Egyptian Journal of Ear, Nose, Throat and Allied Sciences*, vol. 17, no. 2, pp. 111–114, 2016.

[30] T. N. Chao, C. H. Rassekh, S. B. Cannady, and V. A. LiVolsi, "Giant parotid carcinosarcoma arising in a pleomorphic adenoma: facial nerve preservation by retrograde dissection," *OTO open*, vol. 1, no. 3, p. 2473974X1771941, 2017.

[31] H. Alnofaie, T. Alshammeri, Y. Alturkistany, A. Aljabab, and A. Alweteid, "Giant pleomorphic adenoma of parotid gland in Saudi Arabia: a rare case report," *SN Comprehensive Clinical Medicine*, vol. 2, no. 8, pp. 1258–1263, 2020.

[32] Y. K. Pareek, D. Gupta, Y. Aseri, D. S. Rawat, B. K. Singh, and P. C. Verma, "Giant pleomorphic adenomas of parotid gland: a case series," *Indian Journal of Otolaryngology and Head & Neck Surgery*, 2020.

[33] S. Jousse-Joulin, "Chapter 17 - salivary glands," in *Essential Applications of Musculoskeletal Ultrasound in Rheumatology*, R. J. Wakefield and M. A. D'Agostino, Eds., pp. 199–206, W.B. Saunders, Philadelphia, 2010.

[34] D. K. Das and J. T. Anim, "Pleomorphic adenoma of salivary gland: to what extent does fine needle aspiration cytology reflect histopathological features?," *Cytopathology : official journal of the British Society for Clinical Cytology*, vol. 16, no. 2, pp. 65–70, 2005.

[35] M. C. V. Goulart, P. Freitas-Faria, G. R. Goulart et al., "Pleomorphic adenoma with extensive squamous metaplasia and keratin cyst formations in minor salivary gland: a case report," *Journal of Applied Oral Science : Revista FOB*, vol. 19, no. 2, pp. 182–188, 2011.

[36] R. R. Seethala and G. Stenman, "Update from the 4th edition of the World Health Organization Classification of Head and Neck Tumours: tumors of the salivary gland," *Head and Neck Pathology*, vol. 11, no. 1, pp. 55–67, 2017.

[37] J. Seok, S. J. Hyun, W. J. Jeong, S. H. Ahn, H. Kim, and Y. H. Jung, "The difference in the clinical features between carcinoma ex pleomorphic adenoma and pleomorphic adenoma," *Ear, Nose, & Throat Journal*, vol. 98, no. 8, pp. 504–509, 2019.

[38] S. Di Palma, "Carcinoma ex pleomorphic adenoma, with particular emphasis on early lesions," *Head and Neck Pathology*, vol. 7, no. S1, pp. 68–76, 2013.

[39] M. Asahina, T. Saito, T. Hayashi, Y. Fukumura, K. Mitani, and T. Yao, "Clinicopathological effect of plag1 fusion genes in pleomorphic adenoma and carcinoma ex pleomorphic adenoma with special emphasis on histological features," *Histopathology*, vol. 74, no. 3, pp. 514–525, 2019.

18

Metastasis of Renal Cell Carcinoma Causing Significant Facial Asymmetry

Rafael Netto,[1] Silas Antonio Juvencio de Freitas Filho,[2] Wladimir Cortezzi,[3] Flávio Merly,[3] Vitor Marcello de Andrade,[3] and Fábio Ramôa Pires[4]

[1]*Stomatology Service, Department of Oral Diagnosis and Pathology, School of Dentistry, Federal University of Rio de Janeiro, Rio de Janeiro, RJ, Brazil*
[2]*Department of Surgery, Stomatology, Pathology and Radiology (Area of Pathology), Bauru School of Dentistry, University of São Paulo, Bauru, SP, Brazil*
[3]*Oral and Maxillofacial Surgery Service, Federal Hospital of State Servers, Brazilian Government, Rio de Janeiro, RJ, Brazil*
[4]*Department of Oral Pathology, School of Dentistry, State University of Rio de Janeiro, Rio de Janeiro, RJ, Brazil*

Correspondence should be addressed to Rafael Netto; rafanetto@gmail.com

Academic Editor: Yehuda Ullmann

The occurrence of metastatic tumors in the orofacial region is rare and may represent the first clinical manifestation of occult malignant disease. An orofacial lesion diagnosed as a metastatic tumor from a renal cell carcinoma in a 68-year-old man is reported. This metastatic tumor caused significant facial asymmetry involving the parotid gland and mandible regions, and the patient died four months after diagnosis. Here, we discuss the clinical aspects, the diagnostic approach, and the importance of early diagnosis to obtain a better response to treatment and provide longer survival time.

1. Introduction

Oral metastatic tumors are uncommon lesions that can occur at any age and in both genders, which represent the systemic spread of the disease or initial presentation of an unknown malignancy at a distant place [1].

Metastatic lesions to the oral cavity can occur in the jawbones and soft tissues, including salivary glands [2–5]. Oral metastases arise most commonly from the breast, liver, and thyroid for women [2]. In men, the most common origin of oral metastatic tumors is from the lung, kidney, liver, and prostate [2, 4].

The clinical and radiological aspects of metastatic tumors are varied, making diagnosis and therapeutic management challenging [6], so it is highly relevant to investigate the patient's medical history. The lesions may be asymptomatic or painful and may cause paresthesia, tooth mobility, regional lymphadenopathy, local swelling, exophytic growth, modification of the normal aspects of the oral mucosa, and still pathologic fracture in osseous lesions [7].

Histopathological findings are essential and generally reflect the pattern of primary tumors [8]. Due to the rarity of these metastatic tumors in the maxillofacial region and the challenging diagnosis, the immunohistochemical expression is an auxiliary diagnostic tool [7, 8].

Herein, we report and discuss a case of oral metastasis with significant facial asymmetry involving the parotid gland and mandible regions, resulting from a primary renal cell carcinoma.

2. Case Presentation

A 68-year-old male patient was referred by the public health service of his city for specialized care to the Oral and Maxillofacial Surgery Service of the Federal Hospital of Rio de Janeiro State Servers/Brazil for the evaluation of volumetric increase on the right side of the face. Medical history has reported systemic hypertension and gastritis, both conditions under drug control. He also reported having had surgery for an appendectomy at 25 years of age and denied allergies. The

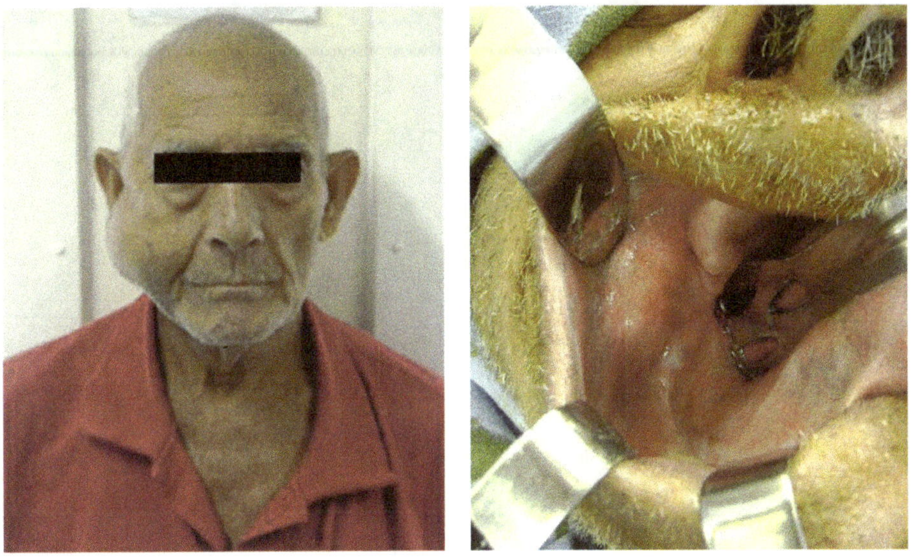

(a) (b)

Figure 1: (a) Extraoral clinical aspect causing significant facial asymmetry. (b) Intraoral clinical aspect shows a slight elevation in the jugal mucosa.

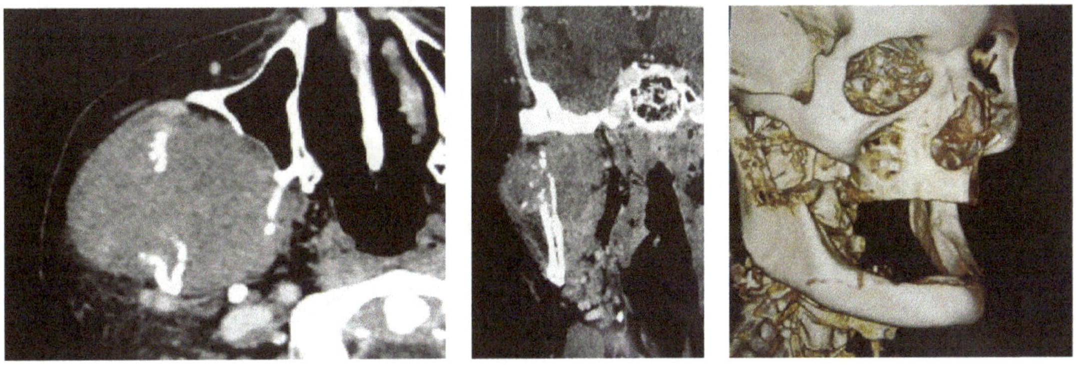

(a) (b) (c)

Figure 2: (a) Axial CT image reveals an expansive lesion in the soft tissue of mixed aspect and regular contours. (b) Coronal CT image shows hyperdense foci among the lesions. (c) 3D reconstruction of CT scan reveals mandibular ramus lytic lesions.

patient reported frequent use of alcohol and smoking for 35 years and having stopped smoking 4 years ago. The patient reported a progressive and painless growth of lesion in the genian region in the last four months.

Extraoral examination revealed a tumor-like lesion, firm consistency, well-defined contours, and significant expansion near the parotid region (Figure 1(a)). On intraoral examination, a slight elevation in the ipsilateral jugal mucosa was noted, corresponding to the expansion of the medial growth tumor (Figure 1(b)).

For an incisional biopsy, computed tomography (CT) images of the face and preoperative laboratory tests were requested. The results showed normal serum levels of most of the requested blood fractions, except for slightly elevated urea and creatinine. The axial CT image (Figure 2(a)) revealed an expansive lesion (approximately 6.0×6.0 cm) in the soft tissue of the mixed aspect and regular contours. In the coronal CT image, hyperdense foci of the lesion were observed (Figure 2(b)), suggestive of calcification or bone lysis. In the three-dimensional reconstruction of the tomography (Figure 2(c)), bone destruction in the mandibular branch was evidenced by possible tumor compression.

An intraoral incisional biopsy was performed. In the first 72 hours after the biopsy, the patient developed significant local edema and volumetric expansion of the lesion, which became inaccurate (Figure 3(a)). On gross examination, three fragments of smooth brown tissue were observed (Figure 3(b)), which were sent for histopathological analysis. After anamnesis and clinical and radiological examinations, our diagnostic hypotheses were Warthin's tumor, pleomorphic adenoma, mucoepidermoid carcinoma, and soft tissue sarcoma.

Microscopically, large neoplastic cells often eosinophilic and pale, sometimes clear, with reticulated cytoplasm, centralized oval nucleus and perinuclear halo, and prominent nucleoli were observed (Figure 4). The diagnosis was strongly suggestive of oral metastasis of chromophobe renal cell carcinoma.

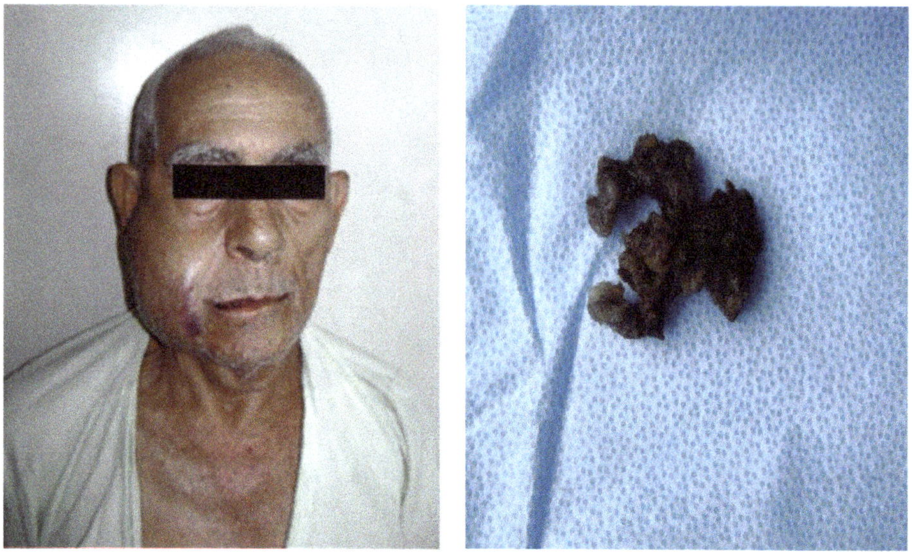

(a) (b)

Figure 3: (a) Clinical aspect 72 hours after an intraoral incisional biopsy showing significant expansion of the lesion. (b) Surgical specimen.

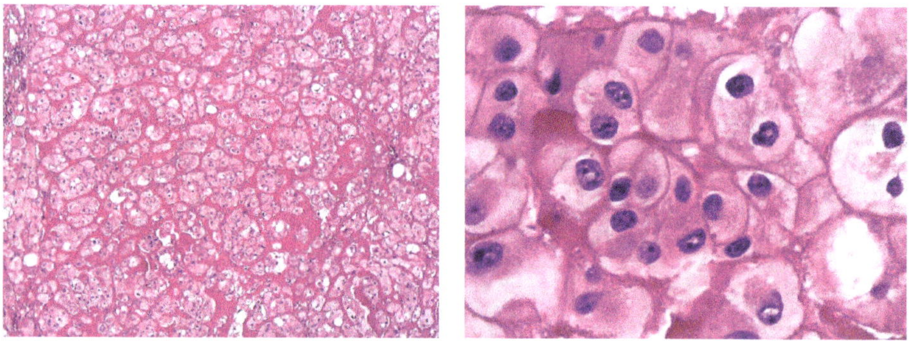

(a) (b)

Figure 4: Microscopic analysis: (a) large neoplastic cells often eosinophilic and pale with reticulated cytoplasm and a centralized oval nucleus; (b) neoplastic cells with a centralized oval nucleus, perinuclear halo, and prominent nucleoli (H and E staining: (a) 100x and (b) 400x).

The patient underwent primary CT scan of the abdomen, which showed the presence of lesion involving the right kidney cortex and parenchyma (Figure 5). The patient was referred to the Referral Oncology Service, where renal cell carcinoma was effectively diagnosed, and then began treatment with chemotherapy for kidney tumor and radiotherapy for orofacial metastatic tumor. The patient died four months after starting treatment.

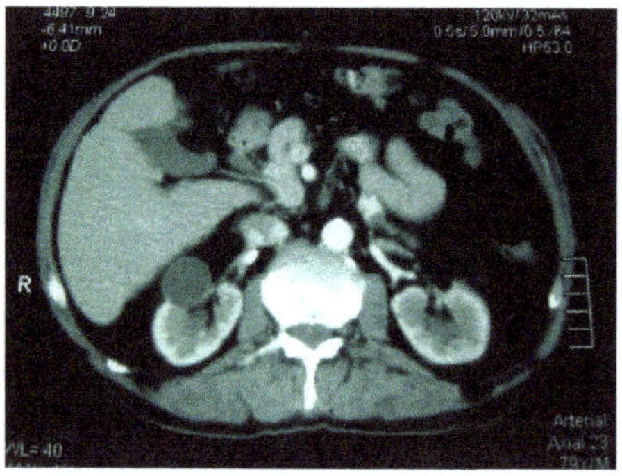

Figure 5: Axial CT image of the abdomen reveals a lesion involving the right kidney cortex and parenchyma.

3. Discussion

Metastases to the oral cavity or head and neck region are extremely rare conditions [7, 9]. Metastatic tumors account for less than 1% of all oral malignancies [7, 10]. Such metastases can affect men and women equally and at any age [11]. According to Hirshberg et al. [4], the kidney is the third most common primary site for oral metastases, although there is underreporting [8]. The incidence of oral metastases and their origins may vary according to the study population [4, 7, 11].

As shown in our case, oral lesions have been reported among the first manifestations of an undiagnosed primary malignant disease [7, 11] or may still be indicative of terminal disease [1]. Initially, our patient had no signs or symptoms for suspected metastatic tumor. Among the main signs and symptoms, pain and swelling of the region with a metastatic tumor have been observed in most patients [2]. Clinically, orofacial metastases of renal cell carcinoma may show the following characteristics: submucosal or jaw mass, jaw or oral pain, lip numbness, gingival swelling, or even an extensive bilobed mass [1]. Other signs may be noted as bleeding, tooth mobility, trismus, paraesthesia, and paralysis [2, 11]. When bone tissue is involved by metastatic tumors, lytic lesions are often observed [4]. Despite the significant size of the lesion, our patient had no painful symptoms, and surprisingly lytic lesions in the mandibular branch were found on radiological examinations, although the lesion mainly involved the maxillary region. In addition, the use of technologies such as PET-CT collaborates in identifying primary or metastatic skeletal tumors [12].

Initially, the location, size, and limits of the lesion led to the clinical hypothesis of a primary neoplastic lesion in the parotid gland, mainly Warthin's tumor due to cigarette use. However, mandibular bone resorption was indicative of aggressiveness of the lesion. After the surgical intervention for an incisional biopsy and worsening of the clinical picture, our team began to consider a malignant or metastatic tumor. However, for cases with a history of cancer, the professional should evaluate the patients' complaint and reflect on the inclusion of metastatic disease among the diagnostic hypotheses [13, 14]. Oral metastases of renal cell carcinoma may show clinical features similar to those of aggressive malignant tumors [15]. For cases with a suspected parotid gland tumor, the surgeon may perform a fine-needle aspiration biopsy, avoiding possible discomfort and complications from an incisional biopsy [8].

In the study by Liu et al. [7], all cases of oral metastasis from CCR had no previous diagnosis, showing that this tumor is insidious in nature. For tumor lesions in the orofacial region, histopathological analysis is mandatory to distinguish the neoplasia and then define the treatment plan and outline the patient's prognosis [16]. Often, the definitive diagnosis with no previous history of cancer is challenging to the pathologist. Thus, an immunohistochemical panel with limited or broader molecules may be useful in establishing the origin of the tumor and the definitive diagnosis [7, 8, 10, 12]. In the present case, due to the experience of the pathological anatomy service with head and neck metastatic tumors associated with the infrastructure provided by the hospital, our patient was submitted to the investigation of primary renal neoplastic injury immediately after microscopic analysis. Also, for cases similar to ours, the immunohistochemistry has not been a frequent technique in establishing a diagnosis [1].

Since metastases reflect the primary tumor pattern [7], microscopic analysis is essential for predicting the neoplasia's biological behavior. Although most of these tumors are clear cell type, a thorough evaluation of other more frequent patterns such as papillary and chromophobe is relevant for understanding the disease. Although the chromophobe pattern of renal cell carcinoma is associated with low mortality, in our case, the late diagnosis was relevant in the outcome of the disease [17]. In addition, Pires et al. [15] affirm the importance of immunohistochemical differentiation between metastatic renal cell carcinoma and mucoepidermoid carcinoma in case of overlapping of histopathological features.

According to Owosho et al. [1], adult patients with oral metastases have a worse prognosis compared to pediatric patients, and in adults, oral soft tissue involvement leads to a shorter survival compared to patients with mandibular bone involvement. For cases similar to ours, the treatment modalities are surgical resection, radiotherapy, and chemotherapy [14], and there may be variation among metastatic tumors of renal cell carcinomas [1]. Moreover, the use of antiangiogenic agents and genome sequencing are promising therapeutic modalities [1]. Our elderly patient with advanced metastatic disease did not respond to treatment and had a shorter survival time than that found in the study by Hirshberg et al. [4]. The conservative and palliative treatment has been recommended for cases with worse prognosis, while the option for surgical removal is restricted to cases with less advanced disease [14].

In summary, the occurrence of metastatic tumors in the orofacial region is rare and may represent the first clinical manifestation of occult malignant disease. These lesions are very serious and have a poor prognosis. Wherever possible, early diagnosis should be performed to obtain a satisfactory response to treatment and provide better patient survival.

References

[1] A. A. Owosho, B. Xu, A. Kadempour et al., "Metastatic solid tumors to the jaw and oral soft tissue: a retrospective clinical analysis of 44 patients from a single institution," *Journal of Cranio-Maxillofacial Surgery*, vol. 44, no. 8, pp. 1047–1053, 2016.

[2] Y. H. Lee and J. L. Lee, "Metastatic carcinoma of the oral region: an analysis of 21 cases," *Medicina Oral Patología Oral y Cirugia Bucal*, vol. 22, no. 3, pp. e359–e365, 2017.

[3] S. A. McClure, R. Movahed, A. Salama, and R. A. Ord, "Maxillofacial metastases: a retrospective review of one institution's 15-year experience," *Journal of Oral and Maxillofacial Surgery*, vol. 71, no. 1, pp. 178–188, 2013.

[4] A. Hirshberg, A. Shnaiderman-Shapiro, I. Kaplan, and R. Berger, "Metastatic tumours to the oral cavity - pathogenesis and analysis of 673 cases," *Oral Oncology*, vol. 44, no. 8, pp. 743–752, 2008.

[5] A. Bhaskaran, S. Harding, and D. Courtney, "An unusual presentation of metastatic colon adenocarcinoma in the oral cavity," *Case Reports in Dentistry*, vol. 2011, Article ID 357518, 2 pages, 2011.

[6] E. Poulias, I. Melakopoulos, and K. Tosios, "Metastatic breast carcinoma in the mandible presenting as a periodontal abscess: a case report," *Journal of Medical Case Reports*, vol. 5, p. 265, 2011.

[7] Y. Liu, R. J. Vargo, and E. A. Bilodeau, "Analytic survey of 57 cases of oral metastases," *Journal of Oral Pathology & Medicine*, vol. 47, no. 3, pp. 275–280, 2018.

[8] Y. Morita, T. Iwagami, C. Kawakita, Y. Kusuyama, A. Niki-Yonekawa, and N. Morita, "Oral metastasis of renal cell carcinoma mimicking recurrence of excised malignant myoepithelioma: a case report," *Molecular and Clinical Oncology*, vol. 9, no. 1, pp. 66–69, 2018.

[9] J. I. Harada, T. Matsutani, N. Hagiwara et al., "Metastasis of hepatocellular carcinoma to the esophagus: case report and review," *Case Reports in Surgery*, vol. 2018, Article ID 8685371, 6 pages, 2018.

[10] D. M. Guimarães, F. S. Pontes, L. A. Miyahara et al., "Metastatic renal cell carcinoma to the oral cavity," *Journal of Craniofacial Surgery*, vol. 27, no. 6, pp. 533-534, 2016.

[11] J. Murillo, J. V. Bagan, E. Hens, J. M. Diaz, and M. Leopoldo, "Tumors metastasizing to the oral cavity: a study of 16 cases," *Journal of Oral and Maxillofacial Surgery*, vol. 71, no. 9, pp. 1545–1551, 2013.

[12] S. Derakhshan, S. Rahrotaban, N. Mahdavi, and F. Mirjalili, "Metastatic renal cell carcinoma presenting as maxillary lesion: report of two rare cases," *Journal of Oral and Maxillofacial Surgery*, vol. 22, no. 1, pp. S39–S43, 2018.

[13] N. J. D'Silva, D. J. Summerlin, K. G. Cordell et al., "Metastatic tumors in the jaws: a retrospective study of 114 cases," *The Journal of the American Dental Association*, vol. 137, no. 12, pp. 1667–1672, 2016.

[14] Y. Israel, A. Rachmiel, K. Gourevich, and R. Nagler, "Non-primary salivary malignancies: a 22-year retrospective study," *Journal of Cranio-Maxillo-Facial Surgery*, vol. 47, no. 9, pp. 1351–1355, 2019.

[15] F. R. Pires, R. S. Azevedo, G. Ficarra et al., "Metastatic renal cell carcinoma to the oral cavity and clear cell mucoepidermoid carcinoma: comparative clinicopathologic and immunohistochemical study," *Oral Surgery, Oral Medicine, Oral Pathology, Oral Radiology, and Endodontology*, vol. 109, no. 4, pp. e22–e27, 2010.

[16] H. Majewska, A. Skálová, K. Radecka et al., "Renal clear cell carcinoma metastasis to salivary glands - a series of 9 cases: clinico-pathological study," *Polish Journal of Pathology*, vol. 67, no. 1, pp. 39–45, 2016.

[17] V. F. Muglia and A. Prando, "Renal cell carcinoma: histological classification and correlation with imaging findings," *Radiologia Brasileira*, vol. 48, no. 3, pp. 166–174, 2015.

19

The Curious Case of Lip Tongue Fusion: A Consequence of Suboptimal Oral Care

Jimmy Xu,[1] **Prateek Biyani**,[2] **Andrew Rajkumar**,[2] **and Robert Orr**[2]

[1]*Royal Derby Hospital, Derby, UK*
[2]*Chesterfield Royal Hospital, Chesterfield, UK*

Correspondence should be addressed to Jimmy Xu; jimmy.xu@nhs.net

Academic Editor: Fabio Roccia

Oral care is an often difficult and an unappreciated part of hospital life. Patients who are unable to provide their own care rely on assistance from hospital personnel. Most sequelae from suboptimal oral care often present over months if not years, in the form of dental caries and periodontal disease. We present an exception, where a 66-year-old patient who experienced widespread ulceration and necrosis from *Capnocytophaga*-related sepsis received suboptimal oral care, resulting in their tongue being fused to their lip. This was later divided by the oral and maxillofacial team resulting in restoration of full function. Future cases can be avoided in patients with similar symptoms, such as Stevens-Johnson syndrome or erythema multiforme, if rigorous oral care can be provided.

1. Introduction

Good mouth care in an intensive care setting is crucial; however, unfortunately, it is often carried out in a suboptimal manner. This is understandable due to patients being more complicated to manage, with multiple other morbidities including confusion and lack of cooperation. We present a case of a patient whose tongue, as a result of suboptimal oral care, has granulated onto their lip.

2. Case Presentation

A 66-year-old male attended a neighbouring accident and emergency department with an unknown cause of sepsis and multiorgan failure. The patient had no relevant medical history apart from asplenia as a result of splenectomy after a previous postfundoplication complication. He was socially independent.

Initially presenting to a neighbouring hospital due to shortness of breath, fever, confusion, and feeling unwell for 24 hours, our patient was admitted under a medical ward briefly before starting to rapidly desaturate on room air and oxygen. A CT chest-abdomen-pelvis showed bilateral mild pleural effusion with a mildly dilated common bile duct, and a CT head showed no abnormalities. Blood, sputum, urine, and bronchoalveolar lavage cultures proved negative, and meropenem was started empirically. He later developed septic cardiomyopathy with an ejection fraction of 10%, and later, complete anuria. The patient had developed multiorgan failure and was eventually mechanically ventilated via an endotracheal tube at the neighbouring hospital.

The patient was later transferred to the intensive care unit at Chesterfield Royal Hospital five days after initial presentation where he was placed on norepinephrine, continuous venovenous hemofiltration, and continued on continuous positive airway pressure. A tracheostomy was later provided and sedation weaned off when symptoms started to improve. Upon presentation at our hospital, the skin to the majority of his body was extremely mottled, bleeding, and blistered, with severe purpura and peripheral ischemia, especially peripherally. This had apparently developed 2 days before transfer. The mottled purple appearance of his skin gave the initial impression of vasculitis secondary to infection; however, the presence of blisters was unusual for this as it was also on undamaged skin. Both haematological

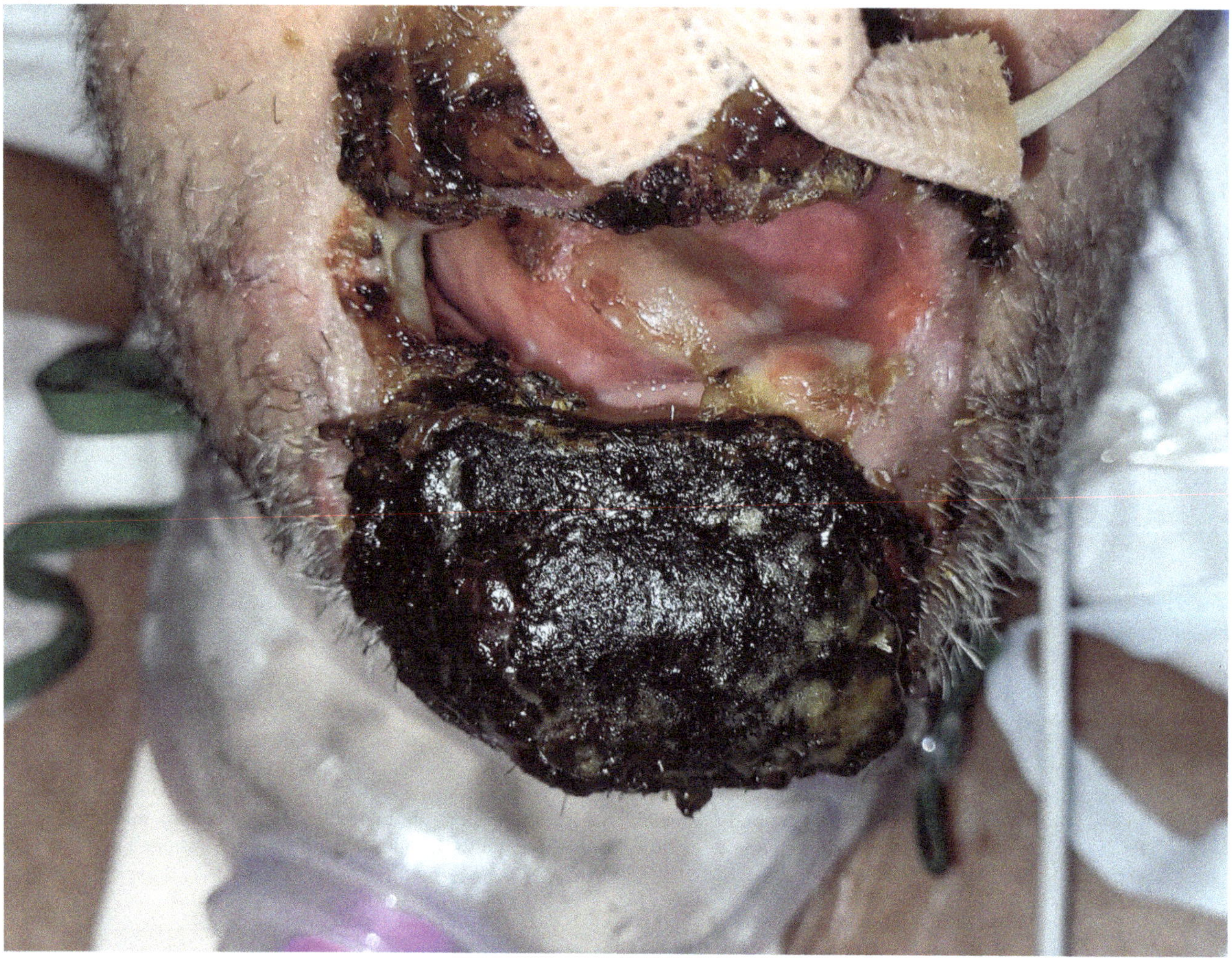

Figure 1: Tongue tethered to lower left lip due to granulation and associated extensive necrosis.

screening and skin biopsies later proved negative for vasculitis. After a subsequent positive blood culture, it was discovered that this patient had *Capnocytophaga*-related fulminant sepsis, a rare complication arising from a calf wound licked by his dog several days before initial presentation. Microbiology had recommended both Tazocin and Teicoplanin based on sensitivity. As the patient's symptoms were already improving, antibiotics had already been stopped a week prior.

The normal mouth care regimen at our hospital involves cleaning all intraoral surfaces with a solution of 0.2% chlorhexidine using a soft brush approximately every 4 hourly and to brush teeth twice daily for those in critical care. Unfortunately, mouth care was not always performed intraorally due to the patient not being able to open his mouth when asked to. Additionally, staff were hesitant to clean intraorally whilst the patient was intubated due to the severity of the necrosis, resulting in bleeding when attempted. Intraoral care was therefore done very reluctantly, if at all. Our oral and maxillofacial surgery department was later involved when speech and language therapy noted the patient's tongue tip was fused to the left side of his lip resulting in impaired swallowing. They had initially used a toothbrush to lightly rub a pale coating between the tongue and the lip as it was thought to be dried secretions, but instead the area started to bleed, leading to the finding. This was discovered just under 3 weeks after admission, but approximately 2 weeks after oral blistering started. Upon further examination by our team, the tongue appeared to have granulated into the patient's lip as a result of the generalised necrosis in the oral cavity, along with previous lack of tongue movement (Figure 1). The attachment was later carefully divided under local anaesthetic using 2% lidocaine with 1 : 80000 adrenaline and a 15 blade without any complications (Figure 2). The patient regained full range of movement and restoration of function immediately after. Unfortunately, the patient started deteriorating approximately a week later, also acquiring pseudomonas and coagulase negative staphylococci bacteraemia, and has now passed away.

3. Discussion

This case not only demonstrates the difficulty of managing *Capnocytophaga*-related sepsis, but also the significant importance of good oral care in intensive care patients.

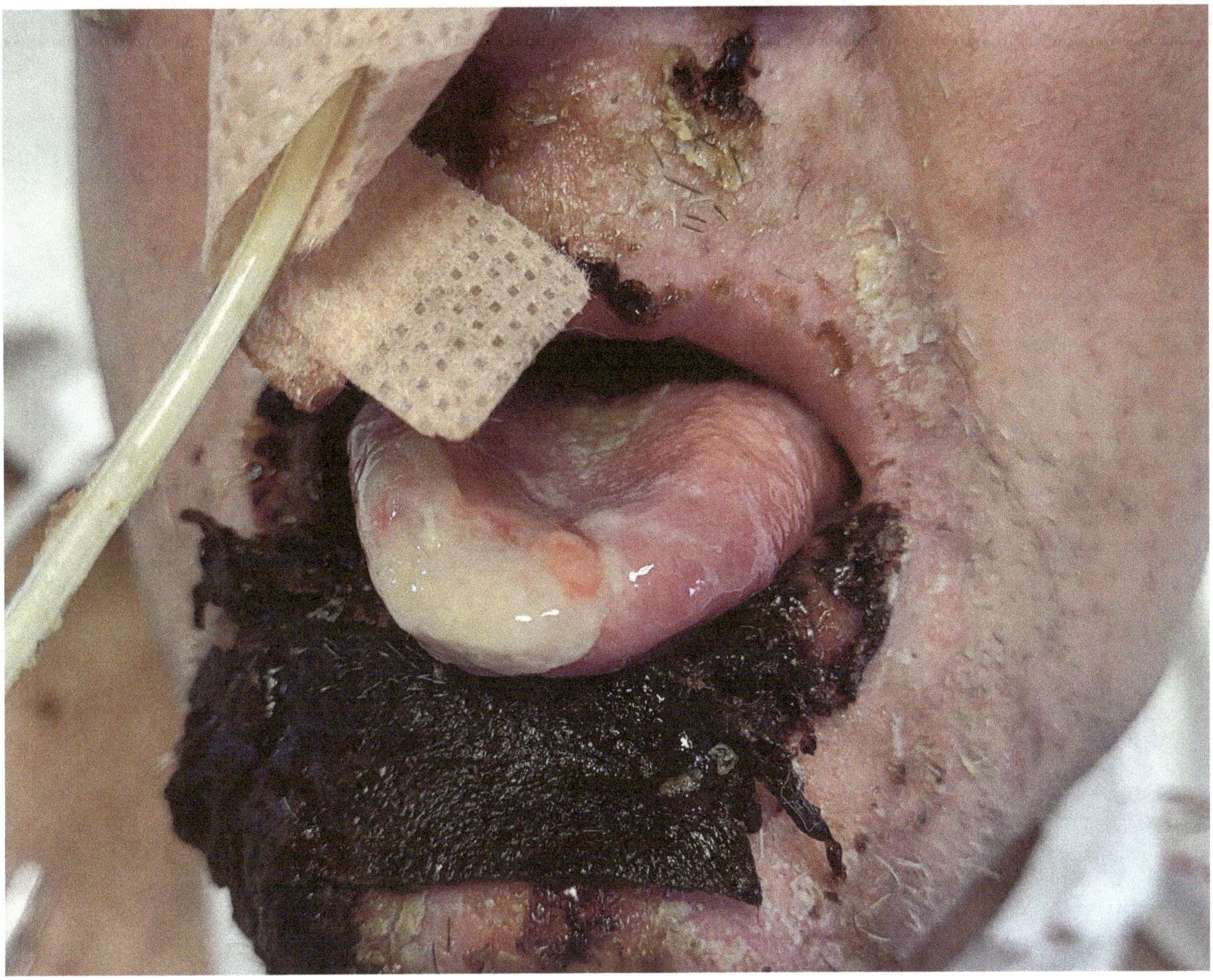

FIGURE 2: Tongue after division of fused tissues with full range of movement.

Capnocytophaga spp are an opportunistic genus of gram-negative bacteria which can cause a varied presentation of infections [1]. *Capnocytophaga canimorsus*, specifically, can be transferred to humans via saliva in dogs or cats, especially in open wounds. Immunocompromised patients are therefore at a high risk of developing serious complications such as sepsis, meningitis, and respiratory distress from this condition [2]. Patients who have had their spleens removed are therefore more prone to serious infections including to *Capnocytophaga* and appear to develop more serious symptoms than those who are splenic [3–5]. Other at risk groups include patients with diabetes, liver cirrhosis, and those with a history of alcohol abuse [6].

The mainstay of treatment for *Capnocytophaga*-related sepsis are antibiotics. The current consensus appears to be penicillins with beta-lactamase inhibitors, due to increasing incidence of penicillin resistant strains [7]. Patients with dermatological symptoms, such as purpura fulminans or thrombocytopenia purpura, appear to not be uncommon [8], and this can evidently have an impact on mouth care if present in the perioral and intraoral tissues.

In the intensive care setting, cleaning the mouth is recognised as especially important for plaque control, and potentially reducing systemic infection [9]. Furthermore, the reduction in bacterial load and disrupting the biofilm is critical in reducing dental caries [10] and periodontal disease for those individuals unable to take care of themselves. Despite this, the priority is often low amongst staff, especially with uncooperative and confused patients [11].

There are no current reports in the literature of such extensive ulceration and necrosis on the mucosal tissues causing fusion intraoral tissues. The combination of severe generalised ulceration along with immobility to intraoral tissues for at least several days appears to be an exceptionally rare occurrence. Nonetheless, our case report helps to demonstrate that such an event can occur and highlights one of the rare complications of not only *Capnocytophaga*-related sepsis but also other conditions which could result in widespread necrosis and ulceration, such as Stevens-Johnson syndrome and erythema multiforme. This situation could have ultimately been avoided through more rigorous oral care practices.

References

[1] J. Zajkowska, M. Król, D. Falkowski, N. Syed, and A. Kamieńska, "Capnocytophaga canimorsus - an underestimated danger after dog or cat bite - review of literature," *Przegląd Epidemiologiczny*, vol. 70, no. 2, pp. 289–295, 2016.

[2] C. Pers, B. Gahrn-Hansen, and W. Frederiksen, "Capnocytophaga canimorsus septicemia in Denmark, 1982-1995: review of 39 cases," *Clinical Infectious Diseases*, vol. 23, no. 1, pp. 71–75, 1996.

[3] T. Butler, "Capnocytophaga canimorsus: an emerging cause of sepsis, meningitis, and post-splenectomy infection after dog bites," *European Journal of Clinical Microbiology & Infectious Diseases*, vol. 34, no. 7, pp. 1271–1280, 2015.

[4] L. Shahani and N. Khardori, "Overwhelming Capnocytophaga canimorsus infection in a patient with asplenia," *BMJ Case Reports*, vol. 2014, article bcr2013202768, 2014.

[5] P. Langguth, L. Leissner, G. Zick et al., "Why Asplenic patients should not take Care of the Neighbour's dog? A fatal course of *Capnocytophaga canimorsus* sepsis," *Case Reports in Infectious Diseases*, vol. 2018, Article ID 3870640, 5 pages, 2018.

[6] S. Chesdachai, D. B. G. Tai, Z. A. Yetmar, A. Misra, N. Ough, and S. O. Abu, "The characteristics of *Capnocytophaga* infection: 10 years of experience. Open forum," *Infectious Diseases*, vol. 8, no. 7, article ofab175, 2021.

[7] A. Jolivet-Gougeon, J. L. Sixou, Z. Tamanai-Shacoori, and M. Bonnaure-Mallet, "Antimicrobial treatment of _Capnocytophaga_ infections," *International Journal of Antimicrobial Agents*, vol. 29, no. 4, pp. 367–373, 2007.

[8] C. Lion, F. Escande, and J. C. Burdin, "Capnocytophaga canimorsus infections in human: review of the literature and cases report," *European Journal of Epidemiology*, vol. 12, no. 5, pp. 521–533, 1996.

[9] K. Kite and L. Pearson, "A rationale for mouth care: the integration of theory with practice," *Intensive and Critical Care Nursing.*, vol. 11, no. 2, pp. 71–76, 1995.

[10] P. D. Marsh, "Microbiology of dental plaque biofilms and their role in oral health and caries," *Dental Clinics of North America*, vol. 54, no. 3, pp. 441–454, 2010.

[11] T. Costello and I. Coyne, "Nurses' knowledge of mouth care practices," *British Journal of Nursing*, vol. 17, no. 4, pp. 264–268, 2008.

20

Orbital Prosthetic Rehabilitation in "ADAM Complex" Multiple Orofacial-Cleft Disruption Syndrome

Aparna Barabde,[1,2] Shailesh M. Barabde,[3] Ashish Bhagat,[1] and Amar Thakare[1]

[1] *Department of Prosthetic Dentistry, V.Y.W.S. Dental College & Hospital, Amravati 444 602, India*
[2] *Dr Barabde Dental Clinic, Badnera Road, Rajkamal Square, Amravati 444 601, India*
[3] *Department of Obstetrics & Gynaecology, P.D.M. Medical College, Amravati 444 602, India*

Correspondence should be addressed to Aparna Barabde; draparnabarabde@yahoo.com

Academic Editors: R. Mofidi and F. Roccia

To be human is great; to look human is wonderful! It is nature's greatest gift! Mother nature's womb is the safest place on earth for any life, but the calamity strikes and no one knows how Hence, Treasure your exceptions!, since nature seems nowhere accustomed more openly to display, its secret mysteries than in cases where it shows traces of its workings apart from the beaten path. A dismorphological pattern of congenital oro-craniofacial and limb defects which is a rare form of amniotic rupture sequence required persistent coordinated efforts of multiple disciplines and had manifested as bizarre orofacial clefting, cat eye syndrome with an ectopic eye, and aberrant tissue band lesions on limb. The challenge was to meet the child's clamour for functional demands on premature exposure to open world and was overcome through a phased treatment implementation. Anophthalmos resulting from multiple ophthalmic surgeries for aberrant ectopic left eye and cat eye syndrome of right eye required a staged sequential preemptive planning for a successful outcome. Every phase of fabrication of orbital prosthesis comes with an impending challenge. Thus, a well-defined technique eliminating the common errors and creating a natural looking prosthesis, in the face of limitations, is imperative.

1. Introduction

The naturally vibrant and dynamically variable region of the orbit poses innumerable challenges in making an indiscernible replica of the opposing eye. Simulation of nature through rehabilitation forms the primary goal for state-of-art restoration in these genres of maxillofacial prosthodontic modelling.

Dr. Leisely, Sweden, 1991 has said no matter how accurate your diagnosis is, no matter how effective your prognosis; the entire success in disease management depends upon the patient's will to come out of the odd.

Thus, to create the perfect esthetic illusion of normal eye poses multiple challenges as we are attempting to restore a moving organ with a static prosthesis. An interdisciplinary case report provides the perfect medium for determining plausible solutions to overcome the challenges posed at every step of the wall till we achieve a successful outcome, thus, turning a distressing scenario of nightmare into a metaphysical reality.

2. Clinical Features

"Adam complex" disruption syndrome [1] is a rare, complex, fetal, fatal spectrum of malformations portraying as dismorphological pattern of congenital orofacial and limb defects involving all three basic types of anomalies, that is, disruptions, deformations, and malformations, whereas the mnemonic term "ADAM" complex stands for A: Amnion, D: Deformity, A: Adhesion, and M: Mutilation.

The clinical features include:

(1) craniofacial defect-facial clefts CL(L) and (P), asymmetric microphthalmia (Figures 1, 2, and 3),

(2) visceral defect—gastroschisis, omphalocele,

(3) limb defect—constriction ring or amputations (Figure 2).

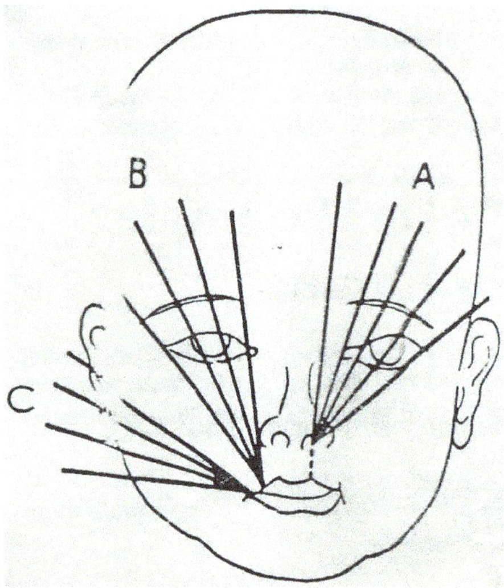

FIGURE 1: Oblique facial clefts.

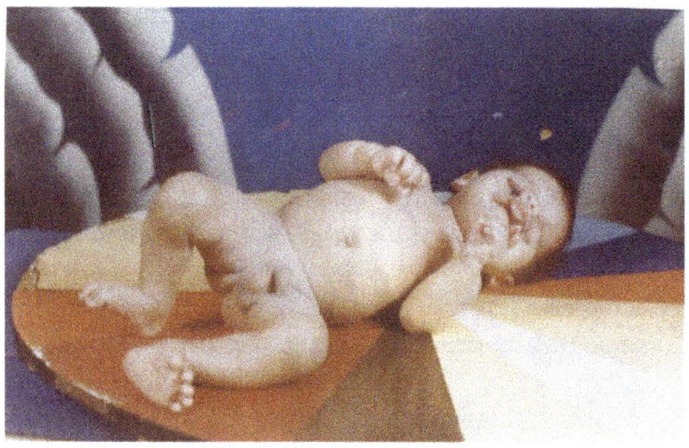

FIGURE 2: Gaurav at birth.

Epidemiology. 1 : 1,200–1 : 15,000 live births, extremely rare congenital abnormality. Also known as Amniotic band syndrome [2].

Etiology. Remains unclear. Factors postulated are based upon Streeter's endogenous [3] and Torpin's exogenous theory [4]. Early amnion rupture due to genetic, toxic, congenital, endocranial factors may determine the process (Figure 4).

Antenatal Diagnosis. Second trimester of pregnancy by elevated amniotic α-fetoprotein levels, or specialised, genetic consultation, ultrasound.

Differential Diagnosis. One needs to exclude similar conditions like Meckel's syndrome, Frontonasal dysplasia, and so forth, to confirm the diagnosis.

A remarkable feature is that the general intelligence is normal.

Due to complexity of this association a complete study and adequate treatment requires multidisciplinary collaboration. Thus defects in oral and craniofacial tissues, resulting from congenital abnormalities present a formidable challenge. At birth surgical removal of ectopic left eye leads to Anophthalmos whereas respiratory distress required prompt resuscitation.

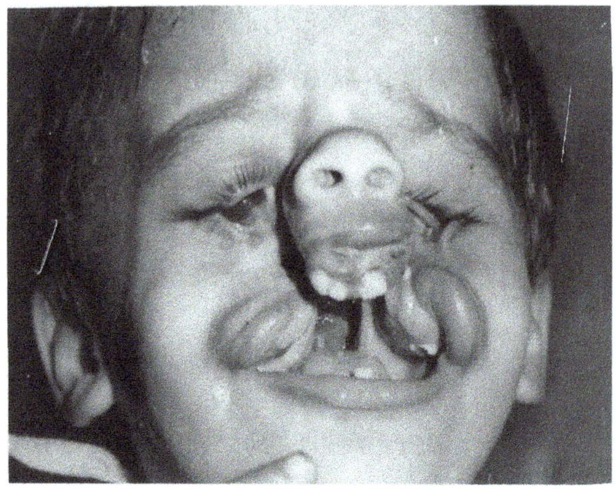

FIGURE 3: ADAM-complex features.

3. Clinical Report

A 7-year-old male child "Gaurav" reported to the Department of Prosthodontics with chief complaint of missing left eye and inadequate vision of right eye. He is the first child of a healthy nonconsanguineous parents with no family history of any congenital defect. His mother gave history of bacterial infection and he was born prematurely in 30th week of gestation. At birth surgical removal of ectopic left eye and prompt resuscitation for respiratory distress were required.

Medical and dental history revealed that he is operated for ectopic left eye. He has undergone repeated surgeries (8 times) for correction of intraoral, extraoral, and limb defect.

Examination revealed Anophthalmos with left eye, leading to symptoms of postenucleation socket syndrome like superior sulcus deepening and lower lid laxity; coloboma of right eye with multiple scar marks and variable degree of cleft fragment approximation along with surgically repaired bilateral oblique facial cleft, bilateral maxillary cleft lip (and palate), and floating premaxilla is seen. An extensive pigmentation on right forearm for constriction band lesion correction is evident (Figure 5).

Oroocular cleft type I (medial to infraorbital formen, according to Boo Chai's classification) and cleft number 4 (Tessier classification) mixed group for all facial clefts was determined.

Postsurgical radiograph showed that both the maxillary antrum were hypoplastic but not cleft and there was funnelling of orbital floor (Figure 6).

Intraoral examination revealed bilateral fibrous band from lips to canine area to palate and proclinated anterior teeth causing typical gold fish appearance.

The most miraculous learning occurs when an infant turns into an eloquent child and no one knows how! It is by imitation at its pristine best! At 7 years of age, apart of missing eye Gaurav's chief complaint was flat cheeks, drooping eye lids, and cleft alveolar ridge and palate.

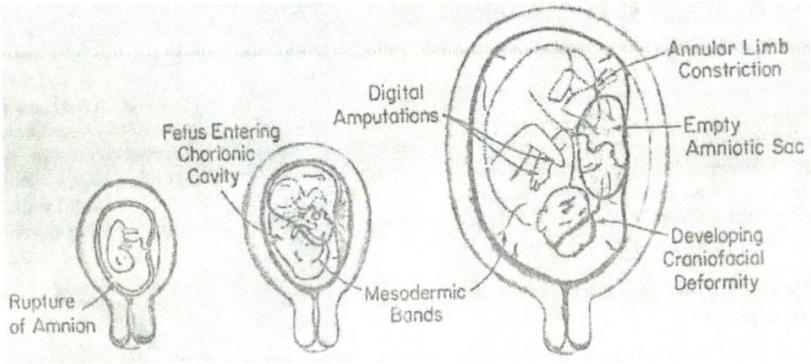

FIGURE 4: Torpin's exogenous theory.

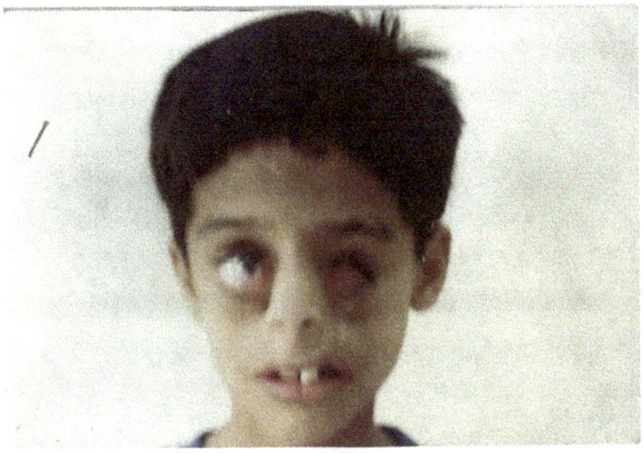

FIGURE 5: Frontal view showing ocular defect.

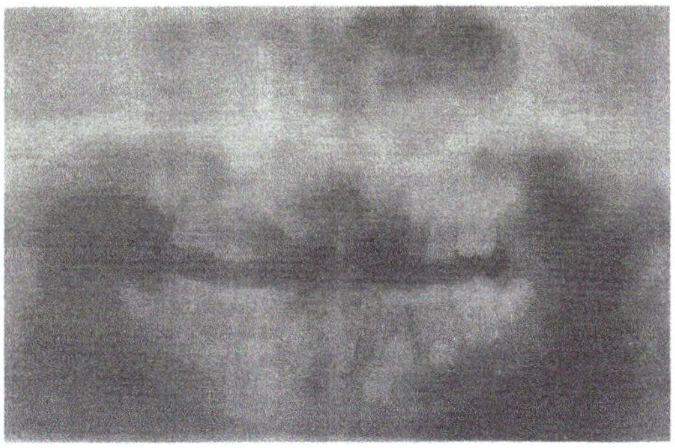

FIGURE 6: Postsurgical OPG view.

"He had but one eye; but the pocket of prejudice lies in favour of two." The crippling effect of the defect on the growing child's mind cannot be overemphasized but this positive attitude was evident.

4. History and Review of Literature

Although interest in congenital malformations dates back to antiquity, a recognizable pattern of anomalies associated with oblique facial cleft was described as early as in 18th century in Latin—by Von Kolmus (1732) [1] known as father of dysmorphology and later by Walter Dick (1837) [1].

George Bartisch [5] in 1583 first described removal of the orbital contents.

Artificial eyes, ears, and noses have been found in Egyptian mummies (Popp 1939).

Ambroise pare (1560) pioneer in maxillofacial prosthesis suggested use of glass and porcelain eyes for the first time.

Pierre Fauchard (1728) father of modern dentistry used prosthesis for a French soldier whose face was mutilated in war and called as "Gunner with as silver mask."

Until World War II, the glass eye was most popular eye manufactured but was difficult to manufacture and hazardous and cannot be modified.

M. U. Ludwig (1835) fabricated eyes for dolls later used for patients.

Muller Uri in 19th century suggested vulcanite, cellulose and glass eyes.

Sykes [6] in 1944 used acrylic physiologic ocular prosthesis.

Niiranen (1947) suggested modified acrylic eyes; K. E. Brown advocated characterization with rayon fibres. James et al. [7] (1976) suggested Graphic ocular locator. Chalian et al. [8] mentioned hollowup of prosthesis. Taicher et al. [9] approved of modified stock eyes and prefabricated eye shell customization. R. S. Schmerber (1986) regarding Iowa wax for modified impression for ocular prosthesis; are some of pioneers for suggested procedure [10].

4.1. Recent Improvements in Art of Ocular Rehabilitation [11]

(1) Garonzick (US patent number 6530953) used method of magnetically coupling prosthesis with ocular implant.

(2) Self-lubricating ocular prosthesis (dispensing button on demand).

(3) Ocular prosthesis to simulate human pupil dilation.

(4) Use of a light cure urethane dimethacrylate to minimize allergy.

(5) Digitization by scanning the eye socket, digital impression, iris photographs, and discs deposited on posterior scleral portion and joint to anterior scleral portion.

(6) CAD/CAM software to generate geometric models.

(7) Use of photo editing software for change in colour, size, diameter, and multiple depth layer correction of eye.

(8) Digital model with milling flanges and exported STL files.

(9) Motility implant and use of ball and sphere in implants.

(10) Bioeye, hydroxyapatite coralline ocular implant (conceived by Arthur C. Pellry, 1980).

5. Treatment Goals for Ocular Sclupture

The ocular prosthesis is aimed to provide the following benefits:

(1) life like appearance and function,

(2) protection and preservation of tissues,

(3) therapeutic and healing effect,

(4) intimate adaptation, equal distribution of pressure to tissue surface, massaging effect, and lubricating effect,

(5) noninvasive procedure,

(6) functional ocular movement, retention, and lid support,

(7) adjustability to customize, reline, or remake to adapt to future growth and development changes,

(8) enhanced natural feel, acceptability and moral upliftment,

(9) comfortable and economical,

(10) restore balance of face.

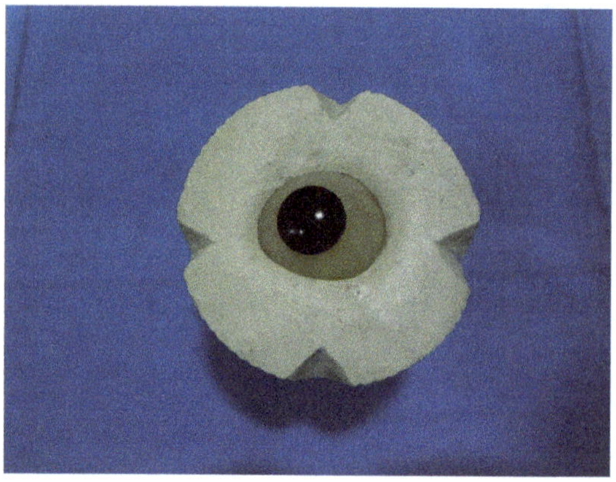

FIGURE 7: Invested eye shell.

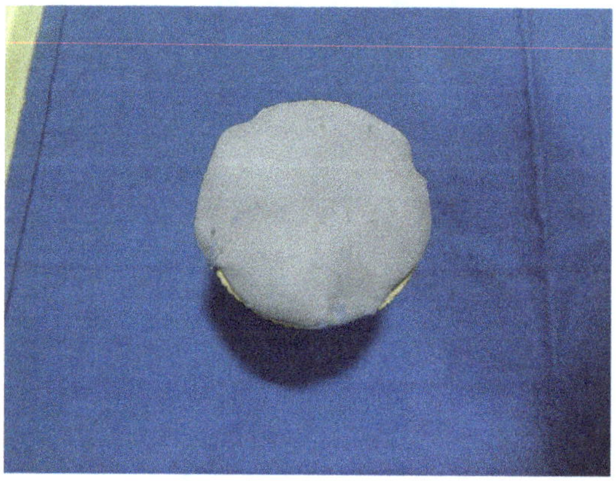

FIGURE 8: PVS cope preparation.

5.1. Ocular Sculpture Methodology. "To extract/remove is human but to restore is Divine!"

Rehabilitation is defined as the combined and coordinated use of medical, social, educational and vocational measure for training and retraining the individual to the highest possible level of functional activity (Park) [12].

The state-of-the art clinical methods and proposed benefits of ocular rehabilitation have changed significantly from those described by the early proponents of the technique.

Conventional processes that are currently in use for manufacturing an ocular prosthesis have been used for more than 6 years. The esthetic and functional outcome of the prosthesis is superior to the stock ocular prosthesis. They traditionally begin with the preparation of an impression of the anophthalmic eye socket. A confining impression tray is selected and placed into the socket anterior to the globe and posterior to the eyelids.

Unfortunately, following multiple ophthalmic invasive surgeries, lack of postoperative socket care led to constriction of the eye socket.

(1) Surgical dipping procedure of eye socket is carried out and after six weeks of healing period an impression for ocular conformer is made. In order to maintain the orbit volume an acrylic conformer is placed to form the cul-de-sac for lid pocket to hold the eye in place.

(2) *Ocular tray fabrication.* To fabricate an ocular tray to make an impression of eye socket, a prefabricated stock eye that optimally fits the socket is selected. The tissue surface of the eye is lubricated and invested in dental plaster to the height of contour. After plaster was set notches are made on its edges. Polyvinyl siloxane putty (Reprosil, Type I Dentsply, Germany) is mixed and adapted over the top of invested prosthesis into notched edges (Figures 7 and 8). After putty was set, it was removed and a bevelled sprue hole is made in the centre of the polyvinyl siloxane cope.

The eye shell is then removed from the mould, plaster surface is lubricated and putty cope is replaced on the mould. The mould is filled with self-cure acrylic resin (DPI RR Cold Cure Bombay Burma trading Corp. Ltd.) mix (Figure 9). Thus, formed clear acrylic ocular tray is removed from the mould. Multiple perforations are made, polished, trimmed, and disinfected. It is tried in patient for overextension and orientation.

(3) *Fabrication of conformer.* The tray is marked for iris and sclera portion for better handling. An acrylic stick is attached to the iris (centre) to act as a handle to facilitate removal of the ocular tray. Appropriate increments by low

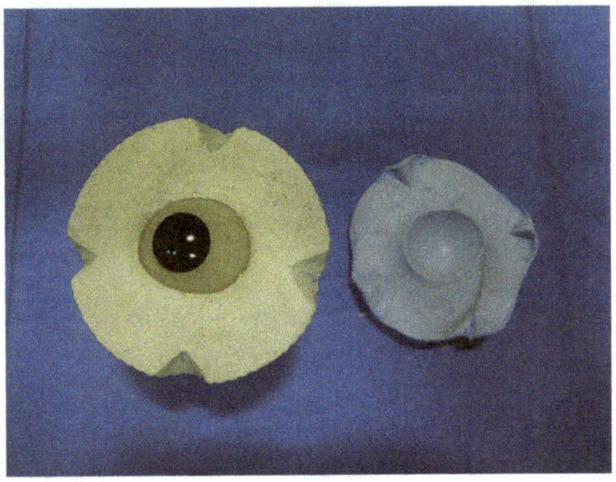

(a)

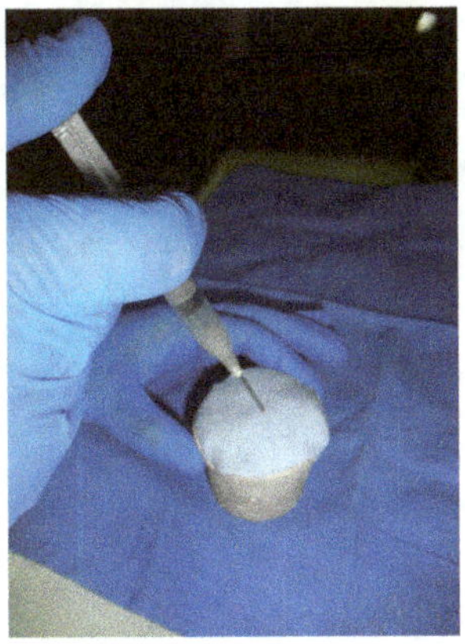

(b)

FIGURE 9: Fabrication of clear acrylic ocular tray.

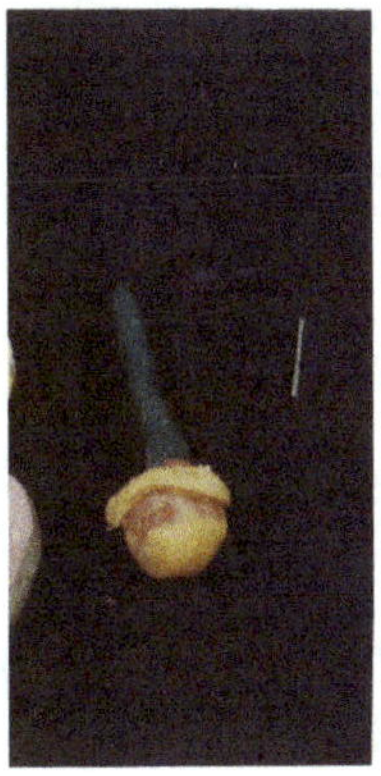

(a) Impression for conformer

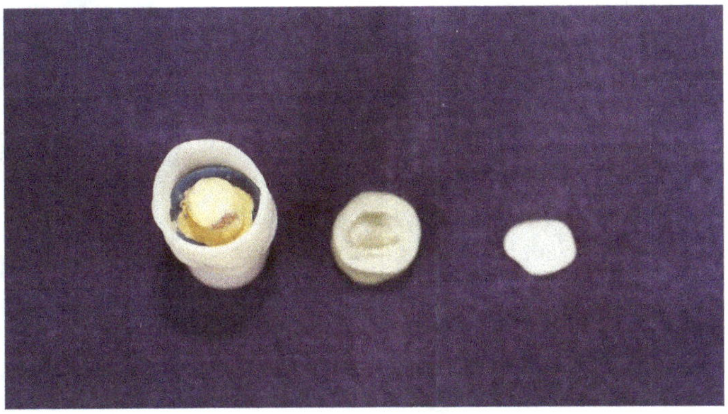

(b) Processing of conformer

FIGURE 10: Fabrication of conformer.

fusing impression compound were added to restore normal opening and to provide support to iris. The patient was asked to move his natural eye in various directions till material had set to obtain a functional impression. Subsequently a wash impression was made in light bodied elastomeric impression material. The entire assembly is flasked and the conformer prosthesis was processed in heat cure clear acrylic resin (DPI RR Heat Cure Bombay Burma trading Corp. Ltd.) and was polished, disinfected, and checked for fit. The conformer is retained in all times for 8 weeks therapeutic period to maintain socket volume (Figure 10).

(4) *Selection and orientation of eye shell.* A stock eye is selected that matches the colour and size of the sclera and iris-pupil complex of contralateral natural eye. It was modified by trimming and staining to match and resemble natural eye and rechecked for precise fit to the socket.

Ocular prosthesis was positioned to simulate the right eye with a reference mark placed at the midline and a Boley's gauge [8] was used to verify and confirm the mediolateral placing.

(5) *Fabrication of acrylic portion of eye prosthesis.* First, a conforming impression tray is prepared as before using the selected eye and placed into the socket anterior to the globe and posterior to the eyelid. A syringe with needle (shortened length 10 mm) is secured to ocular tray with cold cure acrylic resin (Figure 11). The syringe is loaded with low viscosity poly-vinyl siloxane (Reprosil, type I, Dentsply, Germany).

An impression material is then introduced into the eye socket via a tube protruding from the anterior surface of the impression tray and projecting out between the lids by means of a syringe connected to the tube (Figure 12).

The impression material is injected with the tray into the eye socket, patient is instructed to perform all movement of eye to maintain orientation, opening and closing, and support to lids. After removal of impression material stock eye shell replaces the ocular tray and rechecked in eye socket.

The complete assembly together is first invested with dental plaster till the height of contour and then with the stone (Tpye-3, Goldstone Asian Chemicals) and dental plaster to get a three-piece mould. A rounded acrylic elevation is attached at the junction of sclera and iris portion of the eye to

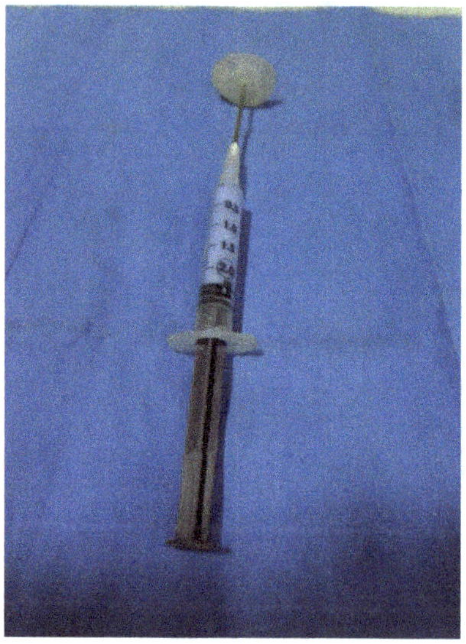

FIGURE 11: Ocular impression tray.

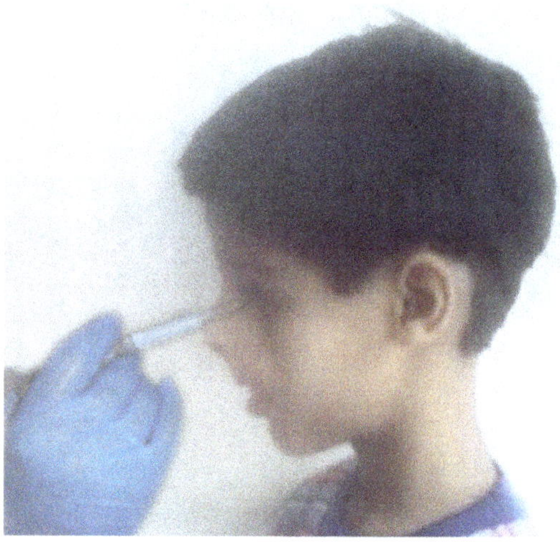

FIGURE 12: Impression for ocular prosthesis.

allow reorientation of the shell during processing. (Figure 13). Thus obtained ocular prosthesis is then customized.

(6) *Orbital prosthetic sculpture and customization*. A few veins are added to the sclera to improve the match. Silk fibres are added to duplicate the veining patterns of the contralateral eye with a thin layer of tooth coloured resin to hold. The prosthesis is then placed in a drying oven to prepare it for placement of clear acrylic resin over the anterior surface.

The bulge of eye and additional wax carving is gained as of contralateral eye by addition of wax (Wax number 2, Dental products, A.P.) onto tissue surface. The tissue surface of the prosthesis is again relined with soft tissue conditioner (Coe-soft GC America, Inc.) and placed into the socket to record functional ocular movement of eye; thus, retained tissue site of ocular prosthesis is invested, dewaxed, and packed with heat cure acrylic resin (DPI RR HC Bombay Burma trading Corp. Ltd.) (Figure 14).

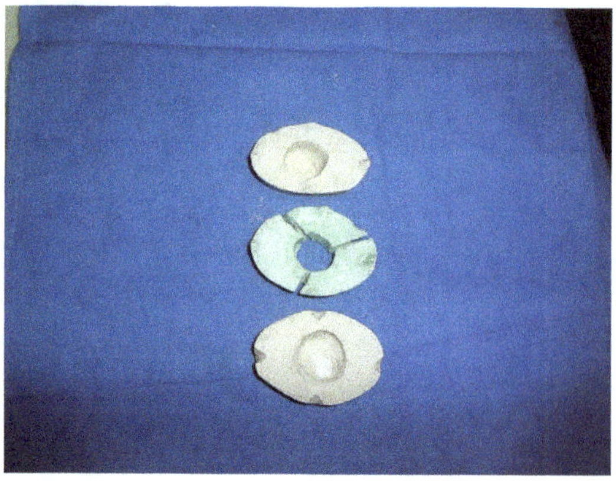

FIGURE 13: Three-piece dental stone mould (middle piece intentionlly fractured).

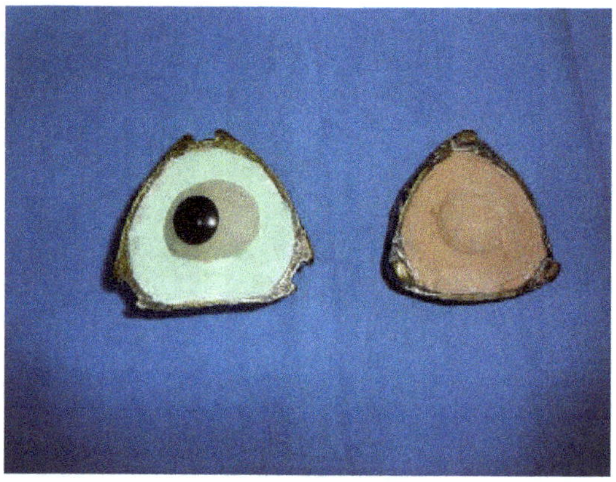

FIGURE 14: Processing for customized ocular prosthesis.

The final assessment of position of eye, anatomic contour, and shaping is carried out.

The entire assembly is cured in 70°C water bath for one and half hour, followed by 100°C water bath for 20 minutes. After deflasking it is polished thoroughly and is disinfected in 0.5% chlorhexidine and 70% isopropyl alcohol for 5 minutes and rinsed in sterile saline solution and inserted.

Thus, customized ocular prosthesis is based on patient's existing socket volume and anatomy and conformed accurately to socket with intimate adaptation to internal tissue surface of socket hence increases the movement of the prosthesis and enhances its natural appearance (Figure 15).

TLC principles in child management: parental counselling and education regarding nature, functioning and limitations of orbital prosthesis, care, maintenance protocol, nutritional therapy and also awareness for importance of periodic checkups were made before start of the treatment. The prior laid down goals of sculpture are thus achieved.

6. Discussion

The importance of an orbital prosthesis with acceptable esthetics and reasonable motility in restoring the natural

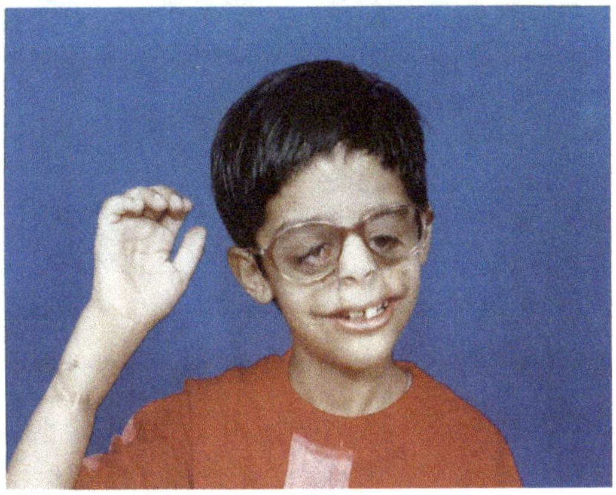

FIGURE 15: Child with customized ocular prosthesis in position.

appearance in patients with anophthalmia is recognized since long [13].

Beumer et al. [14] state that a prefabricated resin eye should not be used because of lack of intimate contact.

This is true if a prefabricated eye shell is selected and ground to close fit.

However, when prosthesis is customized to the patient using proper impression technique, distribution of pressure and intimate adaptation of the modified prosthesis to the tissue surface of the defect provide movement to and aesthetics to rehabilitation. Traditionally chosen customization of prefabricated acrylic eye shell (Taicher et al. [9]) method is based expounding on the virtues of clinical experience.

Organic insult, loss of function, and appearance have serious harmful effects on the total adjustment of the patient to his life situation.

Early treatment is important not only due to esthetic and functional concern but also for the positive psychological impact it has on the child. The treatment planning in this deformity is dependent upon the age, socio-economic status, type and severity of defect and the intra-oral situation at the time the treatment is planned. In recent times there has been a paradigm shift to enhance outcome by moulding for the growth and development than the surgery alone.

The challenge was to meet the infants clamour for functional demands on premature exposure to open world and was overcome through phased treatment implementation. Prosthodontic protocol involved expedient feeder prosthesis at birth with presurgical orofacial orthopaedics (PSIO), naso-alveolar moulding (PNAM), and maxillary expansion prosthesis apart from orbital prosthesis. Early PNAM represents a paradigm shift from traditional methods of PSIO, whereas surgical protocol involves removal of ectopic eye, coloboma of right eye, limb corrections, and craniofacial reconstructive correction for facial clefts, floating premaxilla and nasal deformities.

The components of ongoing treatment include future consideration for an artificial eye implant placement. The astuded guidance by obstetrician, paediatric plastic surgeon, syndromologist, speech therapist, and child psychotherapist was mandatory.

After initial surgeries inadequate parental counselling returned the child and was lost to followup for not less than 7 years of age. Final justification of these creations depends on the quality of life they prolong.

Thus it would be only when multiple disciplines together called forth and regard devotional care can we merit the most profound reverence towards life like restorations.

7. Conclusion

A well-made properly planned and functionally molded stock eye prosthesis maintains its orientation as patient performs various eye movements. Defects in orbitocraniofacial tissues resulting from congenital origin present a formidable challenge and restoration of these tissues is a subject of clinical, basic science, and engineering concern. Hence, primary goal of team work is not only to remove and prepare early replacement for diseased organ but to permit the person rather than the organ perse to function in a relatively normal manner.

Orbital sculpture with digital concept and motility implants is emerging rapidly on the hi-tech horizon. Also prosthesis to simulate human pupil dilation is no longer a distant dream. Hence, this field of dentistry knows no bounds; it crosses the realms of oral cavity, to the extraoral structure and ventures beyond the horizon to restore other facial structures including eyes creating the so-called "healthy beauty".

"The eyes are the windows of the soul." The spark in Gaurav's eyes truly reflects his envisioned soul. This in turn is our inspiration and the golden reward.

References

[1] K. Boo-Chai, "The oblique facial cleft: a 20-year follow-up," *British Journal of Plastic Surger*, vol. 43, no. 3, pp. 355–358, 1990.

[2] J. W. Seeds, R. C. Cephalo, and W. N. Herbert, "Amniotic band syndrome," *American Journal of Obstetrics & Gynecology*, vol. 144, no. 3, pp. 243–248, 1982.

[3] G. L. Streeter, "Focal deficiencies in fetal tissues and their relation to intra-uterine amputation," *Contributions to Embryology*, vol. 22, pp. 1–44, 1930.

[4] R. Torpin, "Amniochorionic mesoblastic fibrous strings and amnionic bands: associated constricting fetal malformations or fetal death," *American Journal of Obstetrics & Gynecology*, vol. 91, pp. 65–75, 1965.

[5] K. P. Dholam et al., *Journal of Prosthetic Dentistry*, p. 57, January 2008.

[6] L. M. Sykes, "Custom made ocular prostheses: a clinical report," *Journal of Prosthetic Dentistry*, vol. 75, no. 1, pp. 1–3, 1996.

[7] H. James, J. R. Ellis, and W. S. Foulds, "A method of artificial eye manufacture," *British Journal of Ophthalmology*, vol. 60, no. 2, pp. 153–155, 1976.

[8] V. A. Chalian, J. B. Drane, and S. M. Standish, *Maxillofacial Prosthodontics Multidisciplinary Practice*, Williams & Wilkins, Baltimore, Md, USA, 1971.

[9] S. Taicher, H. M. Steinberg, I. Tubiana, and M. Sela, "Modified stock-eye ocular prosthesis," *The Journal of Prosthetic Dentistry*, vol. 54, no. 1, pp. 95–98, 1985.

[10] R. L. Schneider, "Modified ocular prosthesis impression technique," *The Journal of Prosthetic Dentistry*, vol. 55, no. 4, pp. 482–485, 1986.

[11] F. K. Shah et al., *Journal of Prosthetic Dentistry*, vol. 8, no. 2, p. 67, April 2008.

[12] *Park—Textbook of Preventive & Social Medicine*, 9th edition.

[13] I. Artopoulou, P. Montogomery, and P. J. Wesley, "Digital imaging in fabrication of ocular prosthesis," *Journal of Prosthetic Dentistry*, vol. 95, no. 4, pp. 327–330, 2006.

[14] J. Beumer, T. A. Curtis, M. T. Marunick et al., *Maxillofacial Rehabilitation Prosthodontics & Surgical Consideration*, C.V. Mosby, St. Louis, Mo, USA, 1979.

21

Massive Submandibular Sialolith: Complete Radiographic Registration and Biochemical Analysis through X-Ray Diffraction

Ademir Franco,[1] Mayara Jessica de Carvalho Mattos,[1] Francine Ferrari,[1] José Manoel dos Reis Neto,[2] Luiz Carlos Carta Gambus,[1] Paulo Henrique Couto Souza,[1] and Soraya de Azambuja Berti-Couto[1]

[1] *Departamento de Estomatologia, Escola de Saúde e Biociências, Pontifícia Universidade Católica do Paraná, Imaculada Conceição 1155, Prado Velho, 80215-901 Curitiba, PR, Brazil*
[2] *Laboratório de Análise de Minerais e Rochas, Departamento de Geologia, Universidade Federal do Paraná, Centro Politécnico 19062, Jardim das Américas, 81615-980 Curitiba, PR, Brazil*

Correspondence should be addressed to Ademir Franco; franco.gat@gmail.com

Academic Editor: David J. Bentrem

Sialolithiasis is a pathologic condition that affects 60 million people per year, which is caused by the presence of calcified structures, named sialoliths, inside the salivary glands and their salivary ducts. Despite the large incidence of sialolithiasis, its etiology is still unknown. In the present case report, a 47-year-old female patient, presenting with local pain and hampered mouth opening, underwent a surgical approach for the removal of a 20 mm sialolith, which was further analyzed through X-ray diffraction. In parallel, a radiographic registration of 8 years, covering all the period for sialolith formation, is presented along the case report.

1. Introduction

The salivary calculi are calcified structures often referred to as sialoliths, which consist of minerals such as calcium phosphate and hydroxyapatite, as well as other substances such as magnesium, potassium, and ammonia [1]. Sialoliths often lead to sialolithiasis, which is a common disease, affecting around 60 million people per year [1]. Mostly, sialolithiasis is clinically characterized by local pain and edema, reduced salivary flow, hampered mouth opening, spontaneous bleeding, and purulent discharge [2]. Radiographically, rounded or cylindrical radiopaque structures are observed near to the salivary glands, or their ducts, especially in panoramic and occlusal radiographs [3].

Small sialoliths can be spontaneously expelled through the stimulation of the salivary flow by performing local massage or using mechanical or chemical sialogogues, such as bubble gums and citric acid, respectively [4]. On the other hand, multiple or massive sialoliths often require major approaches, such as lithotripsy, sialadenectomy, sialotomy, and sialodochoplasty [3].

The present study aims to report the case of a 47-year-old female patient, who was diagnosed with sialolithiasis based on clinical and radiographic signs. Specifically, the present case is illustrated by a minimally invasive surgical procedure, a radiographic registration of 8 years covering the entire period of a massive sialolith formation, and a biochemical analysis through X-ray diffraction.

2. Case Report

In August 2012, a 47-year-old, white Caucasian, female patient was referred, by an orthodontist, to the Stomatology Department of the Pontifícia Universidade Católica do Paraná, Brazil, presenting with extreme signs of local pain in the submandibular region and speaking limitations due to hampered mouth opening. Clinically, left submandibular lymphadenopathy was detected, as well as edema in the left

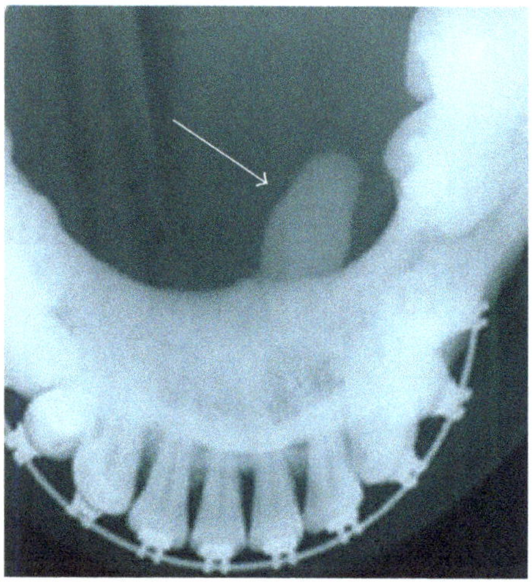

FIGURE 1: Occlusal radiograph of the massive sialolith (arrow).

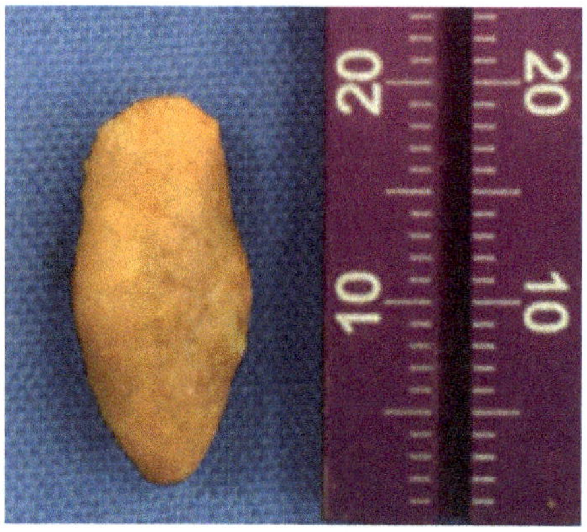

FIGURE 2: Clinical view of the sialolith after surgical removal.

side of the floor of the mouth, with a purulent discharge. In addition, a yellowish structure of hard consistency was observed near to the sublingual caruncle. An occlusal radiograph revealed a cylindrical radiopaque sialolith-compatible image, measuring approximately 2 × 1 cm, in the lower left canine region, confirming the diagnosis of submandibular sialolithiasis (Figure 1).

During the anamnesis, the patient did not report systemic diseases and reported being allergic to Penicillin. Further, the surgical excision was executed in the same day due to the exacerbated symptoms and the favorable position, in which the sialolith took place after a submandibular massage. Under local anesthesia, a 5 mm incision was performed on the mucosa, over the sialolith. In order to move the sialolith close to the incision, the submandibular massage in the posteroanterior direction was repeated. Using forceps, a 20 mm sialolith (Figure 2) was removed from the floor of the mouth. After the sialolith removal, it was possible to see the reinstatement of salivary flow and also the reduction of the purulent discharge. The patient was medicated with Azithromycin 500 mg, Ibuprofen 600 mg, and Paracetamol 750 mg.

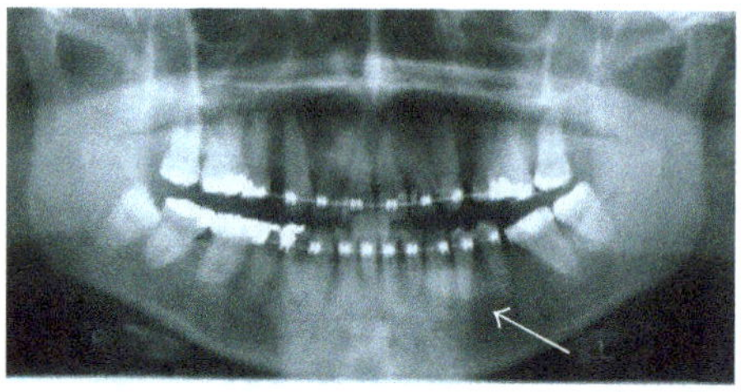

FIGURE 3: The last panoramic radiograph previously obtained for orthodontic purposes indicating the massive sialolith (arrow).

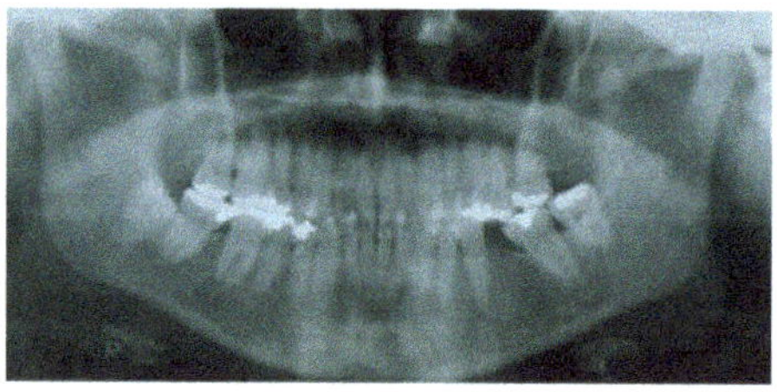

FIGURE 4: An additional panoramic radiograph retrieved from the patient's file revealing no sign of sialolith formation.

In the following week, the patient returned without edema and local inflammation. The submandibular gland function was tested performing local massage, indicating normal salivary flow. Surprisingly, the patient provided a previous panoramic radiograph, dating from March 2011 (Figure 3), representing the last radiographic exam for conclusion of orthodontic treatment. Despite slight morphological alteration, the orthodontic radiograph allowed for the detection of the sialolith. Based on the lack of early detecting the sialolith on the orthodontic radiograph, a deeper investigation in the patient's dental files was carried out revealing an additional panoramic radiograph, dating from June 2004, in which no sign of sialolith was detected (Figure 4). Clinical and radiographic followup were performed 6 months after the surgery revealing no alterations.

3. Biochemical Analysis

The sialolith was referred to the Laboratory for Analysis of Minerals and Rocks, Geology Department, Universidade Federal do Paraná, Brazil (LAMIR-UFPR), for biochemical analysis through X-ray diffraction. The stone weighted 0,593 g. An Empyrean Diffractometer (PANalytical, Almelo, the Netherlands) processed the powdered sialolith. The measured scattered pattern produced out of the interaction between the X-ray beam and the sialolith surface indicated hydroxyapatite Ca5(PO4)(CO3)3(OH) as the only mineral present (Figure 5).

4. Discussion

The medical literature reports the submandibular salivary glands as the most commonly related pair of glands in cases of sialolithiasis (around 80% of prevalence) [5–7], specially involving massive sialoliths [8]. It is explained by

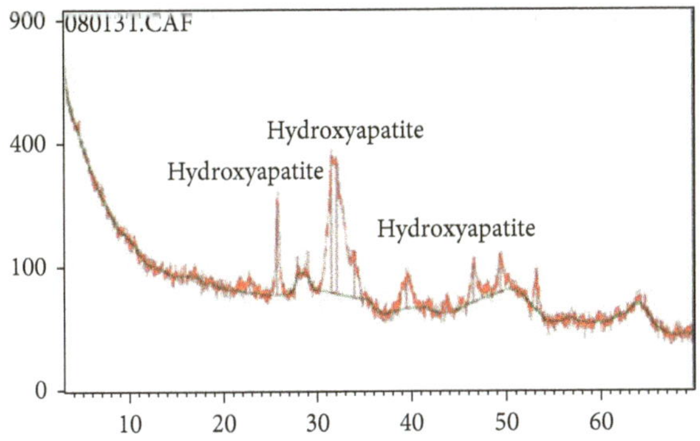

FIGURE 5: Outcome from the analysis through X-ray diffraction indicating hydroxyapatite as mineral structure of the massive sialolith.

the submandibular salivary duct morphology, a tortuous structure which links the salivary gland to the oral cavity. The most narrowed path of the referred duct is named "comma area," which is located near to the duct's outfall and facilitates the deposition of minerals, such as calcium, creating a proper nidus for sialolith formation [8, 9]. In addition, the submandibular salivary gland presents an alkaline environment with high concentration of phosphate, which contributes for the formation of hydroxyapatite. In previous studies [10, 11], hydroxyapatite was detected through X-ray diffraction and classified as the main mineral structure in 24 out of 27 sialoliths. The remaining sialoliths were composed of organic structures such as epithelial cells and bacteria. Accordingly, the present study indicates that even massive sialoliths predominantly consist of hydroxyapatite. Moreover, detailed investigations indicate that levels of phytate and magnesium are decreased in patients with sialoliths [11]. Phytate and magnesium are potent crystallization inhibitors of calcium, strongly related to the daily diet, especially present in plant seeds and wheat bran, respectively. In the present study, the long-term radiographic registration suggests that the time lapse for a massive sialolith formation was less than 8 years, indicating a potential correlation with the patient's routine diet. Thus, possible evidences for the study of the etiology of massive sialoliths are addressed. Further on, deeper investigations on the biochemical formation of sialoliths are not often performed in the daily dental practice due to the high costs and limitations in accessing necessary facilities. However, biochemical investigations are relevant to the search of potential internal and external factors associated with the sialoliths formation, such as the hormonal influence. Specifically in the present case, no especial diet or systemic alterations were reported by the patient. An additional advantage of knowing the composition of a sialolith concerns the possibility of an individualized treatment, advising the patient to avoid certain dietary components, enabling an optimal postoperative follow-up.

In the present study, as consequences of the sialolithiasis, local pain, lymphadenopathy, edema, and purulent discharge were detected. Based on these findings, the patient was medicated with antibiotics during a week. Similarly, Overton et al. [12], 2012, and Combes et al. [13], 2009, treated their patients with antibiotic therapy in the immediate postoperative week. Specifically in the preset report, considering the presence of purulent discharge and the patient's allergy to Penicillin, Azithromycin 500 mg was prescribed for antibiotic coverage in combination with anti-inflammatory (Ibuprofen 600 mg) and analgesic (Paracetamol 750 mg) drugs.

Differently from the case reports already described in the medical literature, the present study is highlighted by the registration of the entire sialolith formation once no sign of ectopic mineralization was detected within the radiographs obtained out of the patient's dental records. These radiographs support the need for correctly recording dental interventions and updating patient's files, as well as early and accurately diagnosing sialolithiasis, for an optimal treatment outcome.

References

[1] M. Rai and R. Burman, "Giant submandibular sialolith of remarkable size in the comma area of Wharton's duct: a case report," *Journal of Oral and Maxillofacial Surgery*, vol. 67, no. 6, pp. 1329–1332, 2009.

[2] R. Rauso, G. Gherardini, P. Biondi, G. Tartaro, and G. Colella, "A case of a giant submandibular gland calculus perforating the floor of the mouth," *Ear, Nose, & Throat Journal*, vol. 91, no. 6, pp. E25–27, 2012.

[3] M. Gonçalves, E. Hochuli-Vieira, C. Lugão, M. S. Monnazzi, and A. Gonçalves, "Sialolith of unusual size and shape," *Dentomaxillofacial Radiology*, vol. 31, no. 3, pp. 209–210, 2002.

[4] R. El Gehani, B. Krishnan, and M. I. L. Shehoumi, "Submandibular giant sialoliths: report of two cases and review of the literature," *Ear, Nose and Throat Journal*, vol. 89, no. 6, pp. 1–4, 2010.

[5] S. Singh and S. Singh, "Submandibular gland megalith eroding the floor of the mouth: a case report," *Ear, Nose & Throat Journal*, vol. 92, no. 12, pp. 17–19, 2013.

[6] T. T. Boynton and S. E. Lieblich, "Unusual case of a sialolith: a case report," *Oral Surgery, Oral Medicine, Oral Pathology and Oral Radiology*, vol. 117, no. 1, pp. e9–e10, 2014.

[7] L. Ardekian, H. H. Klein, S. Araydy, and F. Marchal, "The use of sialendoscopy for the treatment of multiple salivary gland stones," *Journal of Oral and Maxillofacial Surgery*, vol. 72, pp. 89–95, 2014.

[8] C. Pandarakalan, W. M. Goebel, and B. Seyer, "Chronic sclerosing sialodenitis or Küttner's tumor associated with a giant sialolith: a case report," *Oral Surgery, Oral Medicine, Oral Pathology, Oral Radiology*, vol. 115, pp. 33–40, 2013.

[9] L. Y. Zheng, E. Kim, C. Q. Yu, C. Yang, J. Park, and Z. Z. Chen, "A retrospective case series illustrating a possible association between a widened hilum and sialolith formation in the submandibular gland," *Journal of Craniomaxillofacial Surgery*, vol. 41, no. 7, pp. 648–651, 2013.

[10] O. Kasaboğlu, N. Er, C. Tümer, and M. Akkocaoğlu, "Micromorphology of sialoliths in submandibular salivary gland: a scanning electron microscope and X-ray diffraction analysis," *Journal of Oral and Maxillofacial Surgery*, vol. 62, no. 10, pp. 1253–1258, 2004.

[11] F. Grases, C. Santiago, B. M. Simonet, and A. Costa-Bauzá, "Sialolithiasis: mechanism of calculi formation and etiologic factors," *Clinica Chimica Acta*, vol. 334, no. 1-2, pp. 131–136, 2003.

[12] A. Overton, J. Combes, and M. McGurk, "Outcome after endoscopically assisted surgical retrieval of symptomatic parotid stones," *International Journal of Oral and Maxillofacial Surgery*, vol. 41, no. 2, pp. 248–251, 2012.

[13] J. Combes, K. Karavidas, and M. McGurk, "Intraoral removal of proximal submandibular stones—an alternative to sialadenectomy?" *International Journal of Oral and Maxillofacial Surgery*, vol. 38, no. 8, pp. 813–816, 2009.

22

Aplasia Cutis Congenita of the Scalp with a Familial Pattern

Waleed AlShehri, Sara AlFadil, Alhanouf AlOthri, Abdulaziz O. Alabdulkarim, Shabeer A. Wani, and Sari M. Rabah

Department of Plastic & Reconstructive Surgery, King Fahad Medical City, Riyadh 11525, Saudi Arabia

Correspondence should be addressed to Sara AlFadil; sara.alfadil@hotmail.com

Academic Editor: Yueh-Bih Tang

Aplasia Cutis Congenita (ACC) is a condition characterized by congenital absence of skin, usually on the scalp. ACC can occur as an isolated condition or in the presence of other congenital anomalies. Here we describe a case of a 16-day-old baby girl with an isolated ACC of the scalp. Her elder two siblings have been diagnosed with ACC with concomitant cardiac or limb anomalies. The patient was managed conservatively until the defect has formed scar tissue 6 months later.

1. Introduction

Cutis aplasia or Aplasia Cutis Congenita (ACC) is an uncommon and rare congenital abnormality involving variant layers of the skin, mostly as a solitary lesion involving the midline over the skull vertex and, less commonly, underlying periosteum and bone [1]. It may occur in other sites as well such as the chest, abdomen, or limbs [2, 3]. Of lesions on the scalp, 20% involve the cranium, exposing the underlying dura membrane. ACC could also be found in other congenital anomalies; since it was first described in 1767 by Cordon, around 500 similar cases have been reported so far [4]. Frieden classified the different anomalies into 9 groups based on the number and the presence or absence of other anomalies (Table 1) [5]. The lesions in those cases are quite variable, ranging from only local absence of skin to a complete absence of epidermis, subcutaneous tissue, bone, or in some cases the dura [6–8]. The incidence of ACC is estimated as 1 per 10,000 live births [1]. This failure of formation is frequently more observed in females. The etiology remains unclear so far; however, both genetic and environmental causes have been implicated, including vascular blood supply, a sudden arrest of midline embryological development, and failure in neural tube closure, and syphilis has at one time contributed as the cause [1, 9]. Rupture of amniotic membrane in an early time, forming amniotic bands, may also be from the cause [5]. A number of teratogenic drugs such as Methimazole, a Thiomidazole derivative used as an antithyroid agent, have shown to be involved [10–13]. There are similar cases, classified as being of an autosomal-dominant inheritance [14]. Establishing a diagnosis is usually based on the findings of the clinical examination, typically presenting as a hairless, smooth skin defect covered up by atrophic tissue or a dark-colored eschar. Superficial defects presenting as an ulcer are usually treated conservatively. Extensive or deep defects may require reconstruction of the scalp area or the use of bone transplants. However, hairless or scarcely haired scars mandate excision of the lesion and covering it with local flap from the scalp [9, 15–20].

2. Case Report

A 16-day-old newborn Female from Saudi Arabia presented to the clinic with a skin defect localized to the scalp since birth. The baby did not suffer from any ailments, and her medical history was unremarkable. Her mother, 32 years old, denied any history of illnesses during her pregnancy, infection, or drug intake taking including Nonsteroidal Anti-Inflammatory Drugs (NSAID) or Methimazole. She completed 38 weeks of gestation and delivered her baby via a normal vaginal delivery. The newborn did not sustain any birth injury and did not suffer from any other abnormalities or feeding difficulties. She did not require any intensive care and went home from hospital with her mother. Upon

Table 1: Classification for ACC.

	Group	Associated anomalies	Inheritance
1	Scalp ACC without multiple anomalies	Cleft lip and palate, tracheoesophageal fistula, patent ductus arteriosus, omphalocele, mental retardation, polycystic kidneys	Autosomal dominant or sporadic
2	Scalp ACC with limb abnormalities	Limbs reduced, syndactyly, clubfoot, encephalocele, nail dystrophy or absence, persistent cutis marmorata	Autosomal dominant
3	Scalp ACC with skin/organoid nevi	Epidermal nevi, organoid nevi, corneal opacities, scleral dermoids, eyelid colobomas, mental retardation, seizures	Sporadic
4	ACC overlying embryologic malformations	Meningomyelocele, spinal dysraphia, cranial stenosis, leptomeningeal angiomatosis, gastroschisis, congenital midline porencephaly, ectopia of ear, omphalocele	Depends upon underlying condition
5	ACC with fetus papyraceus or placental infarcts	Single umbilical artery spastic developmental delay, spastic paralysis, clubbed hands and feet, amniotic bands	Sporadic
6	ACC associated with epidermolysis bullosa	Blistering of skin and/or mucous membranes, deformed nails, pyloric or duodenal atresia, abnormal ears and nose, ureteral stenosis, renal anomalies, amniotic bands	Depends upon type of epidermolysis bullosa
7	ACC localized to extremities without blistering	None	Autosomal dominant or recessive
8	ACC caused by teratogens	Imperforate anus (methimazole), other signs of intrauterine infection with varicella or herpes simplex	Not inherited
9	ACC associated with congenital syndromes	Trisomy 13, 4p-syndrome, ectodermal dysplasia, focal dermal hypoplasia, amniotic band disruption complex, XY gonadal dysgenesis, Johanson-Blizzard syndrome	Depends upon syndrome

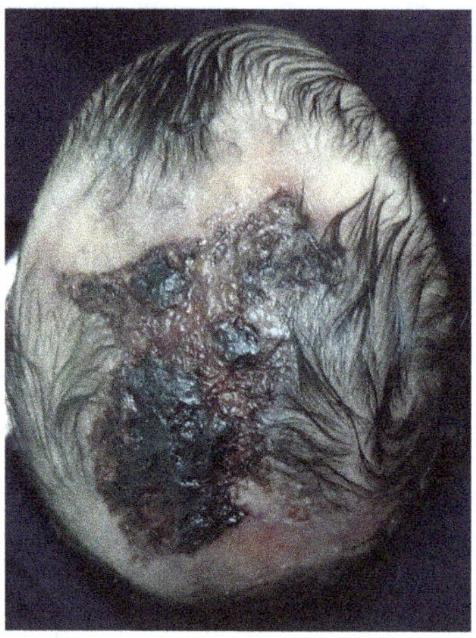

Figure 1: The newborn presented with skin defect of the scalp with an overlying crust.

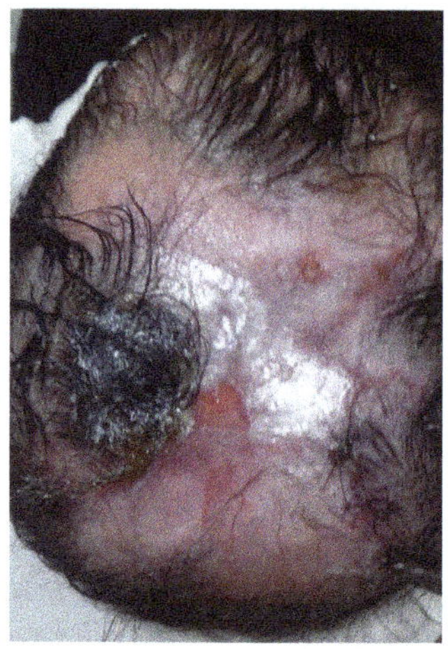

Figure 2: Six-month follow-up shows scar formation over the affected area.

local examination, the defect was solitary, localized with an irregular shape and approximately 6 × 6 cm in size (Figure 1). The lesion involved the epidermis and the upper dermis only. Neurosurgical team was involved in the care of this patient. A CT scan of the head was performed, and no deep tissue involvement was noted. Reconstruction solutions were offered to the parents but they insisted on nonsurgical intervention. Therefore, the patient was treated with noninvasive debridement of the lesion and local therapy, including gentle water cleansing and the application of topical antibiotic ointment. Six months later, the patient has returned for a follow-up. Scar tissue has formed over the defect (Figure 2). Family history revealed that none of her parents had the same condition; however, two of her sisters did and were diagnosed with cutis aplasia. The elder one is currently 4 years of age, with right unilateral terminal reduction of the first and second toes (Figure 3). The other sister was born prematurely and died shortly after birth due to cardiac anomalies.

3. Discussion

ACC occurs as a solitary defect; it can happen alone or in the presence of syndromic congenital anomalies. The involvement of the scalp area may lead to the understanding of the etiology. Upon our review to the literature available, cases were often characterized by an entire absence of skin

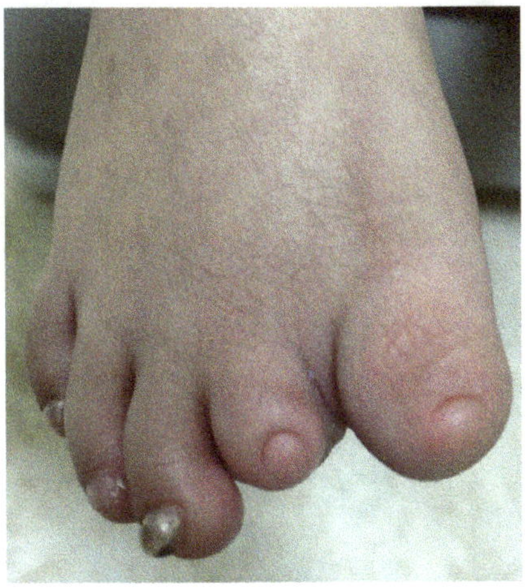

FIGURE 3: Unilateral terminal reduction of the right first and second toe.

and subcutaneous tissues. Histologically, we found that most of the lacking tissues belonged to epithelial ectoderm. The condition could be associated with chromosomal defects [21]. Some researches show the association with gestational conditions such as an intrauterine vascular ischemia, amniotic adherences, and viral infections [22, 23]. A rise of alpha-fetoprotein levels and a distinct amniotic fluid acetylcholinesterase band were found in recent article as markers for ACC [24]. Also, a number of drugs have been linked to ACC. For example, the use of cocaine during pregnancy can lead to vasoconstriction of the placenta or disruption of the fetus vascularity, causing the cranial defects and anomalies of the central nervous system (CNS) [25]. Methimazole, a drug used for the treatment of hyperthyroidism, may show some skin affection. Benzodiazepines use is also linked with ACC as described by Martínez-Lage et al. [7]. Surgical treatment requires careful preoperative planning [26]. Minimal superficial lesions are treated conservatively to heal gradually by reepithelialization and result with a hypertrophic or atrophic scar. Tissue expander insertion may be necessary in extensive lesions reaching the scalp, whereas the one deep enough to reach the brain, bone, and meningeal transplants may be indicated [9, 15, 20, 27]. Deep defects overlying the sagittal sinus are indicators for urgent surgical intervention to prevent potentially lethal infections or hemorrhage [28–30]. Grafting [31] and temporary use of biological dressings [32] and silver sulfadiazine dressings while waiting for the processes of skin and bony ingrowth [3] have been published with variable degree of success.

4. Conclusion

Aplasia Cutis Congenita is a rare congenital disorder characterized by absence of skin, most frequently overlying the scalp. ACC can be associated with many anomalies. We report a case of a newborn with isolated scalp ACC, which was treated conservatively. Although neither of the parents had ACC, two of the patient's siblings have ACC of the scalp with concomitant cardiac or limb anomalies.

References

[1] M. Bajpai and K. Pal, "Aplasia cutis cerebri with partial acrania—total reconstruction in a severe case and review of the literature," *Journal of Pediatric Surgery*, vol. 38, no. 2, article e4, 2003.

[2] J. K. O'Neill, M. Carter, and R. P. Warr, "Aplasia cutis congenita. A case of scalp defect repair using two opposing bipedicled local flaps," *Journal of Plastic, Reconstructive and Aesthetic Surgery*, vol. 63, no. 3, pp. e242–e244, 2010.

[3] K. Blunt, V. Quan, D. Carr, and B. A. Paes, "Aplasia cutis congenita: a clinical review and associated defects," *Neonatal Network*, vol. 11, no. 7, pp. 17–27, 1992.

[4] M. Cordon, "Extrait d'une lettre au sujet de trois enfants de la meme mere nex avec partie des extremites denuee de peau," *Journal de Médecine, Chirurgie, Pharmacie*, vol. 26, pp. 556–557, 1767.

[5] I. J. Frieden, "Aplasia cutis congenita: a clinical review and proposal for classification," *Journal of the American Academy of Dermatology*, vol. 14, no. 4, pp. 646–660, 1986.

[6] L. P. Lassman and D. G. Sims, "Congenital midline scalp and skull defect," *Archives of Disease in Childhood*, vol. 50, no. 12, pp. 958–960, 1975.

[7] J. F. Martínez-Lage, M. J. Almagro, F. L. Hernández, and M. Poza, "Aplasia cutis congenita of the scalp," *Child's Nervous System*, vol. 18, pp. 634–637, 2002.

[8] H. Aloulou, W. Chaari, S. Khanfir et al., "Aplasia cutis congenita of the scalp (5 observations)," *Archives de Pediatrie*, vol. 15, no. 4, pp. 382–387, 2008.

[9] L. C. Argenta and R. O. Dingman, "Total reconstruction of aplasia cutis congenita involving scalp, skull, and dura," *Plastic and Reconstructive Surgery*, vol. 77, no. 4, pp. 650–653, 1986.

[10] M. Inoue, N. Arata, G. Koren et al., "Hyperthyroidismduring pregnancy," *Canadian Family Physician*, vol. 55, pp. 701–703, 2009.

[11] H. Iwayama, H. Hosono, H. Yamamoto, M. Oshiro, and N. Ueda, "Aplasia cutis congenita with skull defect in a monozygotic twin after exposure to methimazole in utero," *Birth Defects Research Part A: Clinical and Molecular Teratology*, vol. 79, no. 10, pp. 680–684, 2007.

[12] M. Abe, T. Syuto, Y. Yokoyama, and O. Ishikawa, "Aplasia cutis congenita after methimazole exposure *in utero* successfully treated with basic fibroblast growth factor," *International Journal of Dermatology*, vol. 49, no. 3, pp. 334–335, 2010.

[13] S. K. Baid and D. P. Merke, "Aplasia cutis congenita following in utero methimazole exposure," *Journal of Pediatric Endocrinology and Metabolism*, vol. 20, no. 5, pp. 585–586, 2007.

[14] M. R. Chitnis, R. Carachi, and P. Galea, "Familial aplasia cutis congenita," *European Journal of Pediatric Surgery*, vol. 6, no. 2, pp. 100–101, 1996.

[15] M. F. Attalla and A. M. El-Sayed, "Scalp aplasia cutis congenita: closure by the L-shaped flap," *Child's Nervous System*, vol. 8, no. 5, pp. 287–288, 1992.

[16] G. Borgnolo, F. Longo, G. Olivo, and G. Guidobaldi, "Aplasia cutis congenita: report of 4 additional cases and review of the literature," *La Pediatria Medica e Chirurgica*, vol. 16, no. 6, pp. 559-563, 1994 (Italian).

[17] J. Kruk-Jeromin and E. Lewandowicz, "Congenital aplasia of scalp skin," *Przeglad Dermatologiczny*, pp. 73908–73911, 1986 (Polish).

[18] D. A. Ross, S. W. S. Laurie, C. J. Coombs, and K. L. Mutimer, "Aplasia cutis congenita: failed conservative treatment," *Plastic and Reconstructive Surgery*, vol. 95, no. 1, pp. 124–129, 1995.

[19] L. M. Field, "Scalp flaps," *The Journal of Dermatologic Surgery and Oncology*, pp. 17190–17199, 1991.

[20] J. G. McCarthy, Ed., *Plastic Surgery*, Saunders, Philadelphia, Pa, USA, 1990.

[21] L. H. Honoré, F. J. Dill, and B. J. Poland, "Placental morphology in spontaneous human abortuses with normal and abnormal karyotypes," *Teratology*, vol. 14, no. 2, pp. 151–166, 1976.

[22] F. L. Mannino, K. L. Jones, and K. Benirschke, "Congenital skin defects and fetus papyraceus," *The Journal of Pediatrics*, vol. 91, no. 4, pp. 559–564, 1977.

[23] M. E. Evers, P. M. Steijlen, and B. C. Hamel, "Aplasia cutis congenital and associated disorders: an update," *Clinical Genetics*, vol. 47, pp. 295–301, 1995.

[24] Y. Dror, Z. Gelman-Kohan, Z. Hagai, A. Juster-Reicher, R. N.-B. Cohen, and B. Mogilner, "Aplasia cutis congenita, elevated alpha-fetoprotein, and a distinct amniotic fluid acetylcholinesterase electrophoretic band," *American Journal of Perinatology*, vol. 11, no. 2, pp. 149–152, 1994.

[25] C. B. Whitley and R. J. Gorlin, "Adams-oliver syndrome revisited," *American Journal of Medical Genetics*, vol. 40, no. 3, pp. 319–326, 1991.

[26] C. Goldberg, G. Fenelon, N. S. Blake, F. Dowling, and B. F. Regan, "Diastematomyelia: a critical review of the natural history and treatment," *Spine*, vol. 9, no. 4, pp. 367–372, 1984.

[27] D. Dyall-Smith, A. Ramsden, and S. Laurie, "Adams-Oliver syndrome: aplasia cutis congenita, terminal transverse limb defects and cutis marmorata telangiectatica congenita," *Australasian Journal of Dermatology*, vol. 35, no. 1, pp. 19–22, 1994.

[28] L. A. Peer and J. V. Duyn, "Congenital defect of the scalp: report of a case with fatal termination," *Plastic and Reconstructive Surgery*, vol. 3, no. 6, pp. 722–726, 1948.

[29] E. J. Kosnik and M. P. Sayers, "Congenital scalp defects: aplasia cutis congenita," *Journal of Neurosurgery*, vol. 42, no. 1, pp. 32–36, 1975.

[30] L. A. Sargent, "Aplasia cutis congenita of the scalp," *Journal of Pediatric Surgery*, vol. 25, no. 12, pp. 1211–1213, 1990.

[31] M. F. B. Bailie, "Aplasia cutis congenita of neck and shoulder requiring a skin graft: a case report," *British Journal of Plastic Surgery*, vol. 36, no. 1, pp. 72–74, 1983.

[32] J. Lambert, P. Govaert, and J. M. Naeyaert, "What syndrome is this?" *Pediatric Dermatology*, vol. 14, no. 4, pp. 330–332, 1997.

23

An Asymptomatic Foreign Body in the Nose in an Eighteen-Year-Old Patient: Button Battery

Merih Onal, Gultekin Ovet, and Necat Alatas

Konya Education and Training Hospital, Department of Otorhinolaryngology, 42090 Konya, Turkey

Correspondence should be addressed to Merih Onal; drmerihonal@gmail.com

Academic Editor: Cheng-Yu Long

Foreign bodies lodged in the upper airway are a common occurrence in children. Many unusual foreign bodies in the nose have been reported as foreign bodies like nuts, plastic toy parts, beads, and so forth. Most of these produce minimal morbidity but button batteries due to their early chemical disintegration require early surgical intervention. Here, we report a case of button battery lodged in the nose for several years with a symptom of nasal obstruction and chronic sinusitis.

1. Introduction

Nasal foreign bodies are generally referred to otorhinolaryngologists [1]. Foul-smelling, purulent nasal flow and epistaxis are typically present in nasal foreign bodies. In particular, stuck nasal foreign bodies may cause morbidities such as chronic sinusitis, septal perforation, or necrosis of bones in the long term obstruction. The button battery is generally used in small devices such as hearing aids, watches, and electronic gadget. Their smooth and shiny surface possibly makes them interesting for children. A button battery in the nose is capable of tissue damage due to its electrochemical content. But sometimes it does not cause any ill effect [2] depending on several factors such as remaining voltage in the battery and chemical composition of the battery [3]. We report a case of 18-year-old young lady who was referred to our clinic with unknown nasal foreign body.

2. Case

18-year-old female patient was referred to our clinic with a diagnosis of foreign body in the nose from another center. The patient had nasal congestion and rhinorrhea. She was admitted to doctor with these complaints many times before and acute sinusitis treatment was given. An otorhinolaryngologist noticed a foreign body in the right nasal passage on her recent admission. He tried to take it out but he failed. He referred the patient to us immediately. She had nasal septal deviation and a prominent maxillary crest on the right side. Between the crest and the hypertrophic inferior turbinate, a black-colored, rigid, and irregular foreign body was impacted. It was thought to be a rhinolith. Forward traction with a curved curette was attempted but the foreign body did not move. Then the foreign body was pushed from the bottom and pulled outward. The object had an irregular and darkish surface, but silver colored button battery can be distinguished in this structure (Figures 1 and 2). She could not remember when she put this button battery into her nose. There was maceration and hemorrhage but no necrosis or perforation was seen, where the battery was removed. Gel foam was placed. One week later, nasal endoscopy revealed a healed nasal mucosa covering the turbinate and septum with a patent nasal passage.

3. Discussion

Cases of foreign body in the nose usually occur in childhood. Foul-smelling discharge and nasal bleeding are symptoms of nasal foreign body. Whatever the object is, it has to be removed as soon as possible when it is noticed [4]. In this case, unlike many other cases, the nasal foreign body may remain asymptomatic for a long time. Our patient had only a complaint of nasal stuffiness and sometimes a runny nose. She has been treated several times for sinusitis.

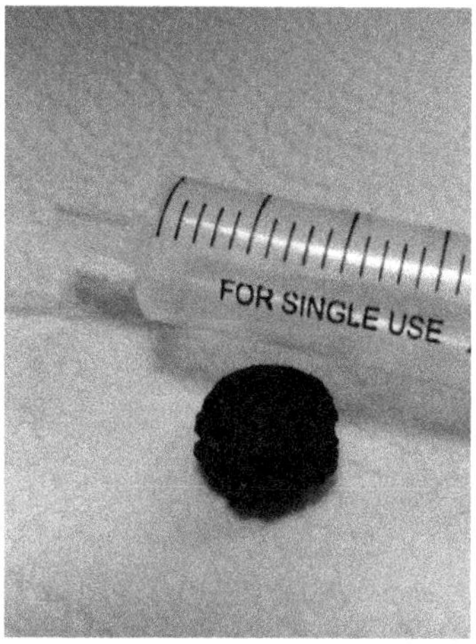

Figure 1: The button battery removed from the nose.

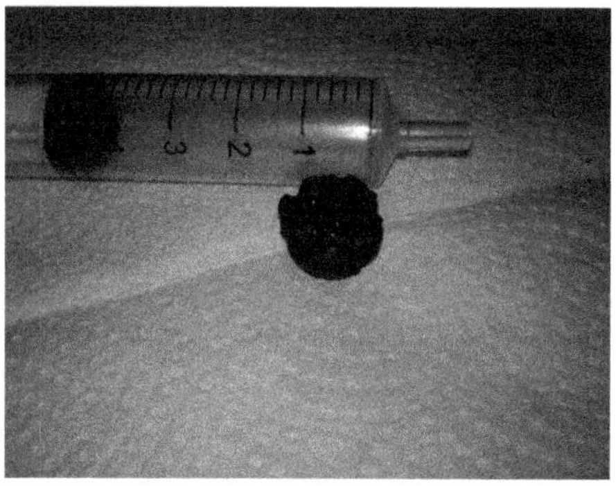

Figure 2: The button battery with its irregular darkish surface.

Probably for the reason of posterior localization and the black color, the foreign body was undetected in previous anterior rhinoscopic examinations. In addition, no imaging method was performed also.

The first report of nasal button battery was published in 1986 [5]. The button battery may irritate the nasal mucosa and cause rhinorrhea. Generally, they are in alkaline structure leading to further chemical disintegration upon contact with saline nasal mucosal discharge. Thus, more capability of additional damage occurs in the nasal mucosa. Secondary to chemical, electrical, and mechanical trauma, ulceration and necrosis of the nasal mucosa and cartilage may be seen, and even perforation may occur. McRae and his colleagues' in vitro studies have showed that spontaneous leakage of electrolyte solution occurs in alkaline batteries which are exposed to moisture. This leaked structure penetrates tissues and causes liquefying necrosis [1, 6]. The current between the battery poles which causes tissue fluids hydrolysis and gives rise to corrosive hydroxides is the primary cause of tissue destruction [7]. The damage of the button battery depends on exposure time. Tong et al. [8] reported that damage to the nasal mucosa has been reported after as few as 3 h and damage leading to perforation after 7 h. Necrosis of the inferior turbinates has occurred also at 24 hours [8]. Foreign bodies in the nose often do not cause significant morbidity or mortality, but this is not valid for button battery cases. The immediate removal is necessary when noticed. Moreover, when a button battery is detected in the nose, saline or vasoconstrictors should not be used because they enhance mucosal necrosis by chemical interaction with alkaline battery [6, 9]. In our patient, button battery does not cause any damage to the nose interestingly. She did not remember when she put it into her nose. Probably the remaining voltage of the battery was diminished. Removal is best accomplished with a right angle hook or ear curette placed behind the battery to pull it forward and out as in our case [10].

4. Conclusion

The button battery should be treated as a life threatening foreign body due to its electrochemical content and rapid tissue damage. Early suspicion and detection of accidental foreign body impaction are the key in the management of foreign bodies. The most effective management of foreign body is prevention. Because of rapid progression of tissue damage, early removal of button batteries must be required. Nonetheless, we see that a button battery can stay in the nose for long periods without specific complaints. But it should be removed when detected [4, 11].

References

[1] A. B. Majumdar, A. Sengupta, and S. S. Paul, "A case series of button batteries as nasal foreign bodies among children," *International Journal of Advances in Medicine*, vol. 1, no. 3, pp. 273–276, 2014.

[2] T. L. Litovitz, "Battery ingestions: product accessibility and clinical course," *Pediatrics*, vol. 75, no. 3, pp. 469–476, 1985.

[3] V. Y. W. Lin, S. J. Daniel, and B. C. Papsin, "Button batteries in the ear, nose and upper aerodigestive tract," *International Journal of Pediatric Otorhinolaryngology*, vol. 68, no. 4, pp. 473–479, 2004.

[4] B. Ince, M. Dadaci, and Z. Altuntas, "Seventeen-year-old asymptomatic foreign body in the nose: case report," *International Medical Journal of Sifa University*, vol. 1, no. 1, pp. 15–17, 2014.

[5] J. M. Capo and F. E. Lucente, "Alkaline battery foreign bodies of the ear and nose," *Archives of Otolaryngology—Head and Neck Surgery*, vol. 112, no. 5, pp. 562–563, 1986.

[6] D. McRae, D. J. Premachandra, and D. J. Gatland, "Button batteries in the ear, nose and cervical esophagus: a destructive foreign body," *Journal of Otolaryngology*, vol. 18, no. 6, pp. 317–319, 1989.

[7] M. Yamashlta, S. Saito, K. Koyama, H. Hattori, and T. Ogata, "Esophageal electrochemical burn by button-type alkaline batteries in dogs," *Veterinary and Human Toxicology*, vol. 29, no. 3, pp. 226–230, 1987.

[8] M. C. F. Tong, C. A. Van Hasselt, and J. K. S. Woo, "The hazards of button batteries in the nose," *Journal of Otolaryngology*, vol. 21, no. 6, pp. 458–460, 1992.

[9] A. Alvi, A. Bereliani, and G. D. Zahtz, "Miniature disc battery in the nose: a dangerous foreign body," *Clinical Pediatrics*, vol. 36, no. 7, pp. 427–429, 1997.

[10] S. Dane, A. J. Smally, and T. R. Peredy, "A truly emergent problem: button battery in the nose," *Academic Emergency Medicine*, vol. 7, no. 2, pp. 204–206, 2000.

[11] M. H. Thabet, W. M. Basha, and S. Askar, "Button battery foreign bodies in children: hazards, management, and recommendations," *BioMed Research International*, vol. 2013, Article ID 846091, 7 pages, 2013.

24

Virtual Surgical Planning and Piezoelectric Surgery in Tumor Extirpative Surgery Aimed at Inferior Alveolar Nerve Preservation

Eric L. Chung,[1] Faizan Alawi,[2] Anh D. Le,[1] and Rabie M. Shanti[1,3]

[1]*Department of Oral and Maxillofacial Surgery and Pharmacology, University of Pennsylvania School of Dental Medicine, Philadelphia, PA, USA*
[2]*Department of Pathology, University of Pennsylvania School of Dental Medicine, Philadelphia, PA, USA*
[3]*Department of Otorhinolaryngology, Head and Neck Surgery, University of Pennsylvania School of Medicine, Philadelphia, PA, USA*

Correspondence should be addressed to Eric L. Chung; eric.chung@uphs.upenn.edu

Academic Editor: Christophoros Foroulis

A myriad of extirpative surgical protocols for the management of benign tumors of the jaws have been presented in the literature. Through significant advancements in computer-aided design and computer-aided manufacturing (CAD/CAM) technology and surgical instrumentation, today surgeons have at their disposal robust technology-driven techniques that are aimed at improving surgical outcomes. Our goal is to investigate the benefits of implementing virtual surgical planning (VSP) in conjunction with piezoelectric surgery (PES) to ensure success while minimizing the risk of complications during extirpation of tumors of the mandible. This case report describes the successful extirpation of an ossifying fibroma of the mandible in an adult patient using both VSP and PES.

1. Introduction

Ossifying fibroma (OF) is a rare and benign fibro-osseous neoplasm found most commonly among the bones of the craniomaxillofacial skeleton. Traditionally, surgical treatments of the OF vary from enucleation and curettage versus resection with high-speed surgical handpieces (rotating burs and reciprocating saws), putting neighboring soft tissue and vital structures at risk for iatrogenic injury. Such procedures were limited in their accuracy in that they required assessment of two-dimensional imaging prior to surgery and performing extirpative procedures with little intraoperative guidance. However, today surgeons are able to employ highly sophisticated technologies that can optimize design of osteotomies for extirpation of bony tumors while still considering adjacent critical structures. Furthermore, the surgical armamentarium of surgeons has expanded with instrumentation that allows for further protection of these critical structures.

2. Case Presentation

A 39-year-old woman initially presented to the office of the senior author (Rabie M. Shanti) for evaluation of an asymptomatic right-sided facial swelling of 2-month duration. The patient's past medical history was noncontributory. On head and neck examination, the patient's face was notable for slight asymmetry, with mild swelling of the lower right side of the face along the angle of the mandible that was consistent with a firm and nontender palpable mass with well-defined margins. Normal cranial nerve exam was noted. There was no evidence of palpable cervical or submandibular lymphadenopathy. Orthopantomogram showed a large mixed well-circumscribed bony lesion along the angle of the right mandible that extended approximately 1 cm beyond the inferior border of the mandible (Figure 1). No involvement of dentition or violation/displacement of the mandibular canal was noted. Computed tomography (CT) scan of the maxillofacial region identified a 22 mm × 24 mm

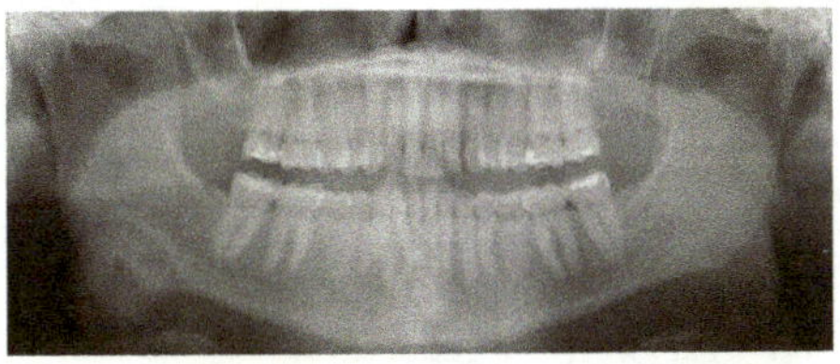

Figure 1: Preoperative orthopantomogram revealing a mixed (radiolucent-radiopaque) lesion, the inferior border of the mandible in the right angle region.

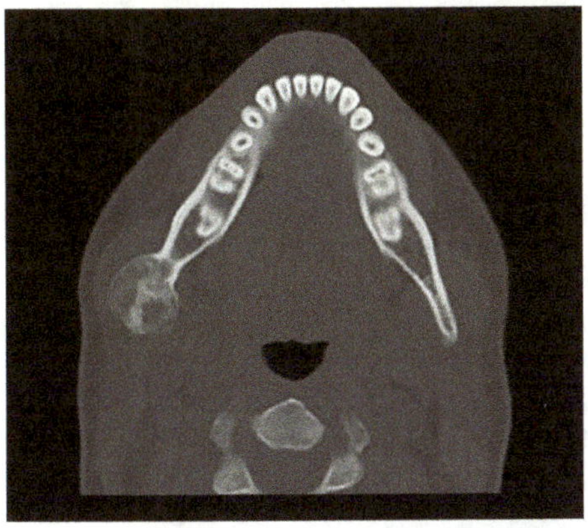

(a)

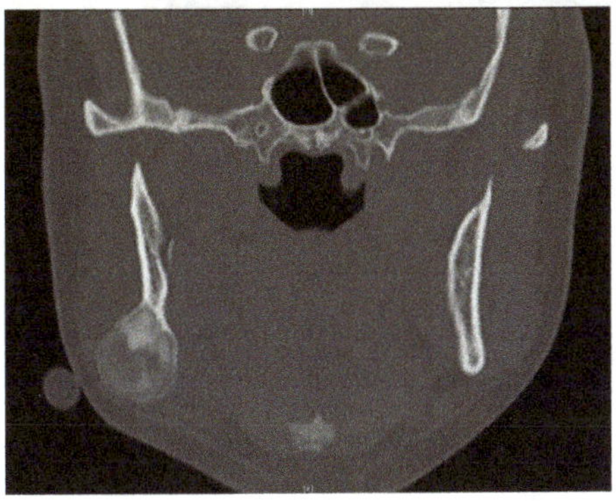

(b)

Figure 2: (a) CT axial cross section and (b) CT coronal cross section of an expansile mixed lesion of the right angle region of the mandible.

mixed (radiolucent-radiopaque), well-circumscribed, expansive lesion at the right mandibular angle region, not involving the dentition (Figures 2(a) and 2(b)). Subsequently, an incisional biopsy via transoral route was performed. The specimen was microscopically diagnosed as a benign fibro-osseous lesion that in correlation with radiographic imaging favored a diagnosis of ossifying fibroma.

Due to the tumor involving the inferior border of the mandible, a recommendation of tumor resection was made. Virtual surgical planning was performed to allow for the fabrication of a cutting guide to ensure a 5 mm surgical bony margin. However, such a margin was noted to overlap with the mandibular canal placing the patient at high risk for transection of the inferior alveolar nerve during tumor extirpation (Figure 3). Therefore, due to the high risk for inferior alveolar nerve injury, a combination of piezoelectric surgery and virtual surgical planning was utilized to allow for preservation and transposition of the nerve, while also maintaining a 5 mm surgical bony margin.

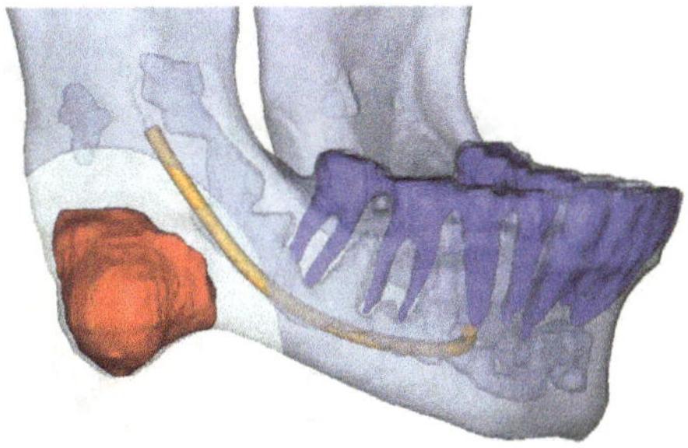

Figure 3: Virtual surgical plan allowing for 5 mm surgical bony margin surrounding the tumor, indicating overlap between surgical margin and mandibular canal.

The patient subsequently underwent right marginal mandibulectomy with 5 mm surgical margin via transcervical route utilizing a customized cutting guide for guidance of osteotomy (Figure 4(a)). Piezoelectric surgical system was used to perform the osteotomy (Figure 4(b)), and following its completion the inferior alveolar nerve was noted to be intact (Figure 4(c)). However, a small superficial laceration to the nerve was noted and was immediately addressed with a 9-0 nylon epineurial suture. Following tumor extirpation (Figure 4(d)), a 2.0 mm reconstruction plate was secured to the mandible, and an autogenous anterior iliac crest bone graft was used to reconstruct the mandibular defect (Figure 4(e)).

Final histologic analysis indicated a diagnosis of ossifying fibroma (fibrous connective tissue with islands of calcifications similar to bone and cementum) (Figure 5). The patient currently is 8 months' status postsurgery and has normal neurosensory function of the right inferior alveolar nerve distribution with a pinpoint area of hypoesthesia along the right lateral lip vermillion border measuring 2×2 mm. Tooth #31 remains vital and asymptomatic. To date, there have been no clinical and/or radiographic signs of local recurrence.

3. Discussion

"Benign fibro-osseous lesions" (BFOLs) is a generic term used to histologically classify bony lesions replaced with benign connective tissue [1]. BFOLs encompass a myriad of lesions and account for 17.6–39.9% of all lesions within the oral cavity [2, 3]. Among BFOLs, ossifying fibroma (OF) is a rare and benign fibro-osseous neoplasm found most commonly among the craniofacial bones. Over 70% of OF lesions of craniofacial skeleton involve the maxilla and mandible, with the latter being the most common [4]. Nonetheless, rare cases of OF have been reported in the long bones, nasal cavity, paranasal sinuses, temporal bone, frontal bone, and skull base [4–6]. It is most commonly observed in females during the second to fourth decade of life as an asymptomatic and asymmetrical mandibular buccal and/or lingual expansion and swelling

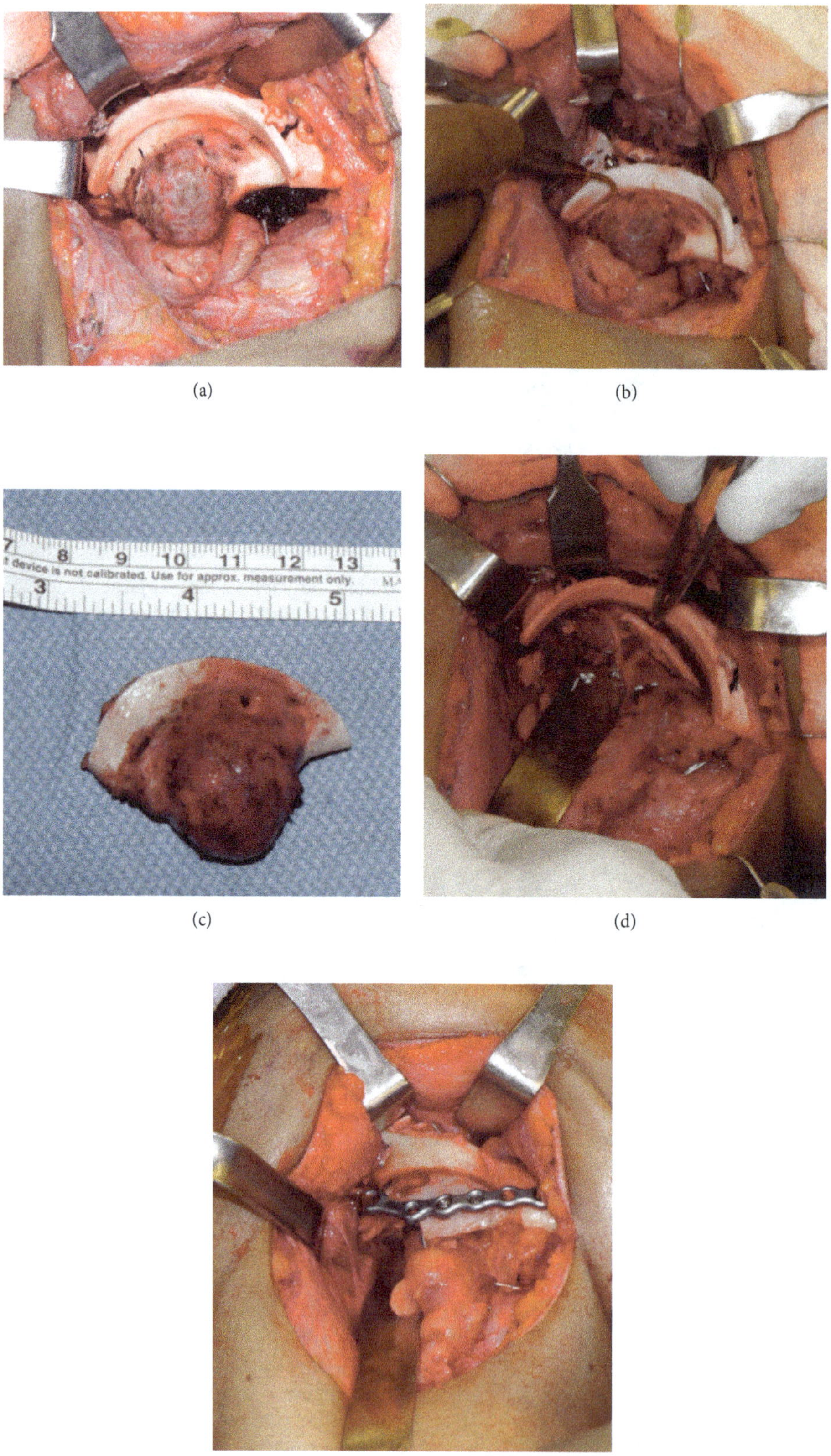

(a) (b) (c) (d) (e)

FIGURE 4: (a) Intraoperative photograph following exposure of tumor and application of custom tumor cutting guide. (b) Piezoelectric handpiece used to perform osteotomy. (c) Resection specimen. (d) View of the inferior alveolar nerve following completion of resection. (e) Autogenous anterior iliac crest bone graft in place.

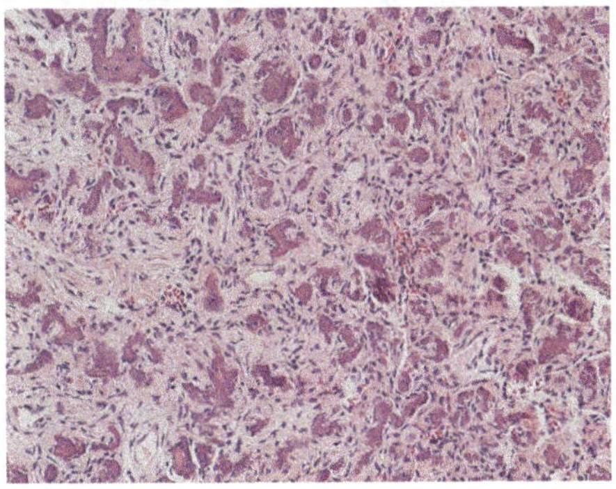

Figure 5: Histologic imaging of gross specimen. Histopathology of the tumor comprised numerous small, round ossicles embedded in cellular fibrous stroma, and occasional osteoclast-like giant cells are identified. The lesion is well demarcated from the surrounding bone. No increased mitotic figures or necrosis is seen. Benign fibro-osseous lesion, consistent with ossifying fibroma of the jaw (hematoxylin and eosin, 100x).

[7, 8]. Despite their normal slow growth process, significant growth potential can be observed if these lesions are left untreated [9]. Although rare, a more aggressive variant, juvenile ossifying fibroma (JOF), can be seen among younger patients (usually younger than 15 years of age). The pathogenesis of OF is largely unknown and has been tied to trauma, infection, neoplastic, and developmental origins. The origin of OF was originally thought to arise from undifferentiated cells of the periodontal ligament tissues [10]; however, reports of histologically similar lesions presenting in other craniofacial bones aside from the maxilla and mandible suggest otherwise.

Traditionally, surgical treatments of OF include enucleation and curettage versus resection with delayed or immediate reconstruction to restore form and function [11]. Small, well-defined lesions can be treated with conservative curettage or enucleation with a favorable prognosis. Due to the morbidity associated with resection of portions of the jaw bones, such extirpative procedures should only be reserved for large, aggressive, lesions involving the inferior border of the mandible and/or extending into the maxillary antrum and/or nasal cavities [11]. Conventionally, extirpative surgical techniques involve the use of traditional bony surgery armamentarium (high-speed surgical handpieces with rotating burs, reciprocating saws, mallets, and chisels), which are a low cost and readily available option in the rapid nonselective cutting of hard tissue at the expense of generating excessive heat and bone fragments, putting surrounding soft tissue vital structures at risk for iatrogenic injury. Due to the inherently compact anatomy of the head and neck, vital anatomic structures are at risk of partial or complete injury during tumor extirpation. Complications that are associated with extirpative procedures of the jaws include but are not limited to incomplete resection, damage to nearby vital structures, severe hemorrhage, hematoma, infection, seroma, malocclusion, dehiscence, and iatrogenic fracture [12].

With the advancement of medical technology, new surgical instruments have been developed in attempts to minimize iatrogenic injury, indirectly increasing the weight of surgeon experience and the presence of nontypical anatomy. Methods to reduce the incidence of iatrogenic injury to adjacent structures include VSP and PES. VSP allows visualization of surrounding and deep anatomy, construction of a comprehensive preoperative plan, and more precise osteotomies and restoration via use of intraoperative surgical cutting jigs as well as custom prebent reconstruction plates. PES was first described in the 1880s with claims of preserving nerves and vessels by controlled and selective cutting of hard tissue [13, 14]. PES utilizes electrical currents to create oscillations of ultrasonic frequency to exclusively cut mineralized tissue while preserving neighboring soft tissue structures. Together, these techniques minimize complications while allowing for more precise osteotomies. Unfortunately, today rotary instruments, such as surgical handpieces with a rotating bur or reciprocating saw, are still the mainstay in head and neck extirpative surgery. Therefore, it is our hope to advance head and neck surgical techniques by presenting a successful extirpative surgery case using these robust technologies.

OF lesions should be treated as conservatively as possibly to preserve aesthetics, occlusion, and function. Small and well-defined OF lesions are typically excised by curettage and enucleation; however, large expansile lesions with aggressive patterns require extirpative surgery with healthy margins (>3 mm) and aesthetic recontouring [11, 15, 16]. The recurrence rate of OF ranges from 0% to 28% with most recurrences occurring among patients treated with curettage alone. Recently, Titinchi and Morkel proposed a protocol for the surgical management of OF lesions (enucleation versus curettage versus resection with reconstruction) [11]. Based on this protocol, our patient underwent resection with reconstruction due to inferior border of mandible involvement. Titinchi and Morkel recommended resection with > 3 mm to <5 mm margins would have caused violation of the IAN canal, so preoperative VSP and utilization of PES played a key role in achieving a successful extirpative surgery [11].

A successful extirpative surgery is classified as complete removal of the infected organ or tissue with negative margins; however, preservation of major anatomical structures should always be attempted. There are many complications that may arise from extirpative surgery. Although rare, these complications should be avoided at all costs. Traditionally, rotating burs and reciprocating saws are used to nonselectively cut bone during resection surgeries, putting surrounding soft tissue structures at significant risk of injury. With the constant advancement of medicine, surgical techniques, and technology, all options should be considered during the preoperative planning stage to help reduce any predictable risks of complications during surgery.

The piezoelectric effect states that when a mechanical stress is applied to certain ceramics and crystals, an electrical charge is generated. First described by Jacque and Pierre Curie in the 1880s, piezosurgery evolved from exploiting the piezoelectric effect and utilizing ultrasonic microvibrations to cut through mineralized tissue [17]. These ultrasonic vibrations create a cavitation phenomenon (mechanical cutting that occurs exclusively on mineralized tissue) when made in contact with bone [14]. PES also allows for increased osteotomy precision due to the predictable force and rate of cutting, while conventional drills and saws are greatly affected by the density of the mineralized tissue. Cavitation method and vibrations produced by piezo handpieces cause blood to naturally be removed, allowing for a cleaner surgical field. This contrasts with conventional rotating burs that create bone dust to accumulate and blood from moving in and out of the surgical area. Altiparmak et al. documented a 0.014% chance of damaging nearby dentition and a statistically significant reduction of postoperative skin and mucosa paresthesia when utilizing PES compared with conventional techniques for surgical graft harvesting of the mandible [18]. Use of the piezoelectric technique has also been reported to cause less postoperative pain, swelling, and recovery time [17]. Several studies have shown that bone harvested with a piezoelectric handpiece had a better chance of success when grafted than bone harvested with a round bur on a traditional surgical handpiece. This was likely due to the ability to preserve osteocytes, causing an overall increased number of remaining osteocytes with less occurrence of nonvital bone. In the present study, no lesions of the mandible nerve were detected with piezosurgery, whereas surgery with rotary instruments resulted in 8% hypesthesia [17]. Schaeren et al. reported that direct exposure of a nerve to piezosurgery would preserve the perineural sheath and never transect or dissect the nerve; therefore, any nerve contacting the piezoelectric handpiece tip should theoretically be able to regenerate [19]. Although the advantages of PES are widely accepted by oral and maxillofacial surgeons, it is seldom used during head and neck surgery. Despite the numerous advantages of piezoelectric surgery, it has been largely criticized for longer intraoperative time. However, a study by Landes et al. discussed the application of PE surgery in 90 orthognathic surgery resulted in similar surgery time and reduced blood loss when comparing to conventional techniques [20]. This study explained that with increased operator PES experience and utilization of the Epker method (creating grooves in bone with a layer of cortical bone using a fissure bur, then pressing the piezoelectric tip into these grooves to cut the cortical bone completely), this disadvantage can be largely prevented [21]. As with all surgical techniques, the precision and overall outcome may vary depending on surgeon's experience and case selection. VSP is an effective tool that allows residents/fellows, attendings, and biomedical engineers a platform to discuss preoperative anatomy, surgical techniques, and potential challenges to help minimize complications while simultaneously maximizing outcomes. VSP helps to control unpredictable variables, optimizes efficiency, and provides an ideal reconstruction plan that can be transferred intraoperatively via surgical cutting guides [22]. Fabrication of intraoperative surgical cutting guides allows for improved accuracy and decreased intraoperative time [23]. Zhang et al. described an overall mean linear difference of 0.81 mm (0.71 mm for the maxilla and 0.91 mm of the mandible) among 30 consecutive double-jaw orthognathic surgery patients planned with VSP (occlusal splints and cutting jigs) [24]. Roser et al. reported accuracies of 2.00 ± 1.12 mm among 19 mandibular osteotomies and 1.30 ± 0.59 mm among 44 independent fibula osteotomies [23]. Roser et al. stated that the accuracy of fibula osteotomies was largely based by the placement of the surgical guide which is ultimately dictated by the location of the flap's perforator vessels [23]. Several studies utilizing VSP for maxillary and mandibular resection surgery with a fibula free flap reconstruction indicated an increased accuracy among fibula osteotomies; likely due to the relative accessibility of long bones in comparison to facial bones. Bernstein et al. reported that the median distance among 224 unnavigated and 244 navigated osteotomies was 2.1 mm and 1.2 mm, respectively [25]. The option of VSP may increase a surgeon's confidence and overall likelihood of treating larger and more complex cases. However, it is important to note that surgeons who are unfamiliar with VSP technology and surgeons who possess less surgical experience may ultimately produce larger variations when comparing pre- and postoperative results [22].

4. Conclusion

In general, many studies have shown the superiority of PE surgery over conventional surgery and the excellent predictability when using preoperative VSP with intraoperative surgical cutting guides. The overall use of VSP and PE surgery is undoubtedly superior to traditional unguided surgery and the use of conventional rotary handpieces and reciprocating saws. With continued use and study, our long-term goal is to develop new standards for the management of head and neck extirpative surgeries. In conclusion, VSP and PE surgery should always be considered whenever performing surgery in a compact anatomical zone such as the head and neck region.

References

[1] Y. Liu, H. Wang, M. You et al., "Ossifying fibromas of the jaw bone: 20 cases," *Dentomaxillofacial Radiology*, vol. 39, no. 1, pp. 57–63, 2010.

[2] S. Godhi, S. Goyal, G. Giraddi, and S. Goyal, "Cementifying fibroma of the mandible: a case report," *Journal Oral Health Community Dentistry*, vol. 2, pp. 42–45, 2008.

[3] A. Williams, R. Browne, and J. Akinosi, "Fibro-osseous lesions of the jaw in Nigeria," *Journal of the National Medical Association*, vol. 66, no. 3, pp. 185–191, 1974.

[4] B. Cakir and N. Karaday, "Ossifying fibroma in the nasopharynx: a case report," *Clinical Imaging*, vol. 15, no. 4, pp. 290–292, 1991.

[5] M. Mitrani, K. Remsen, W. Lawson, and H. Biller, "Giant ossifying fibroma of the paranasal sinuses," *Ear Nose Throat Journal*, vol. 67, pp. 186–192, 1988.

[6] P. Levine, R. Wiggin, R. Archibald, and R. Britt, "Ossifying fibroma of the head and neck: involvement of the temporal bone—an unusual and challenging site," *Laryngoscope*, vol. 91, no. 5, pp. 720–725, 1981.

[7] P. Speight and R. Carlos, "Maxillofacial fibro-osseous lesions," *Currenty Diagnostic Pathology*, vol. 12, no. 1, pp. 1–10, 2006.

[8] R. Eversole, L. Su, and S. ElMofty, "Benign fibro-osseous lesions of the craniofacial complex. A review," *Head Neck Pathology*, vol. 2, no. 3, pp. 177–202, 2008.

[9] H. Spjut, H. Dorfman, R. Fechner, and L. Ackerman, "Tumors of bone and cartilage," *Atlas of Tumor Pathology, Second Series Fat 5*, pp. 260-261, Armed Forces Institute of Pathology, Rawalpindi, Pakistan, 1983.

[10] A. Krausen, P. Pullon, S. Gulmen, N. Schenk, and J. Ogura, "Cementomas–aggressive or innocuous neoplasm?," *Archives of Otolaryngology–Head & Neck Surgery*, vol. 103, no. 6, pp. 349–354, 1977.

[11] F. Titinchi and J. Morkel, "Ossifying fibroma: analysis of treatment methods and recurrence patterns," *Journal of Oral Maxillofacial Surgery*, vol. 74, no. 12, pp. 2409–2419, 2016.

[12] L. Muscatello, R. Lenzi, R. Pellini, M. Guidice, and G. Spriano, "Marginal mandibulectomy in oral cancer surgery: a 13-year experience," *European Archives Otorhinolaryngology*, vol. 267, no. 5, pp. 759–764, 2010.

[13] H. Seshan, K. Konuganti, and S. Zope, "Piezosurgery in periodontology and oral implantology," *Journal of Indian Society Periodontology*, vol. 13, no. 3, pp. 155-156, 2009.

[14] E. Crosetti, B. Battiston, and G. Succo, "Piezosurgery in head and neck oncological and reconstructive surgery: personal experience on 127 cases," *Acta Otorhinolaryngologica Italica*, vol. 29, no. 1, pp. 1–9, 2009.

[15] R. Marx and S. Diane, *Oral and Maxillofacial Pathology: A Rationale for Diagnosis and Treatment*, pp. 789–795, Quintessence, Chicago, IL, USA, 2002.

[16] C. Chang, H. Hung, J. Chang et al., "Central ossifying fibroma: a clinicopathologic study of 28 cases," *Journal of the Formosan Medical Association*, vol. 107, no. 4, pp. 288–294, 2008.

[17] S. Pappalardo and R. Guarnieri, "Randomized clinical study comparing piezosurgery and conventional rotatory surgery in mandibular cyst enucleation," *Journal of Cranio-Maxillo-Facial Surgery*, vol. 42, no. 5, pp. 80–85, 2014.

[18] N. Altiparmak, S. Soydan, and S. Uckan, "The effect of conventional surgery and piezoelectric surgery bone harvesting techniques on the donor site morbidity of the mandibular ramus and symphysis," *International Journal of Oral Maxillofacial Surgery*, vol. 44, no. 9, pp. 1131–1137, 2015.

[19] S. Schaeren, C. Jaquiery, M. Heberer, M. Tolnay, T. Vercellotti, and I. Martin, "Assessment of nerve damage using a novel ultrasonic device for bone cutting," *Journal of Oral Maxillofacial Surgery*, vol. 66, no. 3, pp. 593–596, 2008.

[20] C. Landes, S. Stubinger, J. Rieger, B. Williger, T. Ha, and R. Sader, "Critical evaluation of peizoelectrical osteotomy in orthognathic surgery: operative technique, blood loss, time requirement, nerve and vessel integrity," *Journal of Oral Maxillofacial Surgery*, vol. 66, no. 4, pp. 657–674, 2008.

[21] T. Shirota, T. Kamatani, T. Yamaguchi, H. Ogura, K. Maki, and S. Shintani, "Effectiveness of piezoelectric surgery in reducing surgical complications after bilateral sagittal split osteotomy," *British Journal of Oral and Maxillofacial Surgery*, vol. 52, no. 3, pp. 219–222, 2014.

[22] P. Metzler, E. Geiger, A. Alcon, X. Ma, and D. M. Steinbacher, "Three-dimensional virtual surgery accuracy for free fibula mandibular reconstruction: planned versus actual results," *Journal of Oral Maxillofacial Surgery*, vol. 72, no. 12, pp. 2601–2612, 2014.

[23] S. Roser, S. Ramachandra, H. Blair et al., "The accuracy of virtual surgical planning in free fibula mandibular reconstruction: comparison of planned and final results," *Journal of Oral Maxillofacial Surgery*, vol. 68, no. 11, pp. 2824–2832, 2010.

[24] N. Zhang, S. Liu, Z. Hu, J. Hu, S. Zhu, and Y. Li, "Accuracy of virtual surgical planning in two-jaw orthognathic surgery: comparison of planned and actual results," *Oral Surgery Oral Medicine Oral Pathology Oral Radiology and Endodontics*, vol. 122, no. 2, pp. 143–151, 2016.

[25] J. Bernstein, M. Daly, H. Chan et al., "Accuracy and reproducibility of virtual cutting guides and 3D-navigation for osteotomies of the mandible and maxilla," *PLoS One*, vol. 12, no. 3, article 0173111, 2017.

25

Congenital Intranasal Glioma

Sajad Ahmad Salati[1, 2] and Ajaz Ahmad Rather[3]

[1] *Department of Plastic and Reconstructive Surgery, King Fahad Medical City, Riyadh 11525, Saudi Arabia*
[2] *Department of Surgical Specialties, Sheri Kashmir Institute of Medical Sciences, Soura, Srinagar 190020, India*
[3] *Department of General Surgery, Sheri Kashmir Institute of Medical Sciences (Medical College), Bemina, Srinagar 190018, India*

Correspondence should be addressed to Sajad Ahmad Salati, docsajad@yahoo.co.in

Academic Editor: L. Tacconi

Congenital midline swellings of nose are encountered rarely, and nasal gliomas constitute about 5% of such lesions. Various theories have been suggested to explain the pathogenesis. Imaging preferably by MRI is mandated to study the extent and to rule out intracranial extension. Treatment is complete excision, and the approach depends upon the extent of the lesion and availability of expertise. We present the management of one such case of congenital intranasal glioma without any intracranial extension that presented as a septal polyp.

1. Case Presentation

A three-month-old male baby was brought by parents with complaint of a fleshy mass coming out of right nostril ever since birth. There was history of occasional nasal obstruction, and the mass was growing slowly. There was no history of epistaxis or any other nasal discharge. The baby was first in birth order, product of nonconsanguineous marriage and born at fullterm by a normal vaginal delivery. The family history was unremarkable. On general physical examination, the baby was playful and hemodynamically stable. Examination of nose revealed a lesion protruding through the right external nares like a polyp (Figure 1(a)). The polyp was soft, pedunculated, nonpulsatile, and moving in and out with respiration, and the skin over it had no special features. The pedicle was arising from caudal part of nasal septum. No change in size of the mass was observed during crying or on jugular vein compression (Furstenberg's test). The left nostril was patent. There were no other abnormalities. The parents were counseled, and CT scan was advised to study the nature and extent of the polyp. CT scan revealed a well-defined soft tissue attenuation lesion, about 10 mm × 8 mm in dimensions, at the caudal end of nasal septum in right side with a stalk (Figure 1(b)). No bony defect or intracranial extension or other synchronous lesion was seen. As the base of the pedicle was clearly visible, trans-nasal excision was done under general anesthesia. There were no perioperative complications, and the patient was particularly observed for postoperative bleeding, CSF leak, fever or other features of infection. Histopathological analysis of the specimen revealed nonmalignant gliomatous cells with low proliferative activity. No meningeal or dural tissue was identified. The diagnosis of nasal glioma was hence established. The patient remained under followup for fifteen months and did not show any evidence of recurrence of the lesion.

2. Discussion

Congenital midline nasal masses are rare anomalies that occur in about one in 20000–40000 live births [1]. Nasal gliomas account for approximately 5% of all congenital nasal swellings. These usually arise during infancy or later childhood with relative peaks of occurrence between 5 and 10 years of age. Although the majority of patients present during the first year of life, a later presentation may be due to a specialist's failure to recognize a subclinical lesion in childhood.

The term "nasal glioma" is a confusing misnomer as it implies a neoplastic condition, which it is not. It needs to be

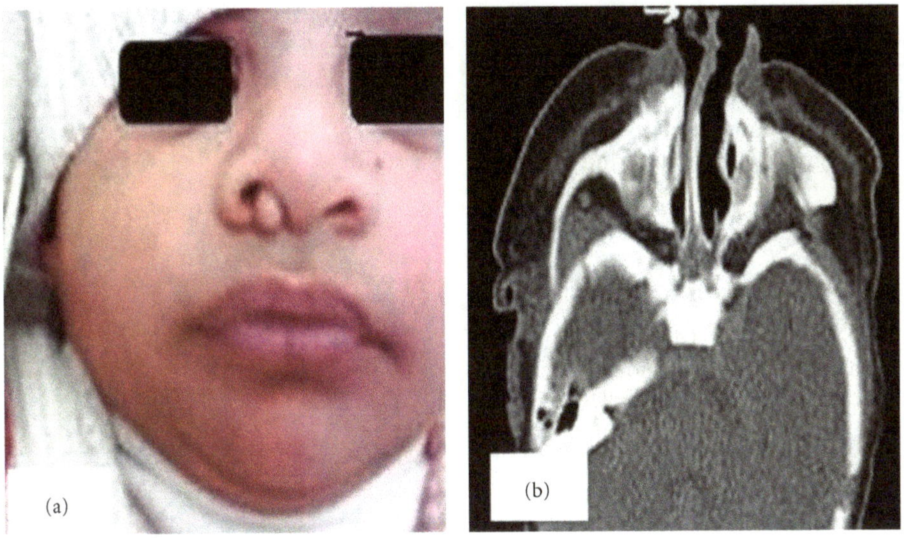

(a) (b)

Figure 1: (a) 3 months old baby with right nasal congenital polyp-glioma. (b) Axial CT scan revealing a soft tissue lesion arising from nasal septum (white arrow).

differentiated from glioma, which is a malignant tumor of the brain [1, 2]. 60% of these gliomas are extranasal, lying external to the nasal bones and cavities; 30% are intranasal lying within the nasal cavity, mouth, or pterygopalatine fossa and 10% are mixed, dumbbell shaped communicating through a defect of the nasal bones [3]. Our case was of an intranasal glioma.

The possible theories of development of nasal gliomas include the following: (a) sequestration of glial tissue of the olfactory bulb entrapped during cribriform plate fusion; (b) ectopic neural tissue cells; (c) encephaloceles with lost intracranial connection and meningeal continuity; (d) inappropriate closure of the anterior neuropore (fonticulus frontalis) [1, 4]. In 15–20% of cases, a fibrous stalk exists to connect them to the intracranial space.

Clinically, these masses are firm in consistency, noncompressible, nonpulsatile, grayish or purple lesions. These masses can protrude through the nostrils and can be confused with a nasal polyp. The patient may suffer from nasal obstruction, epistaxis, cerebrospinal fluid (CSF) rhinorrhoea, nasolacrimal duct obstruction, epiphora, hypertelorism and cosmetic deformity [5].

Histologically, these lesions are made up of astrocytic neuroglial cells interlaced with fibrous and vascular connective tissue [5] that may be covered with skin or nasal respiratory mucosa. True capsule is absent, and mitosis is rare. The glial nature of the cells can be further confirmed by immune-histochemical demonstration of S100 protein and GFAP.

CT scan or MRI forms the mainstay of investigation as fine needle aspiration cytology or excision biopsy carries a significant risk of meningitis or CSF leaks [6]. CT scan demonstrates bony defects, and MRI can demonstrate the characteristics of the soft-tissue mass and its possible intracranial connection. On CT, the mass is usually isodense to brain tissue. On MRI, the lesion is isointense to hypointense relative to gray matter on T1-weighted sequences and hyper-intense on T2-weighted and proton density sequences [5, 7]. Magnetic resonance imaging also has an advantage of minimizing the level of exposure to ionising radiation, particularly in infants.

The clinical differential diagnosis of nasal gliomas includes several disorders, which can present as nasal masses [1, 8]. Some of such important lesions include: (a) nasal dermoids, which constitute the most common congenital nasal anomaly and are cavities or sinus tracts possessing epithelial lining and variable numbers of skin appendages, including hair follicles, sebaceous glands, and eccrine glands; (b) encephaloceles which constitute the lesions caused by herniation of neural tissue through defects in the skull. They may contain meninges (meningocele) or brain matter and meninges (encephalomeningocele), or they may communicate with a ventricle (encephalomeningocystocele). Encephaloceles are etiologically similar to nasal gliomas as per one of the theories; (c) hemangioma which are the most frequent benign vascular tumors in infancy.

The treatment of choice of nasal gliomas is complete surgical excision [1]. Gliomas are benign but incomplete excision results in a 4% to 10% recurrence rate. The approach depends upon the location and extent of the lesion [1] and levels of expertise available. When facilities are available, intranasal endoscopic surgery is considered most appropriate approach for the removal of intranasal glioma having no intracranial extension as this approach allows precise excision with minimal trauma to the surrounding tissues [9]. If however intracranial extension is evident, than frontal craniotomy, multidisciplinary team approach may be required [10] in specialized neurosurgical or craniofacial centers to ensure complete and safe excision of the lesions.

3. Conclusion

Nasal gliomas are rare congenital anomalies. It is mandatory to rule out intracranial extension by cross-sectional imaging, preferably by MRI before performing any invasive procedure. Surgical excision in the mainstay of treatment and the route depend upon the extent of the lesion and the available expertise.

Acknowledgment

The help provided by parents by consenting to use images of the patient for academic purposes is duly acknowledged.

References

[1] V. Nada, V. Dejan, D. Dragan, and J. Ljiljana, "Nasal glioma," *Archive of Oncology*, vol. 14, no. 1-2, pp. 57–59, 2006.

[2] Y. Ducic, "Nasal gliomas," *Journal of Otolaryngology*, vol. 28, no. 5, pp. 285–287, 1999.

[3] M. Cerdá-Nicolás, C. Sanchez Fernandez de Sevilla, C. Lopez-Ginés, A. Peydro-Olaya, and A. Llombart-Bosch, "Nasal glioma or nasal glial heterotopia? Morphological, immunohistochemical and ultrastructural study of two cases," *Clinical Neuropathology*, vol. 21, no. 2, pp. 66–71, 2002.

[4] A. C. Swift and S. D. Singh, "The presentation and management of the nasal glioma," *International Journal of Pediatric Otorhinolaryngology*, vol. 10, no. 3, pp. 253–261, 1985.

[5] S. K. Singhal, R. S. Virk, A. Dass, and S. Bansal, "Amanjit: neonatal nasal glioma: a case report," *Internet Journal of Otorhinolaryngology*, vol. 4, p. 2, 2006.

[6] P. Claròs, R. Bandos, A. Claròs, I. Gilea, A. Claròs, and M. Real, "Nasal gliomas: main features, management and report of five cases," *International Journal of Pediatric Otorhinolaryngology*, vol. 46, no. 1-2, pp. 15–20, 1998.

[7] P. H. Jartti, A. E. Jartti, A. I. Karttunen, E. L. Paakko, R. L. Herva, and T. O. Pirila, "MR of a nasal glioma in a young infant," *Acta Radiologica*, vol. 43, pp. 141–143, 2002.

[8] N. R. Dasgupta and M. L. Bentz, "Nasal gliomas: identification and differentiation from hemangiomas," *The Journal of Craniofacial Surgery*, vol. 14, no. 5, pp. 736–738, 2003.

[9] M. Yokoyama, N. Inouye, and F. Mizuno, "Endoscopic management of nasal glioma in infancy," *International Journal of Pediatric Otorhinolaryngology*, vol. 51, no. 1, pp. 51–54, 1999.

[10] R. Rahbar, V. A. Resto, C. D. Robson et al., "Nasal glioma and encephalocele: diagnosis and management," *Laryngoscope*, vol. 113, no. 12, pp. 2069–2077, 2003.

26

Congenital Agenesis of the Internal Jugular Vein: An Extremely Rare Anomaly

Oguz Kayiran,[1] Caglar Calli,[2] Abdulkadir Emre,[3] and Fatih Kemal Soy[3]

[1]*Department of Plastic and Reconstructive Surgery, Izmir University, 35000 Izmir, Turkey*
[2]*Department of Head and Neck Surgery, Ekol ENT Hospital, 35000 Izmir, Turkey*
[3]*Department of Head and Neck Surgery, Ataturk Training and Research Hospital, 35000 Izmir, Turkey*

Correspondence should be addressed to Oguz Kayiran; droguzk@yahoo.com

Academic Editor: Alexander R. Novotny

Vascular anomalies of major venous vessels are rarely seen. Moreover, congenital absence of internal jugular vein is extremely uncommon. In our case, a female patient presented with primary unknown left cervical mass. Cervical ultrasonography demonstrated absence of right internal jugular vein. In addition, computed tomography and dynamic magnetic resonance imaging scans confirmed this diagnosis. Compensatory left internal jugular vein enlargement mimicked sort of cervical mass. Venous magnetic resonance imaging images revealed the absence of right internal jugular vein with compensatory left internal jugular vein dominance. In the literature, the agenesis of IJV was mentioned in a case with concomitant multiple problems. Here, an asymptomatic case is reported with an incident diagnosis. No interventions were planned upon the patient's request. It should be kept in mind that any kind of anomalies can be seen during venous access and neck surgery.

1. Introduction

Vascular anomalies are divided into two groups as vascular tumors and vascular malformations according to International Society for the Study of Vascular Anomalies (ISSVA) (Table 1) [1–3]. Vascular tumors consist of hemangioma, hemangioendothelioma, and angiosarcoma. Vascular malformations are comprised of abnormally formed channels that are lined by quiescent endothelium. They are categorized according to the predominant channel type and rheological characteristics as slow-flow (capillary, venous, and lymphatic) and fast-flow (arterial, combined). Developmental venous anomalies in general population are seen in about 0.05% to 0.25%. However, rates up to 20% have been reported [4].

2. Case Report

17-year-old female patient was referred to Izmir Ataturk Training and Research Hospital Ear, Nose and Throat Clinic, with a painless mass on her left side of the neck existing since childhood. The examination of the head and neck revealed a suspicious mass without color and heat changes at left midjugular region. The physical examination was uneventful. Ultrasonography did not show any mass in the region; however, CT demonstrated absence of right IJV. Doppler USG and dynamic MRI clearly exhibited the same abnormality (Figures 1, 2, and 3). This observation depended on a developmental agenesis rather than a thrombus.

The patient was informed with the situation and no further treatment was planned upon her request. Follow-up periods continue annually within different facilities concomitantly.

3. Discussion

Vascular anomalies result from embryological developmental deformities. Hemangiomas regress in time while vascular malformations occasionally progress and remain lifetime. Although vascular malformations exist at birth, they may not be detected until adolescence or adulthood [3]. Venous malformations are mostly asymptomatic and are located at head and neck region, frequently [5]. The vascular anomalies in the head and neck region have tendency to coexist with intracranial venous malformations [4].

Table 1: ISSVA classification of vascular anomalies.

Tumors	Malformations
	Slow-flow
	Capillary
Hemangioma	Lymphatic
Hemangioendothelioma	Venous
Angiosarcoma	Fast-flow
Miscellaneous	Arterial
	Combined

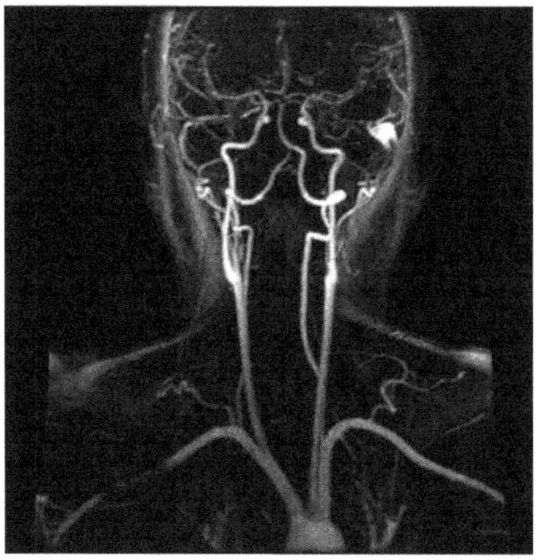

Figure 1: Sagittal view of arterial system (dynamic magnetic resonance image).

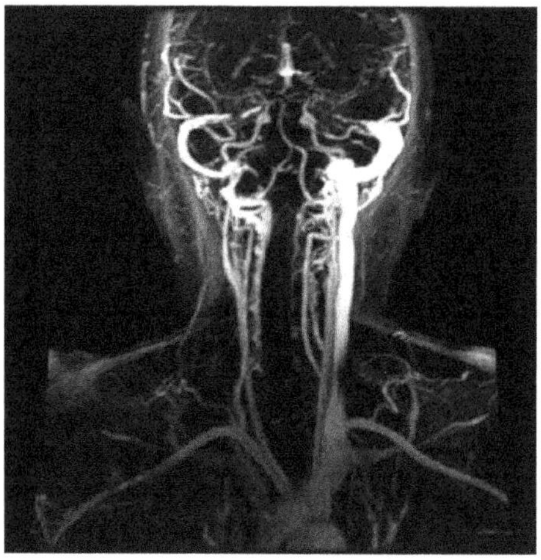

Figure 2: Sagittal view of venous system (dynamic magnetic resonance image). Please note that right filling of IJV with the radiopaque contrast is absent, markedly, from the bifurcation. Moreover, left IJV is seen thickened.

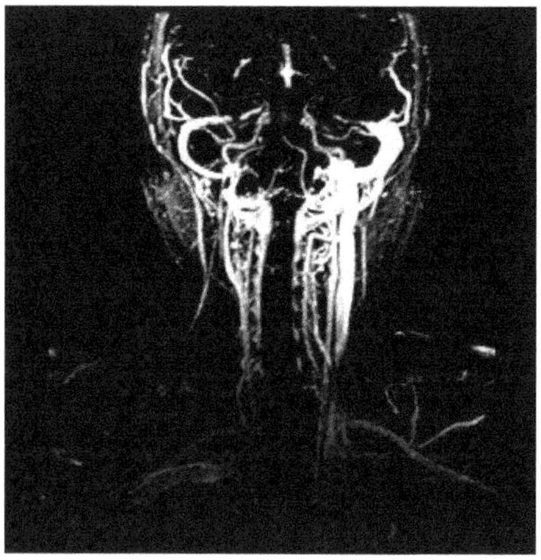

Figure 3: Sagittal view of collateral system (dynamic magnetic resonance image).

IJV runs downwards through the neck within the carotid sheath and behind the sternal end of the clavicle. It then unites within the subclavian vein to form the brachiocephalic vein, which enters the thorax to join vena cava superior.

The information of anatomical variations of IJV is clinically essential for venous applications. In intensive care units, central catheters are frequently applied. Anomalies of IJV may preclude the practitioner resulting in serious complications. The surgeon should be familiar with the anatomy and possible variations of IJV in order to avoid complications. In a study of 93 cadaveric dissections, Asouhidou et al. found that 3 of these dissections showed narrowing of IJV (<6 mm) while the external jugular veins were over normal limits [6]. Duplication of IJV is frequently encountered [7]. Prades et al. showed IJV duplications in 3 of 750 patients during unilateral neck dissections and detected the course of accessory nerve passing through duplicated internal jugular veins [8].

Spontaneous thrombosis of IJV is a very rare condition. In a study of 200 patients whose IJVs were catheterized and examined by two-dimensional ultrasonography, Denys and Uretsky identified nonvisualization of IJV in 5 (2.5%) patients resulting from the thrombosis [9]. The thrombosis of IJV is mostly caused by repeating intravenous injections, drug abuse, polycythaemia, and hypercoagulability, following neck surgery like neck dissection, radiotherapy, deep neck infections, oropharyngeal infections, Lemierre's syndrome, and cervical trauma. Cervical inflammation, mass, or sepsis may also coexist with the thrombosis of IJV [10–12]. Our patient did not have any of the abovementioned conditions and thrombosis antecedently. The ultrasonography, CT, and magnetic resonance imaging did not reveal any thrombosis and showed congenital agenesis of the IJV.

In the literature, one case with the absence of IJV was depicted who also had additional problems [13]. However, further diagnostic analysis and dynamic proofs were not elucidated in this study. In addition, agenesis of both IJVs (right and left) and left external jugular vein has been reported in a cat [14].

Herein, we reported an asymptomatic case of lack of right IJV with compensatory left IJV thickening which was diagnosed accidently. We believe the practitioner should always be aware of possible head and neck anomalies and variations during neck surgeries and vascular interventions.

References

[1] G. M. Legiehn and M. K. S. Heran, "Venous malformations: classification, development, diagnosis, and interventional radiologic management," *Radiologic Clinics of North America*, vol. 46, no. 3, pp. 545–597, 2008.

[2] J. B. Mulliken and J. V. Glowacki, "Hemangiomas and vascular malformations in infants and children: a classification based on endothelial characteristics," *Plastic & Reconstructive Surgery*, vol. 69, no. 3, pp. 412–422, 1982.

[3] H. J. Paltiel, P. E. Burrows, H. P. W. Kozakewich, D. Zurakowski, and J. B. Mulliken, "Soft-tissue vascular anomalies: utility of US for diagnosis," *Radiology*, vol. 214, no. 3, pp. 747–754, 2000.

[4] M. Boukobza, O. Enjolras, J.-P. Guichard et al., "Cerebral developmental venous anomalies associated with head and neck venous malformations," *The American Journal of Neuroradiology*, vol. 17, no. 5, pp. 987–994, 1996.

[5] J. G. Kromhout, V. C. d. Horst, F. Peeters, and M. Gerhard, "The combined treatment of congenital vascular defects," *International Angiology*, vol. 9, no. 3, pp. 203–207, 1990.

[6] I. Asouhidou, K. Natsis, T. Asteri, P. Sountoulides, K. Vlasis, and P. Tsikaras, "Anatomical variation of left internal jugular vein: clinical significance for an anaesthesiologist," *European Journal of Anaesthesiology*, vol. 25, no. 4, pp. 314–318, 2008.

[7] F. C. Uecker, E. Wüstenberg, and T. Zahnert, "High duplication of an internal jugular vein," *Laryngo- Rhino- Otologie*, vol. 86, no. 8, pp. 592–594, 2007.

[8] J. M. Prades, A. Timoshenko, J. M. Dumollard, M. Durand, N. Merzougui, and C. Martin, "High duplication of the internal jugular vein: clinical incidence in the adult and surgical consequences, a report of three clinical cases," *Surgical and Radiologic Anatomy*, vol. 24, no. 2, pp. 129–132, 2002.

[9] B. G. Denys and B. F. Uretsky, "Anatomical variations of internal jugular vein location: impact on central venous access," *Critical Care Medicine*, vol. 19, no. 12, pp. 1516–1519, 1991.

[10] N. Gormus, K. Durgut, U. Ozergin, K. Odev, and H. Solak, "Lemierre's syndrome associated with septic pulmonary embolism: a case report," *Annals of Vascular Surgery*, vol. 18, no. 2, pp. 243–245, 2004.

[11] D. M. Kaplan, D. M. Fliss, Y. Peiser, D. Greenberg, and A. Leiberman, "Internal jugular vein thrombosis in a child due to a 'pencil point injury' of the palate," *International Journal of Pediatric Otorhinolaryngology*, vol. 44, no. 2, pp. 183–187, 1998.

[12] E. E. Ünsal, C. Karaca, and S. Ensarí, "Spontaneous internal jugular vein thrombosis associated with distant malignancies," *European Archives of Oto-Rhino-Laryngology*, vol. 260, no. 1, pp. 39–41, 2003.

[13] B. R. Miller, "Absence of a right internal jugular vein detected by ultrasound imaging," *Paediatric Anaesthesia*, vol. 21, no. 1, p. 91, 2011.

[14] G. Bertolini and A. Zotti, "Imaging diagnosis: absence of the left external and both internal jugular veins in a cat," *Veterinary Radiology and Ultrasound*, vol. 47, no. 5, pp. 468–469, 2006.

27

Bilateral Chylothorax after Falling from Height

Vildan Akpinar,[1] Fulya Yilmaz Duran,[1] Elif Duman,[2] Murat Yasar Özkalkanli,[1] Özgür Duran,[3] and Burcu Horsanali[1]

[1] *Anaesthesiology and Reanimation Department, Bozyaka Training and Research Hospital, İzmir, Turkey*
[2] *Thoracic Surgery Department, Bozyaka Training and Research Hospital, İzmir, Turkey*
[3] *Emergency Medicine Department, Bozyaka Training and Research Hospital, İzmir, Turkey*

Correspondence should be addressed to Fulya Yilmaz Duran; drfulya@mynet.com

Academic Editor: Angelo Carretta

Chylothorax is accumulation of chyle in the pleural cavity due to disruption of the thoracic duct. The causes can be classified as neoplastic, traumatic (iatrogenic or noniatrogenic), congenital, sporadic, spontaneous, and miscellaneous. A 22-year-old man with no feature in his history and family history was referred to emergency department with the case of falling from height. Abdominal computed tomogram (CT) revealed laceration of liver, grade 5 splenic laceration, fracture of the left acetabulum, and dislocation of the left hip. He was optimized for emergency splenectomy and close left hip reduction. On the 2nd day of the operation, bilateral chylotorax revealed. The treatment depends on its etiology, the amount of drainage, and the clinical picture. Treatment can be classified into 3 categories treatment of the underlying condition, conservative management (such as bed rest, nil by mouth or low fat medium chain triglycerides by mouth and total parenteral nutrition), and surgical management by ligation or clipping of the thoracic duct with open thoracotomy or video-assisted thoracoscopic surgery. The main purpose of surgical treatment is to stop the chylous leak.

1. Introduction

Chylothorax is accumulation of chyle in the pleural cavity due to disruption of the thoracic duct [1–4]. Chylothorax is rare following blunt trauma; its diagnosis is usually delayed until the puncture or drainage of posttraumatic pleural effusion and its cause is not clear [5, 6]. The causes can be classified as neoplastic, traumatic (iatrogenic or noniatrogenic), congenital, sporadic, spontaneous, and miscellaneous [1, 3, 4]. We assumed bilateral chylothorax in this case was related to the fall from height.

2. Case Report

A 22-year-old man was referred to our hospital after falling from height. He has no feature in his history and family history. He was conscious and cooperative. Vital signs and laboratory tests were within normal limits. Abdominal ultrasonography revealed free fluid in perisplenic and perihepatic areas and Morrison pouch. It is more prominent in the perisplenic area. Abdominal computed tomogram (CT) revealed laceration of liver, grade 5 splenic laceration, fracture of the left acetabulum, and dislocation of the left hip; brain CT revealed air-fluid level in right maxillary sinus and both sphenoid sinuses, upper and medial wall fracture of right orbita; thorax CT revealed parenchymal laceration and contusional changes. He was optimized for emergency splenectomy and close left hip reduction.

Preoperative laboratory findings were as follows: WBC: 23600/mm^3, Hb: 12.6 g/dL, Htc: % 44, platelets: 292000/mm^3, glucose: 141 mg/dL, BUN: 22 mg/dL, Cr: 0.99 mg/dL, Na^+ : 140 mEq/L, K^+ : 2.37 mEq/L, and Cl^- : 105 mEq/L. Postoperatively the patient was admitted to the intensive care unit. On the 2nd day of the operation, he was extubated without any problem. Right pleural fluid was detected in control chest X-ray after extubation (Figure 1). The patient was examined by thoracic surgeon and chest tube was placed on the right side. The appearance of the fluid was chylous which was later confirmed on biochemical analysis (triglyceride level: 90 mg/dL; cholesterol level: 7 mg/dL). Conservative

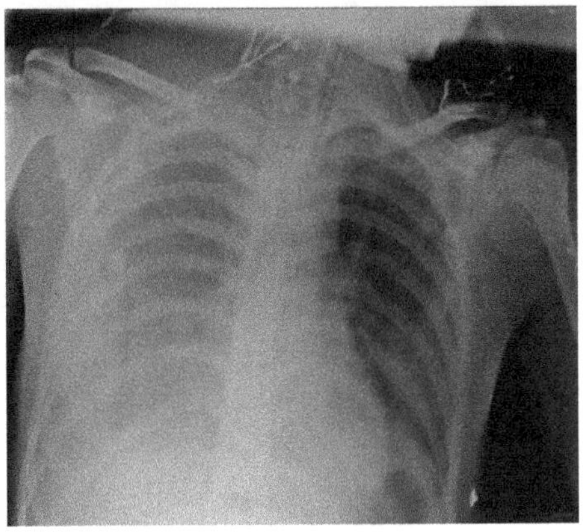

FIGURE 1

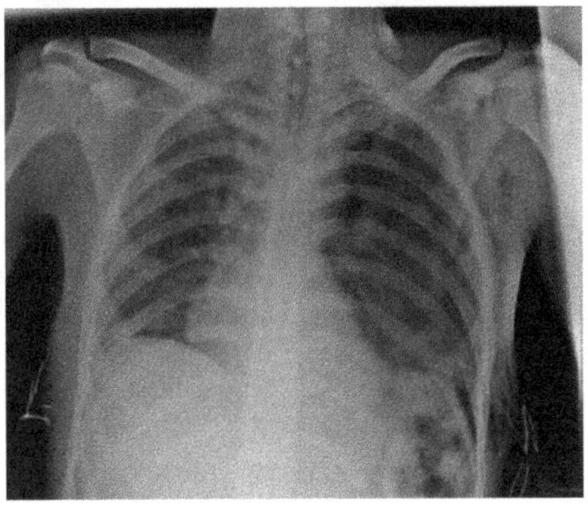

FIGURE 2

treatment for chylothorax with nothing by mouth and total parenteral nutrition (TPN) was instituted. On the 3rd day of the operation, thorax CT showed right pleural fluid and chest tube was 2 placed on the right side. The appearance of the fluid was chylous which was later confirmed on biochemical analysis (triglyceride level: 245 mg/dL; cholesterol level: 15 mg/dL). On the 4th day of the operation chest X-ray showed left pleural fluid and chest tube was placed on the left side. on the 10th day of the operation, the patient was discharged to the ward. On the 11th day of the operation, although left basal tube was inserted, left total pneumothorax (Figure 2) was developed and left apical tube thoracostomy was performed. Left apical chest tube was removed 6 days after insertion and left basal chest tube was removed 13 days after insertion. On the 18th day of the operation, although right basal tube was inserted, control chest X-ray showed right total pneumothorax and right apical tube thoracostomy was performed. After right apical tube thoracostomy was performed, right basal chest tube was removed 16 days after insertion. Right apical chest tube removed 6 days after insertion. The patient was discharged from hospital on the 28th day of operation without any complication.

3. Discussion

In this paper, a case was reported of a man who fell from height and was operated for splenic laceration and developed bilateral chylothorax on the 2nd day of the operation. Although chylothorax due to blunt trauma was reported in the literature, this patient has developed chylothorax on the left side one day after the detection of right side chylothorax.

Thoracic duct is the main lymphatic duct that binds lymphatic system to venous system. Its function is to transport lipids absorbed from the gastrointestinal tract. Traumatic noniatrogenic chylothorax etiology ratio is 2.6% [6]. The most common form of blunt injury to the thoracic duct is produced by sudden hyperextension of the spine with rupture of the duct just above the diaphragm in the right thorax. Half of the chylothoraces are right-sided, one-third is left-sided, and the remainders are bilateral [4]. This patient encountered trauma after falling from height. Damage to his thoracic duct most likely occurred as a result of sudden hyperextension of the spine. The colour of the pleural fluid is not always indicative of chylothorax. It may not appear chylous if the patient is fasting or the pleural fluid is mixed with blood [4]. There are several techniques [presence of chylomicrons in the pleural fluid [3, 4, 7], lipoprotein analysis [4], bipedal lymphangiography [4], and analysis of the pleural fluid [3, 4, 7]] used in the diagnosis of chylothorax. The exact diagnosis of chylothorax is based on the presence of chylomicrons in the pleural fluid [3, 4]. Important 3 characteristics of the fluid are pH of 7.4 to 7.8 [4], lymphocyte predominance in cell count [7], specific gravity of 1.012 or higher [4], triglyceride levels > 110 mg/dL [3, 4, 7], and low cholesterol level [7]. Clinical features are hypovolemia, respiratory difficulty, malnutrition, immunosuppression, dyspnea, chest pain, and cough [3]. Symptoms of chylothorax typically have a gradual onset. Often, a latency period of 2–7 days exists between the time of injury and clinical evidence of chylothorax [4]. The longest latency period reported in the literature was 20 years [1]. In our case, the latency period is 2 days. However, this patient had developed chylothorax first on the right side and one day later on the left side. The treatment depends on its etiology, the amount of drainage, and the clinical picture [4]. Treatment can be classified under 3 categories: treatment of the underlying condition, conservative management (such as bed rest, nil by mouth or low fat medium chain triglycerides by mouth, and total parenteral nutrition), and surgical management by ligation or clipping of the thoracic duct with open thoracotomy or video-assisted thoracoscopic surgery [3, 4]. Somatostatin and octreotide have proved to be useful in the conservative treatment of chylothorax [3, 7]. Conservative measurements have achieved an 88% success rate [4]. The duration of conservative management varies in the literature anywhere from 1 to 8 weeks [6], but most authors recommend conservative management for no more than 2 weeks [4].

The main purpose of surgical treatment is to stop the chylous leak [6]. In general, surgical intervention offers better results than conservative management when daily chyle leak exceeds 1 L/day for a period more than 5 days or 1.5 L/day in an adult or > 100 mL/kg body weight per day in a child, persistent chyle flow for more than 2 weeks [3, 4]. Surgery is also recommended if here has been a rapid decline in nutritional status despite conservative management [3].

Before the introduction of surgical ligation of the thoracic duct, the mortality rate from chylothorax was approximately 100% [6]. With the advent of TPN and surgical ligation for persistent leaks, the mortality rate of chylothorax became less than 10% [4].

This case is a rare example of bilateral chylothorax resulting from falling from height and onset of bilateral pneumothorax in a patient with open and functioning bilateral basal chest tubes. The mechanism of chylothorax is thought to be a hyperextension injury to the spine. But we cannot explain the onset of bilateral pneumothorax.

The pleural fluid was chylous and contained high triglycerides concentration and low cholesterol level. We performed a conservative approach including tube thoracostomy, nil by mouth, and TPN, which resulted in regression of the chylous fluid and improvement of the patient. Medium chain triglycerides were not given to patient but TPN was applied to prevent malnutrition due to chylothorax and fasting.

In conclusion, early detection of the bilateral chylothorax due to blunt trauma resulted in early management. During the ICU stay daily imaging demonstrated the delay of left-sided chylothorax one day after the right-sided chylothorax. Conservative management resulted in successful treatment.

References

[1] M. Kamiyoshihara, T. Ibe, S. Kakegawa, K. Sato, A. Takise, and I. Takeyoshi, "Late-onset chylothorax after blunt chest trauma at an interval of 20 years: report of a case," *Surgery Today*, vol. 38, no. 1, pp. 56–58, 2008.

[2] M. Chamberlain and C. Ratnatunga, "Late presentation of tension chylothorax following blunt chest trauma," *European Journal Cardio-Thoracic Surgery*, vol. 18, no. 3, pp. 357–359, 2000.

[3] E. E. McGrath, Z. Blades, and P. B. Anderson, "Chylothorax: aetiology, diagnosis and therapeutic options," *Respiratory Medicine*, vol. 104, no. 1, pp. 1–8, 2010.

[4] E. Seitelman, J. J. Arellano, K. Takabe, L. Barrett, G. Faust, and L. D. George Angus, "Chylothorax after blunt trauma," *Journal of Thoracic Disease*, vol. 4, no. 3, pp. 327–330, 2012.

[5] E. Apostolakis, K. Akinosoglou, E. Koletsis, and D. Dougenis, "Traumatic chylothorax following blunt thoracic trauma: two conservatively treated cases: Case reports," *Journal of Cardiac Surgery*, vol. 24, no. 2, pp. 220–222, 2009.

[6] R. Demirhan, A. Çevik, H. Küçük, M. Altıntaş, and N. Kurt, "Traumatic chylothorax: case report," *Türk Göğüs Kalp Damar Cerrahisi Dergisi*, vol. 11, pp. 50–51, 2003.

[7] S. S. Ezer, P. Oğuzkurt, E. İnce, and A. Hiçsönmez, "Bilateral chylothorax after blunt thoracic trauma: a case report," *The Turkish Journal of Pediatrics*, vol. 51, pp. 504–506, 2009.

28

Pterygoid Hamular Bursitis: A Possible Link to Craniofacial Pain

Sameep S. Shetty,[1] Premalatha Shetty,[1] Prit Kiran Shah,[2] Jayanth Nambiar,[3] and Nancy Agarwal[1]

[1]*Department of Oral and Maxillofacial Surgery, Manipal College of Dental Sciences, Manipal Academy of Higher Education, Mangalore 575001, India*
[2]*Consultant Oral and Maxillofacial Surgeon, My Dentist and Bhatia Hospital, Mumbai, India*
[3]*Department of Conservative Dentistry and Endodontics, Sharavathi Dental College, Shiomoga, India*

Correspondence should be addressed to Sameep S. Shetty; sameep.shetty@manipal.edu

Academic Editor: Sibu P. Saha

A striking feature of the skull base is the pterygoid hamulus known for its bizarre morphology and biomechanical location. Pterygoid hamular bursitis is an inflammation of bursae located between the tendon, muscle, and bony prominences. The minimal objective finding in an apparently normal orofacial apparatus and dependence on the subjective symptoms experienced by the patient with widespread referral pattern often perplexes the clinician. Bursitis should be considered in the differential diagnosis of craniofacial neuralgia, temporomandibular joint dysfunction, and chronic craniofacial pain. Clinical signs and symptoms of this intriguing entity are diverse and multifaceted that can sometimes demand services of clinicians across various specialties considering the anatomic density of the region. Care must be taken to avoid delay, misdiagnosis, and overtreatment.

1. Introduction

Chronic orofacial pain is a complex process whose causes originate from the trigeminal nociceptive reflex arcs within the central and peripheral nervous systems. It comprises a highly extensive spectrum of pain disorders because of their unique anatomic, physiologic, and biochemical components.

Patients with persistent orofacial pain do not present with concrete symptoms that allow for a straightforward clinical reasoning. Orofacial pain can have a blend of neurogenic, myogenic, and psychogenic causes entangled amidst the intricate anatomy and high vascular network. This umbrella of uncertainty shades the judgment for every patient to whom we provide care.

The clinical course of a chronic orofacial pain often seems to worsen the quality of life with polypharmacy and doctor shopping that have their own repercussions eventually leading to overdiagnosis and overtreatment.

Pain in the soft palate due to an elongated pterygoid hamulus was first termed by Gores [1]. Hjørting-Hansen and Lous [2, 3] in 1987 designated the term "pterygoid hamulus syndrome" characterized by pain in the palatal and pharyngeal regions, caused by a bizarre shape or an elongated pterygoid hamulus. Pterygoid hamulus bursitis is one such rare entity showing a constellation of symptoms in the orofacial region. The apparently normal clinical picture of the oral cavity can perplex the clinician.

The pterygoid hamulus is a variable anatomical structure with its subdivisions: base, corpus, sulcus, and caput. The average measurements are length 7.2 mm, sagittal breadth 1.4 mm, and transverse breadth of 2.3 mm. The muscle attachment within the hamulus subjects its body to a greater load in the mediodorsal direction, while the head of the hamulus can be freely pulled away laterally and caudally. The bare position of the hamulus at the distal end of the upper dental arch and the presence of a bursa or sliding layer in the sulcus suggest that it could be a possible source for trauma or infection [4].

The symptoms of pterygoid hamulus bursitis cited by Shankland are multifaceted; pain in the hamular region, palatal pain, earache, odynophagia, maxillary pain, dysphagia, and localized erythema [5]. Some of its clinical presentations may mimic glossopharyngeal neuralgia, temporomandibular joint disorders.

Vigilance of this intriguing entity is essential to all health practitioners concerned in the diagnosis and management of orofacial pain. In patients with undiagnosed neck and/or facial sporadic pain, an elongated pterygoid hamulus or a styloid process needs to be included in the diagnostic cascade of orofacial pain. It would be worthwhile to diligently listen to our patients while they narrate their history as this can distill a plethora of maladies involving the orofacial apparatus and adopt a dual axis approach.

The purpose of this article is to present a case of bursitis that was managed by surgical shaving of pterygoid hamulus following a failure of conservative management and discuss its complex pain referral pattern.

2. Case Report

A 42-year-old female presented to us with a primary complaint of pain in the left side of her face for 3 yrs. The pain was spontaneous and oppressive in nature. She had a history of burning, a pricking type of dysesthesia (pins and needles feeling), intermittent in nature and radiated to the left temporal and orbital region. The unremitting nature of pain often made her feel anxious and agitated with lack of sleep. No trigger factors and aggravating or relieving factors were disclosed in the history. She narrated a history of uneventful extraction of a decayed upper third molar and a restoration of carious tooth citing as a possible source of pain by her dentist.

Her medical history was unremarkable except the ingestion of a cocktail of medicines alternating from analgesics, antibiotics, steroids, and antidepressants prescribed by multiple physicians for the unremitting chronic pain she was experiencing. An array of investigations was performed ranging from MRI brain, OPG, and cephalograms that turned out to be inconclusive. Vascular decompression, central pontine dysfunction, skull base, and metastatic tumor were ruled out following the normal slices seen in MRI and CT. Routine chair side diagnostic tests were done to rule out odontogenic pain.

On clinical examination, a sharp localized pain in the hamular region was evident on palpation due to the elongated hamular process that had a knife-edge bony projection (Figure 1). The overlying palatal mucosa had no change in color or texture. A local anesthetic (1 ml of 2% lidocaine) infiltration was injected with subsequent impermanent relief of symptoms in a localized area. Her oral examination was nonremarkable on the affected left side with deep dentinal caries with respect to 18 (Figure 2) and pulp stones with respect to 16 on the right side (Figure 3). Blood investigations carry less significance except in the possible diagnosis of cranial arteritis and for autoimmune disorders such as Sjogren's syndrome.

Following a failure of conservative remedies in the past, a prominent elongated hamular process (18.53 mm) noticed on a cone beam computed tomography: axial section (Figure 4), 3-D reconstructed view (Figure 5), and a positive diagnostic block [6], we opted for a surgical shaving in pursuit of pain relief (Figure 6).

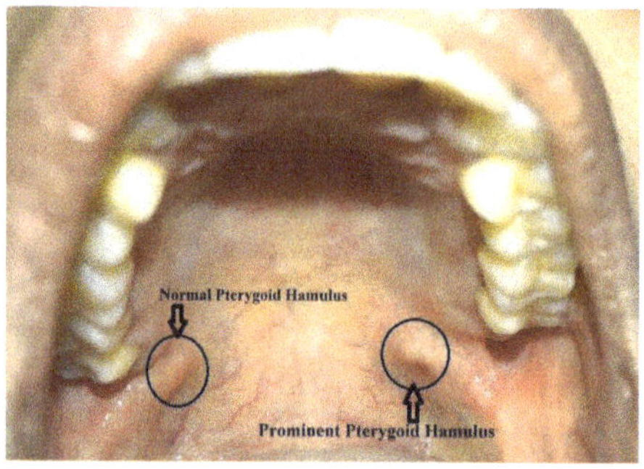

Figure 1: Prominent hamular process with a knife-edge bony projection on the left side.

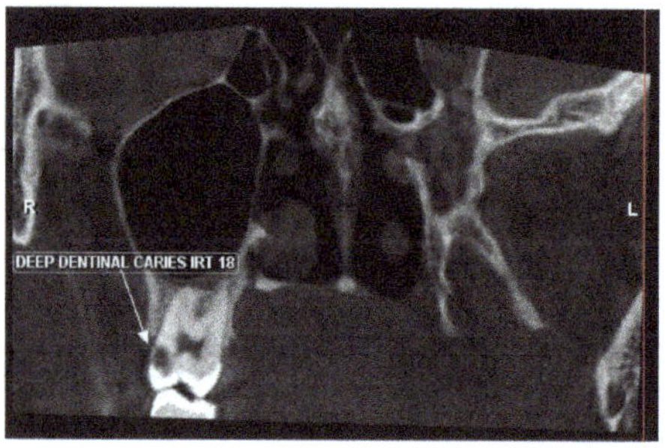

Figure 2: Coronal view showing the presence of dentinal caries on the contralateral side.

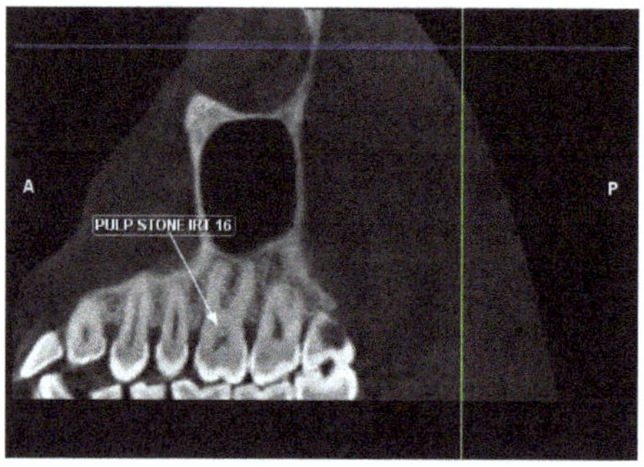

Figure 3: Coronal view showing the presence of pulp stones on the contralateral side.

A longitudinal incision of the mucosa was planned along with dissection up to the pterygoid hamulus followed by resection of the hamulus from its base. The gross specimen measured 13 mm in length and its shape resembled an arrowhead (Figure 7).

3. Discussion

Pain in the orofacial region takes a complex route when it progresses to a chronic state. The neurologic, myogenic, and psychogenic symptoms can overlap in this intricate, innervated anatomic region. A "trigger zone" is a hallmark of both myofascial pain dysfunction and neurologic states.

The "trigger zone" in myofascial pain is a confined tender area on a firm band of skeletal muscle, tendon, or ligament. The pattern of pain referral for each trigger point is

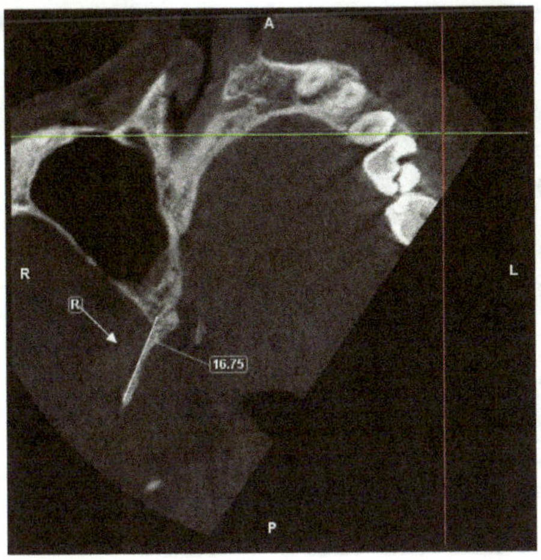

Figure 4: Cone beam computed tomography axial view showing an elongated pterygoid hamulus.

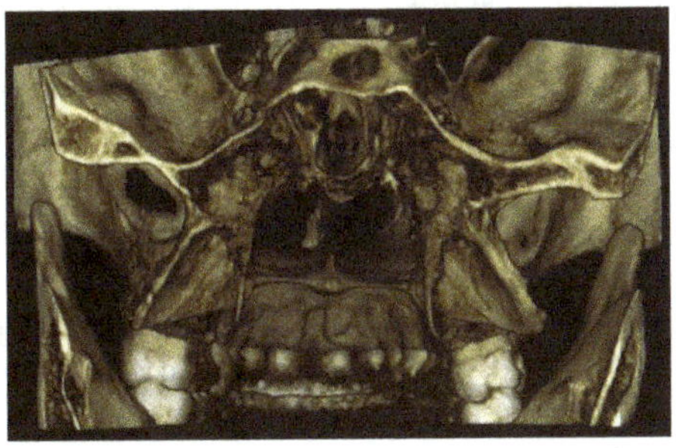

Figure 5: 3-D reconstructed skimmed view showing the elongated pterygoid hamulus.

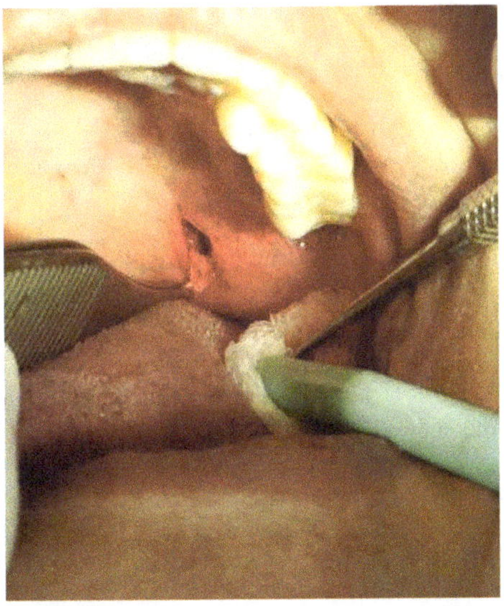

Figure 6: Surgical resection of the elongated and the prominent pterygoid hamulus from its base.

consistent. Contrary to this neurologic pain, states are categorized by voluntary or involuntary activation of painful paroxysms by tactile or thermal stimulation of certain superficial areas supplied by the afflicted nerve [7, 8].

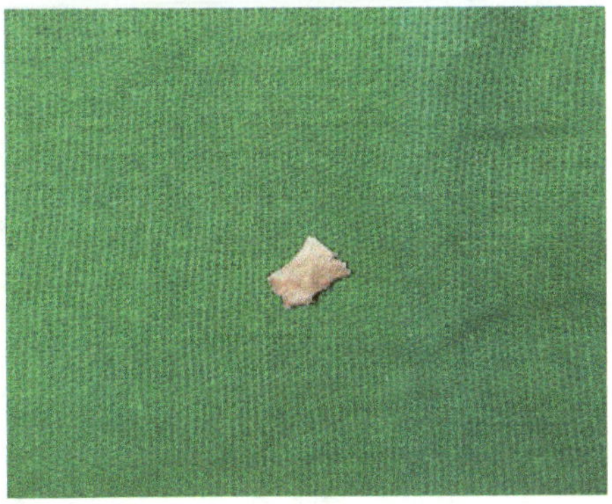

Figure 7: Resected hamular process resembling an arrowhead.

In our case, the absence of tenderness over the muscles of mastication and the spontaneous complex pain referral pattern without any trigger factors made the diagnosis of myofascial pain dysfunction syndrome and craniofacial neuralgia a questionable one [9].

Bursae are fluid-filled compacted sacs with synovial fluid that acts as a cushion between bones, tendons, joints, and muscles. Anaesthesia intubations, swallowing a big bolus, yawning, sustained overextended maxillary prosthesis, traumatic injury while brushing, bulimic patients, and "fellatio" in child sexual abuse are cited as possible perpetuating factors for this intriguing entity [10, 11]. In our patient with no history of major surgery under general anaesthesia and any significant history of comorbidity, a possible etiological factor could be a traumatic injury. Hamular bursitis can trigger referred craniofacial pain, which may mimic a cluster of symptoms as seen in temporomandibular disorders, impacted teeth, trigeminal and glossopharyngeal neuralgia, stylohyoid ligament calcification, stylomandibular ligament inflammation, tumors, and otitis media [12].

Treatment of pterygoid hamulus bursitis per se remains ambiguous with no clear-cut consensus so far. It can be either conservative or surgical. Injection of steroids has been used with a mixed bag of results [5, 13].

The trigeminal nerve innervates anatomically related but functionally diverse anatomic structures such as the meninges, auricle, dentofacial apparatus, and eyes. A large proportion of the sensory cortex > 40% receives the trigeminal input and overlap of trigeminal sensory nucleus with the upper cervical dermatomes in the brain stem [14] seems to be a plausible explanation for the persistent pain in the orofacial region that has functional and psychological consequences.

The baffling nature of the coexisting pain conditions distant from the source of nociception had perplexed us in arriving at a definitive diagnosis. In addition, the bone of contention was "can such a small bony spicule be a source of craniofacial pain?" Although it is inviting to speculate that the intricate vascular and diverse neural networks within the tensor tympani muscle attached to the pterygoid hamulus as a plausible explanation, it cannot be substantiated by the scarcity of reports published in the literature. Sasaki et al. [15] opined that bursitis inhibits the muscular contraction of the tensor veli palatini muscle due to the mechanical stimulation by the bony spicule or osteophyte. This in turn

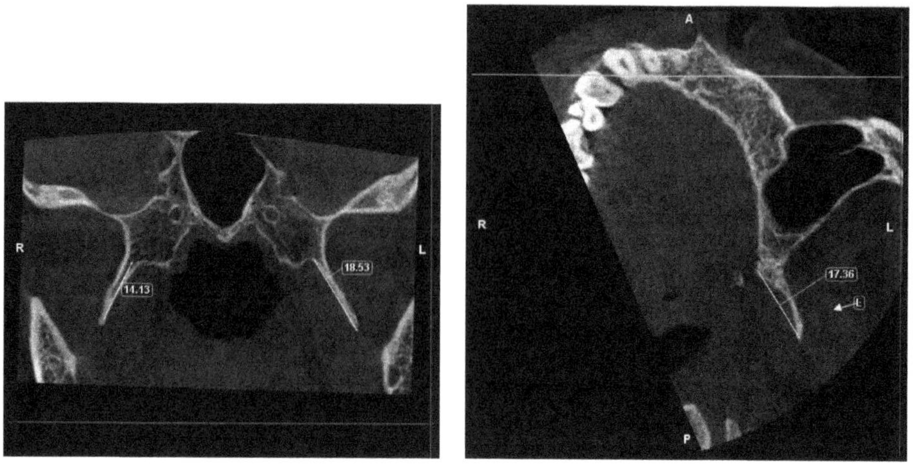

(a) (b)

Figure 8: Axial view depicting an elongated pterygoid hamulus measuring about 18.53 mm on the left side and 14.13 mm on the right side.

may stimulate the branches of the greater and lesser palatine nerve, glossopharyngeal nerve, and facial nerve, which may result in widespread painful sensation following the peripheral distribution of the nerve.

Amongst the growing body of evidence pertaining to the position and morphology of pterygoid hamulus in different populations, the average length was found to be within the range of 4.9 to 7.2 mm [15–20]. This is in contrast to the length of 18.53 mm seen in our case (Figures 8(a) and 8(b)). The prominent bony spicule were suggestive of some mechanical stimulation to the neighbouring tissues by the elongated pterygoid hamulus eliciting pain that perhaps impaired the smooth functioning of the tensor veli palatini muscle. Confirming the elongated pterygoid hamulus radiographically, a reasonable anatomic postulation could have been existed: (1) soft palate mucosa may have been thin and friable than usual; (2) soft palate mucosa may have been much closer than usual to a rather normally located hamulus making it vulnerable to any frictional trauma [21]; and (3) asymmetry of the Pterygoid plates [22].

In addition to the surgical procedure, she also had a session of cognitive behavioral therapy considering the psychosocial aspect of chronic orofacial pain. We had maintained a pain diary that is often considered an indispensable part of assessment of treatment outcome of chronic orofacial pain in terms of pain severity, frequency, and duration of pain. The pain had substantially diminished several months post therapy; this can be attributed to the central sensitization, secondary adjacent muscle hyperactivity, hormonal fluctuations in a female gender, and neuroplasticity, a common phenomenon in chronic pain conditions [23–25]. It should be noted that as the duration of the suffering is protracted, the emotional vector of pain persists despite the inflammatory response to the acute cause of pain has ceased.

4. Conclusion

The superficial location of bursa and its functional orientation predisposes it to traumatic injury and chronic inflammation. A possible diagnosis of hamular bursitis should be considered, while diagnosis of chronic orofacial pain as the management for bursitis is quite inimitable.

This case illuminates the implications of a quiescent pterygoid hamulus that can perplex the clinician by causing craniofacial pain. In addition, the constellation of symptoms mimicking the other maladies of the orofacial apparatus can lead to misdiagnosis and mistreatment. A slice of wisdom allied from this case report is to listen to your patients, amalgamate the information than trivializing it, and always consider multifaceted nature of chronic orofacial pain. There has always been a constant communication between the mind and body, and chronic pain patients need to have a positive outlook. They need to align their thoughts before it malaligns them and their nervous system.

References

[1] R. J. Gores, "Pain due to long hamular process in the edentulous patient. Report of two cases," *The Journal-Lancet*, vol. 84, pp. 353-354, 1964.

[2] R. S. Hertz, "Pain resulting from elongated pterygoid hamulus: report of case," *Journal of Oral Surgery*, vol. 26, no. 3, pp. 209-210, 1968.

[3] E. Hjørting-Hansen and I. Lous, "The pterygoid hamulus syndrome," *Ugeskrift for Laeger*, vol. 149, no. 15, pp. 979–982, 1987.

[4] R. Putz and A. Kroyer, "Functional morphology of the pterygoid hamulus," *Annals of Anatomy - Anatomischer Anzeiger*, vol. 181, no. 1, pp. 85–88, 1999.

[5] W. E. Shankland II, "Pterygoid hamulus bursitis: one cause of craniofacial pain," *The Journal of Prosthetic Dentistry*, vol. 75, no. 2, pp. 205–210, 1996.

[6] G. K. Eyrich, M. C. Locher, T. Warnke, and H. F. Sailer, "The pterygoid hamulus as a pain-inducing factor: a report of a case and a radiographic study," *International Journal of Oral and Maxillofacial Surgery*, vol. 26, no. 4, pp. 275–277, 1997.

[7] J. R. Fricton, R. Kroening, D. Haley, and R. Siegert, "Myofascial pain syndrome of the head and neck: a review of clinical characteristics of 164 patients," *Oral Surgery, Oral Medicine, Oral Pathology*, vol. 60, no. 6, pp. 615–623, 1985.

[8] H. Heyck and N. Datal, *Headache and Facial Pain. Differential Diagnosis, Pathogenesis, Treatment*, Thieme, New York, NY, USA, 4th edition, 1980.

[9] M. Khan, S. E. Nishi, S. N. Hassan, M. A. Islam, and S. H. Gan, "Trigeminal neuralgia, glossopharyngeal neuralgia, and myofascial pain dysfunction syndrome: an update," *Pain Research and Management*, vol. 2017, Article ID 7438326, 18 pages, 2017.

[10] K. L. Moore, *Clinically Orientated Anatomy*, Williams & Wilkins, Baltimore, MD, USA, 1980.

[11] P. C. Salins and G. P. Bloxham, "Bursitis: a factor in the differential diagnosis of orofacial neuralgias and myofascial pain dysfunction syndrome," *Oral Surgery, Oral Medicine, Oral Pathology*, vol. 68, no. 2, pp. 154–157, 1989.

[12] W. E. Shankland II, "Bursitis of the hamular process. Part II: diagnosis, treatment and report of three case studies," *CRANIO®*, vol. 14, no. 4, pp. 306–311, 1996.

[13] J. Y. Cho, K. Y. Cheon, D. W. Shin, W. B. Chun, and H. Lee, "Pterygoid hamulus bursitis as a cause of craniofacial pain: a case report," *Journal of the Korean Association of Oral and Maxillofacial Surgeons*, vol. 39, no. 3, pp. 134–138, 2013.

[14] R. S. Erzurumlu, Y. Murakami, and F. M. Rijli, "Mapping the face in the somatosensory brainstem," *Nature Reviews Neuroscience*, vol. 11, no. 4, pp. 252–263, 2010.

[15] T. Sasaki, Y. Imai, and T. Fujibayashi, "A case of elongated pterygoid hamulus syndrome," *Oral Diseases*, vol. 7, no. 2, pp. 131–133, 2001.

[16] J. Krmpotić-Nemanić, I. Vinter, and A. Marušić, "Relations of the pterygoid hamulus and hard palate in children and adults: anatomical implications for the function of the soft palate," *Annals of Anatomy - Anatomischer Anzeiger*, vol. 188, no. 1, pp. 69–74, 2006.

[17] M. Abe, G. Murakami, M. Noguchi, S. Kitamura, K. Shimada, and G. I. Kohama, "Variations in the tensor veli palatini muscle with special reference to its origin and insertion," *The Cleft Palate-Craniofacial Journal*, vol. 41, no. 5, pp. 474–484, 2004.

[18] K. Orhan, B. U. Sakul, U. Oz, and B. Bilecenoglu, "Evaluation of the pterygoid hamulus morphology using cone beam computed tomography," *Oral Surgery, Oral Medicine, Oral Pathology, Oral Radiology, and Endodontology*, vol. 112, no. 2, pp. e48–e55, 2011.

[19] G. J. Roode and K. W. Bütow, "Pterygoid hamulus syndrome - undiagnosed," *South African Dental Journal*, vol. 69, no. 2, pp. 70-71, 2014.

[20] N. F. Barchetta, R. L. B. de Oliveira, V. Á. S. Silveira, and H. Faig-Leite, "Clinical and morphofunctional aspects of pterygoid hamulus: literature review," *Brazilian Dental Science*, vol. 18, no. 4, pp. 5–11, 2015.

[21] M. E. Guerrero, J. Beltran, A. De Laat, and R. Jacobs, "Can pterygoid plate asymmetry be linked to temporomandibular joint disorders?," *Imaging Science in Dentistry*, vol. 45, no. 2, pp. 89–94, 2015.

[22] T. D. Charbeneau and P. L. Blanton, "The pterygoid hamulus: a consideration in the diagnosis of posterior palatal lesions," *Oral Surgery, Oral Medicine, Oral Pathology*, vol. 52, no. 6, pp. 574–576, 1981.

[23] J. T. T. de Siqueira, H. C. Lin, C. Nasri et al., "Clinical study of patients with persistent orofacial pain," *Arquivos de Neuro-Psiquiatria*, vol. 62, no. 4, pp. 988–996, 2004.

[24] G. B. Rollman and S. Lautenbacher, "Sex differences in musculoskeletal pain," *The Clinical Journal of Pain*, vol. 17, no. 1, pp. 20–24, 2001.

[25] A. J. Barsky, H. M. Peekna, and J. F. Borus, "Somatic symptom reporting in women and men," *Journal of General Internal Medicine*, vol. 16, no. 4, pp. 266–275, 2001.

Permissions

All chapters in this book were first published by Hindawi Publishing Corporation; hereby published with permission under the Creative Commons Attribution License or equivalent. Every chapter published in this book has been scrutinized by our experts. Their significance has been extensively debated. The topics covered herein carry significant findings which will fuel the growth of the discipline. They may even be implemented as practical applications or may be referred to as a beginning point for another development.

The contributors of this book come from diverse backgrounds, making this book a truly international effort. This book will bring forth new frontiers with its revolutionizing research information and detailed analysis of the nascent developments around the world.

We would like to thank all the contributing authors for lending their expertise to make the book truly unique. They have played a crucial role in the development of this book. Without their invaluable contributions this book wouldn't have been possible. They have made vital efforts to compile up to date information on the varied aspects of this subject to make this book a valuable addition to the collection of many professionals and students.

This book was conceptualized with the vision of imparting up-to-date information and advanced data in this field. To ensure the same, a matchless editorial board was set up. Every individual on the board went through rigorous rounds of assessment to prove their worth. After which they invested a large part of their time researching and compiling the most relevant data for our readers.

The editorial board has been involved in producing this book since its inception. They have spent rigorous hours researching and exploring the diverse topics which have resulted in the successful publishing of this book. They have passed on their knowledge of decades through this book. To expedite this challenging task, the publisher supported the team at every step. A small team of assistant editors was also appointed to further simplify the editing procedure and attain best results for the readers.

Apart from the editorial board, the designing team has also invested a significant amount of their time in understanding the subject and creating the most relevant covers. They scrutinized every image to scout for the most suitable representation of the subject and create an appropriate cover for the book.

The publishing team has been an ardent support to the editorial, designing and production team. Their endless efforts to recruit the best for this project, has resulted in the accomplishment of this book. They are a veteran in the field of academics and their pool of knowledge is as vast as their experience in printing. Their expertise and guidance has proved useful at every step. Their uncompromising quality standards have made this book an exceptional effort. Their encouragement from time to time has been an inspiration for everyone.

The publisher and the editorial board hope that this book will prove to be a valuable piece of knowledge for researchers, students, practitioners and scholars across the globe.

List of Contributors

Rocco Narciso
Plastic Surgery Resident, Graduate School of Plastic Reconstructive and Aesthetic Surgery, "Tor Vergata" University, Rome, Italy

Emanuela Basile
Department of Plastic and Reconstructive Surgery, Policlinico Casilino Hospital, Rome, Italy
Sapienza Università di Roma, Via del Policlinico, Roma, Italy

Davide Johan Bottini
Reconstructive and Aesthetic Surgery University "Tor Vergata" of Rome, Department of Plastic and Reconstructive Surgery, Policlinico Casilino Hospital, Rome, Italy

Valerio Cervelli
Department of Surgical Sciences, University "Tor Vergata", Rome, Italy

C. J. Salgado, H. AlQattan, A. Nugent, D. Gerth, W. Kassira, C. S. McGee and L. Wo
Division of Plastic, Reconstructive, Transgender, and Aesthetic Surgery, University of Miami Leonard M. Miller School of Medicine, Miami, FL, USA

Luca Guarda-Nardini
Section of Dentistry and Maxillofacial Surgery, Treviso Hospital, Treviso, Italy

Diletta Trojan, Giulia Montagner and Elisa Cogliati
Treviso Tissue Bank Foundation, Treviso, Italy

Matteo Bendini
Section of Neuroradiology, Treviso Hospital, Treviso, Italy

Daniele Manfredini
School of Dentistry, Department of Neuroscience, University of Padova, Padova, Italy

Umberto Autorino, Claudia Borbon, Maria Chiara Malandrino, Giovanni Gerbino and Fabio Roccia
Division of Maxillofacial Surgery, Surgical Science Department, Città della Salute e delle Scienza Hospital, University of Turin, Corso A.M. Dogliotti 14, 10126 Torino, Italy

Katheleen Miranda, André Sander Carneiro, Jennifer Tsi Gerber and Suyany Gabriely Weiss
School of Health Science, Positivo University, Curitiba, Brazil

Beatriz Sobrinho Sangalette
Department of Biological Sciences-Anatomy, Bauru School of Dentistry, University of São Paulo-FOB/USP Alameda Octávio Pinheiro Brisola, n° 9-75, Zip Code, 17012-901 Bauru-SP, Brazil

Rafaella Ferrari Pavoni
State University of North Paraná-UENP. Av. Getúlio Vargas, no. 850, Zip Code, 86400-000 Jacarezinho, PR, Brazil

Thayna da Silva Emídio and Tiago Levatti
Marília University-UNIMAR. Av. Higino Muzi Filho, n° 1001, Zip Code, 17525-902 Marília, SP, Brazil

Marcos Capelari
Oral Maxillofacial Surgery Department, Santa Casa da Misericórdia de Santa Cruz do Rio Pardo. Av. Dr. Ciro Melo Camarinha, n° 530, Zip Code, 18900-000 Santa Cruz do Rio Pardo, SP, Brazil

Cláudio Maldonado Pastori
Department of Bucomaxilofacial Surgery, University Center of Adamantina-UNIFAI. Av. Francisco Bellusci, n° 1000, CEP, 17800-000 Adamantina, SP, Brazil

Gustavo Lopes Toledo
Oral Maxillofacial Surgery Department, State University of North Paraná-UENP. Av. Getúlio Vargas, no. 850, Zip code, 86400-000 Jacarezinho, PR, Brazil

Johannes Müller
Department of Prosthodontics and Biomaterials, Danube Private University, Krems, Austria
Deputy Medical Director, Danube Private University, Krems, Austria

Rüdiger Junker
Department of Prosthodontics and Biomaterials, Danube Private University, Krems, Austria

Alexandre Meireles Borba
Post-Graduation Department, Faculty of Dentistry, University of Cuiaba (UNIC), 3100 Manoel Jose de Arruda Street, 78065-480 Cuiaba, MT, Brazil
Department of Oral and Maxillofacial Surgery, College of Dentistry, University of Illinois (UIC), 801 South Paulina Street, Chicago, IL 60612-7211, USA
Division of Dentistry, University General Hospital, 2101 Treze de Junho Street, 78025-000 Cuiaba, MT, Brazil

André Luis Fernandes da Silva, Niverso Rodrigues Simão, Fábio Luis Miranda Pedro and Alvaro Henrique Borges
Post-Graduation Department, Faculty of Dentistry, University of Cuiaba (UNIC), 3100 Manoel Jose de Arruda Street, 78065-480 Cuiaba, MT, Brazil

Michael Miloro
Department of Oral and Maxillofacial Surgery, College of Dentistry, University of Illinois (UIC), 801 South Paulina Street, Chicago, IL 60612-7211, USA

Shiv Prasad Sharma
Zulfi General Hospital, Ministry of Health, Saudi Arabia

Akshay Nigam
Radiation Oncology, G.R. Medical College, Gwalior, India

J. S. Vieira, F. R. Deliberador, J. C. Zielak, A. F. Giovanini and T. M. Deliberador
Graduate Program in Dentistry, Positivo University, Curitiba, PR, Brazil

E. M. Brandão-Filho
Private Practice, Balneário Camboriú, SC, Brazil

Jessica Blanchard, Julia Palmer, Enamul Ali and Leo Cheng
Department of Oral and Maxillofacial Surgery, Homerton University Hospital, Homerton Row, London E9 6SR, UK

Sebahattin Destek
Department of General Surgery, Bezmialem Vakif University School of Medicine, Istanbul, Turkey

Vahit Onur Gul
Edremit State Hospital General Surgery Department, Edremit, 10300 Balikesir, Turkey

Serkan Ahioglu
Edremit State Hospital Biochemistry Department, Edremit, 10300 Balikesir, Turkey

G. Turatti and M. Giordano
Odontostomatology OU, Martini Hospital, Via Tofane 71, Turin 10141, Italy

A. Bruni
CIR Dental School, Department of Surgical Sciences, Università degli Studi di Torino, Via Nizza 230, Turin 10126, Italy
Department of Mechanical and Aerospatial Engineering (DIMEAS), Politecnico di Torino, C.so Duca degli Abruzzi 24, Turin 10129, Italy

M. Savoini and G. Gerbino
Division of Maxillofacial Surgery, Department of Surgical Sciences, Università degli studi di Torino, Città della Salute e delle Scienza Hospital, Corso A.M. Dogliotti 14, Turin 10126, Italy

Aline Monise Sebastiani
Department of Stomatology, Department of Oral and Maxillofacial Surgery, Federal University of Paraná, Curitiba, Brazil
Cleft Lip and Palate Integral Care Center, Trabalhador Hospital, Curitiba, Brazil
School of Health Sciences, Department of Oral and Maxillofacial Surgery, Positivo University, Curitiba, Brazil
School of Health Science, Federal University of Paraná, Curitiba, Brazil

Isabela Polesi Bergamaschi, Bernardo Olsson, Nelson Luis Barbosa Rebellato and Delson Joao da Costa
Department of Stomatology, Department of Oral and Maxillofacial Surgery, Federal University of Paraná, Curitiba, Brazil

Guilherme dos Santos Trento
Cleft Lip and Palate Integral Care Center, Trabalhador Hospital, Curitiba, Brazil

Leandro Eduardo Klüppel
Department of Stomatology, Department of Oral and Maxillofacial Surgery, Federal University of Paraná, Curitiba, Brazil
Oral and Maxillofacial Surgery Department, Federal University of Parana, Curitiba, Brazil
Cleft Lip and Palate Integral Care Center, Trabalhador Hospital, Curitiba, Brazil
School of Health Science, Positivo University, Curitiba, Brazil
School of Health Science, Federal University of Paraná, Curitiba, Brazil

Rafael Correia Cavalcante, Fabiano Galina and Marina Fanderuff
Oral and Maxillofacial Surgery Department, Federal University of Parana, Curitiba, Brazil

Rafaela Scariot
Oral and Maxillofacial Surgery Department, Federal University of Parana, Curitiba, Brazil
School of Health Science, Federal University of Paraná, Curitiba, Brazil
Department of Stomatology, Department of Oral and Maxillofacial Surgery, Federal University of Paraná, Curitiba, Brazil
Cleft Lip and Palate Integral Care Center, Trabalhador Hospital, Curitiba, Brazil

School of Health Sciences, Department of Oral and Maxillofacial Surgery, Positivo University, Curitiba, Brazil

Piero Cascone, Valentino Vellone and Valerio Ramieri
Sapienza Università di Roma, Via del Policlinico, Roma, Italy

Achille Tarsitano and Claudio Marchetti
Department of Biomedical and Neuromotor Sciences, Maxillofacial Surgery Unit, S. Orsola-Malpighi Hospital, Alma Mater Studiorum University of Bologna, Bologna, Italy

Mohammed AlKindi, Sundar Ramalingam and Lujain Abdulmajeed Hakeem
Department of Oral and Maxillofacial Surgery, College of Dentistry, King Saud University, Riyadh, Saudi Arabia

Manal A. AlSheddi
Department of Basic Sciences, College of Dentistry, Princess Nourah Bint Abdulrahman University, Riyadh, Saudi Arabia

Rafael Netto
Stomatology Service, Department of Oral Diagnosis and Pathology, School of Dentistry, Federal University of Rio de Janeiro, Rio de Janeiro, RJ, Brazil

Silas Antonio Juvencio de Freitas Filho
Department of Surgery, Stomatology, Pathology and Radiology (Area of Pathology), Bauru School of Dentistry, University of São Paulo, Bauru, SP, Brazil

Wladimir Cortezzi, Flávio Merly and Vitor Marcello de Andrade
Oral and Maxillofacial Surgery Service, Federal Hospital of State Servers, Brazilian Government, Rio de Janeiro, RJ, Brazil

Fábio Ramôa Pires
Department of Oral Pathology, School of Dentistry, State University of Rio de Janeiro, Rio de Janeiro, RJ, Brazil

Jimmy Xu
Royal Derby Hospital, Derby, UK

Prateek Biyani, Andrew Rajkumar and Robert Orr
Chesterfield Royal Hospital, Chesterfield, UK

Aparna Barabde
Department of Prosthetic Dentistry, V.Y.W.S. Dental College & Hospital, Amravati 444 602, India
Dr Barabde Dental Clinic, Badnera Road, Rajkamal Square, Amravati 444 601, India

Shailesh M. Barabde
Department of Obstetrics & Gynaecology, P.D.M. Medical College, Amravati 444 602, India

Ashish Bhagat and Amar Thakare
Department of Prosthetic Dentistry, V.Y.W.S. Dental College & Hospital, Amravati 444 602, India

Ademir Franco, Mayara Jessica de Carvalho Mattos, Francine Ferrari, Luiz Carlos Carta Gambus, Paulo Henrique Couto Souza and Soraya de Azambuja Berti-Couto
Departamento de Estomatologia, Escola de Saúde e Biociências, Pontifícia Universidade Católica do Paraná, Imaculada Conceicão 1155, Prado Velho, 80215-901 Curitiba, PR, Brazil

José Manoel dos Reis Neto
Laboratório de Análise de Minerais e Rochas, Departamento de Geologia, Universidade Federaldo Paraná, Centro Politécnico 19062, Jardim das Américas, 81615-980 Curitiba, PR, Brazil

Waleed AlShehri, Sara AlFadil, Alhanouf AlOthri, Abdulaziz O. Alabdulkarim, Shabeer A. Wani and Sari M. Rabah
Department of Plastic & Reconstructive Surgery, King Fahad Medical City, Riyadh 11525, Saudi Arabia

Merih Onal, Gultekin Ovet and Necat Alatas
Konya Education and Training Hospital, Department of Otorhinolaryngology, 42090 Konya, Turkey

Eric L. Chung and Anh D. Le
Department of Oral and Maxillofacial Surgery and Pharmacology, University of Pennsylvania School of Dental Medicine, Philadelphia, PA, USA

Faizan Alawi
Department of Pathology, University of Pennsylvania School of Dental Medicine, Philadelphia, PA, USA

Rabie M. Shanti
Department of Oral and Maxillofacial Surgery and Pharmacology, University of Pennsylvania School of Dental Medicine, Philadelphia, PA, USA
Department of Otorhinolaryngology, Head and Neck Surgery, University of Pennsylvania School of Medicine, Philadelphia, PA, USA

Ajaz Ahmad Rather
Department of General Surgery, Sheri Kashmir Institute of Medical Sciences (Medical College), Bemina, Srinagar 190018, India

Sajad Ahmad Salati
Department of Plastic and Reconstructive Surgery, King Fahad Medical City, Riyadh 11525, Saudi Arabia
Department of Surgical Specialties, Sheri Kashmir Institute of Medical Sciences, Soura, Srinagar 190020, India

Oguz Kayiran
Department of Plastic and Reconstructive Surgery, Izmir University, 35000 Izmir, Turkey

Caglar Calli
Department of Head and Neck Surgery, Ekol ENT Hospital, 35000 Izmir, Turkey

Abdulkadir Emre and Fatih Kemal Soy
Department of Head and Neck Surgery, Ataturk Training and Research Hospital, 35000 Izmir, Turkey

Vildan Akpinar, Fulya Yilmaz Duran, Murat Yasar Özkalkanli and Burcu Horsanali
Anaesthesiology and Reanimation Department, Bozyaka Training and Research Hospital, İzmir, Turkey

Elif Duman
Thoracic Surgery Department, Bozyaka Training and Research Hospital, İzmir, Turkey

Özgür Duran
Emergency Medicine Department, Bozyaka Training and Research Hospital, İzmir, Turkey

Sameep S. Shetty, Premalatha Shetty and Nancy Agarwal
Department of Oral and Maxillofacial Surgery, Manipal College of Dental Sciences, Manipal Academy of Higher Education, Mangalore 575001, India

Prit Kiran Shah
Consultant Oral and Maxillofacial Surgeon, My Dentist and Bhatia Hospital, Mumbai, India

Jayanth Nambiar
Department of Conservative Dentistry and Endodontics, Sharavathi Dental College, Shiomoga, India

Index

www.ingramcontent.com/pod-product-compliance
Lightning Source LLC
LaVergne TN
LVHW082234200926
848484LV00008B/2353